RECENT ADVANCES IN GASTROINTESTINAL PATHOLOGY

CLINICS IN GASTROENTEROLOGY
SUPPLEMENT I

RECENT ADVANCES IN GASTROINTESTINAL PATHOLOGY

Edited by
RALPH WRIGHT, MA, DPhil, MD, FRCP

Professor of Medicine, University of Southampton Medical School and Medical Unit; Honorary Consultant Physician, Southampton General Hospital, Southampton

on behalf of
THE ROYAL COLLEGE OF PATHOLOGISTS

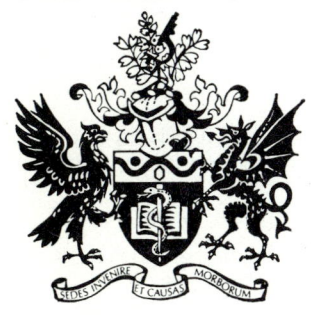

1980

W. B. Saunders Company Ltd   London · Philadelphia · Toronto

W. B. Saunders Company Ltd: 1 St Anne's Road
Eastbourne, East Sussex BN21 3UN

West Washington Square
Philadelphia, PA 19105

1 Goldthorne Avenue
Toronto, Ontario M8Z 5T9

British Library Cataloguing in Publication Data
Clinics in gastroenterology
  Supplement 1: Recent advances in gastrointestinal pathology
  1. Digestive organs — Diseases
  I. Wright, Ralph
  616.3   RC801   80-49802
ISBN 0 7216 9611 2

© 1980 by W. B. Saunders Company Ltd. All rights reserved. This publication is protected by copyright. No part of it may be reproduced, stored in a retrieval system, or transmitted in any form or by any means, electronic, mechanical, photocopying, recording, or otherwise, without permission from the publisher.

Supplements to Clinics in Gastroenterology do not form part of a subscription: they are occasional publications in gastroenterology or related fields of special interest to subscribers. Clinics in Gastroenterology is published three times each year by W. B. Saunders Company Ltd, and is available on subscription.

The editor of this publication is William Wolvey, W. B. Saunders Company Ltd, 1 St Anne's Road, Eastbourne, East Sussex BN21 3UN.

Printed and bound by W &J Mackay Limited, Chatham.

Contributors

R. BASU, MD, Formerly Lecturer, All India Institute of Medical Sciences, New Delhi, India; currently Senior Registrar in Cytology and Histopathology, New Charing Cross Hospital, London, and St Stephen's Hospital, Chelsea, London SW10 9TH.

A.J. BLACKSHAW, MA, MB, BChir, MRCPath, Senior Registrar, Department of Histopathology, St Bartholomew's Hospital, London, and St Mark's Hospital, City Road, London EC1V 2PS.

S.R. BLOOM, MD, FRCP, Reader in Medicine, Royal Postgraduate Medical School, London; Consultant Endocrinologist, Hammersmith Hospital, Du Cane Road, London W12 0HS.

H.J.R. BUSSEY, BSc, PhD, Consulting Research Fellow, St Mark's Hospital, City Road, London EC1V 2PS.

JOHN RICHARD CLAMP, BSc, PhD, MD, MB ChB, FRIC, MRCP, Professor of Experimental Medicine, University of Bristol Medical School, University Walk, Bristol BS8 1TD; Consultant in Medicine, Bristol Royal Infirmary, Bristol.

PAULA COOK-MOZAFFARI, MA, BLitt, Medical Research Council External Staff, Department of Social and Community Medicine, University of Oxford, 9 Keble Road, Oxford OX1 3QG.

D.W. DAY, MA, MB, BChir, MRCPath, Senior Lecturer in Pathology, University of Liverpool; Honorary Consultant Pathologist, Liverpool Area Health Authority (Teaching), Royal Liverpool Hospital, Prescot Street, Liverpool L7 8XW.

ANNE FERGUSON, PhD, FRCP, MRCPath, Senior Lecturer, Gastrointestinal Unit, University of Edinburgh; Honorary Consultant Physician, Western General Hospital, Crewe Road, Edinburgh EH4 2XU.

J. GRAINGER, MRCPath, Consultant Pathologist and Cytologist, National Women's Hospital, Epsom, Auckland 3, New Zealand.

J.D. HARDCASTLE, MA, MChir, FRCS, MRCP, Professor of Surgery, University of Nottingham Medical School; Honorary Consultant Surgeon, General and University Hospitals, Nottingham, and City Hospital, Hucknall Road, Nottingham NG5 1PB.

M.J. HILL, PhD, Director, Bacterial Metabolism Research Laboratory, Central Public Health Laboratory, Colindale Avenue, London NW9 5HT; Consultant to the Research Department, St Mark's Hospital, London.

A.V. HOFFBRAND, DM, FRCP, FRCPath, Professor of Haematology, Royal Free Hospital and School of Medicine, London; Honorary Consultant, Royal Free Hospital, Pond Street, London NW3 2QG.

O.A.N. HUSAIN, MD, FRCPath, FRCOG, Recognized Teacher, Charing Cross Hospital Medical School, London; Consultant Pathologist, Department of Cytology, Westminster Hospital Teaching Group, Charing Cross Hospital, London, and St Stephen's Hospital, Chelsea, London SW10 9TH.

K.S. IBRAHIM, MBChB, Registrar in Cytology, Charing Cross Hospital, London, and St Stephen's Hospital, Chelsea, London SW10 9TH.

v

CONTRIBUTORS

PETER ISAACSON, DM, MRCPath, Senior Lecturer, Department of Pathology, University of Southampton Medical School, Southampton SO9 4XY.

F. KONISHI, MD, Research Fellow, St Mark's Hospital, City Road, London EC1V 2PS.

H.P. LAMBERT, MA, MD, FRCP, Professor of Microbial Diseases, St George's Hospital Medical School, London; Consultant Physician, St George's Hospital, Blackshaw Road, London SW17 0QT.

DONALD J.R. LAURENCE, MA, PhD, Head of Biochemistry Department, Ludwig Institute for Cancer Research (London Branch), Royal Marsden Hospital, Sutton, Surrey SM2 5PX.

J.E. LENNARD-JONES, MD, FRCP, Professor of Gastroenterology, The London Hospital Medical College; Consultant Gastroenterologist, St Mark's Hospital, City Road, London EC1V 2PS.

C.R. MADELEY, MD, MRCPath, Professor of Clinical Virology, University of Newcastle upon Tyne; Consultant Virologist, Newcastle Area Health Authority (Teaching), Royal Victoria Infirmary, Queen Victoria Road, Newcastle upon Tyne NE1 4LP.

D.Y. MASON, DM, MRCPath, University Lecturer in Haematology, University of Oxford; Honorary Consultant Haematologist, Oxford Area Health Authority (Teaching), John Radcliffe Hospital, Headington, Oxford OX3 9DU.

B.C. MORSON, DM, FRCP, FRCPath, Consultant Pathologist and Director of the Research Department, St Mark's Hospital, City Road, London EC1V 2PS.

ALLAN MOWAT, BSc(Hons), MB ChB, Research Fellow, Gastrointestinal Unit, University of Edinburgh; Honorary Registrar in Medicine, Western General Hospital, Crewe Road, Edinburgh EH4 2XU.

A. MUNRO NEVILLE, PhD, MD, MRCPath, Professor of Pathology, Ludwig Institute for Cancer Research (London Branch), Royal Marsden Hospital, Sutton, Surrey SM2 5PX.

R.A. PARKINS, MD, FRCP, Recognized Teacher, Charing Cross Hospital Medical School, University of London; Consultant Physician and Gastroenterologist, Charing Cross Hospital, Fulham Palace Road, London W6 8RF, and Royal Masonic Hospital, London.

JUAN PIRIS, DPhil, MB, MRCPath, Senior Lecturer in Pathology, University of Edinburgh Medical School; Honorary Consultant Pathologist, Royal Infirmary, Lauriston Place, Edinburgh EH3 9YW.

JULIA M. POLAK, MD, MRCPath, Senior Lecturer in Histochemistry, Royal Postgraduate Medical School, London; Consultant Histopathologist, Hammersmith Hospital, Du Cane Road, London W12 0HS.

ASHLEY B. PRICE, MA, BM BCh, MRCPath, Consultant Histopathologist, Northwick Park Hospital and Clinical Research Centre, Watford Road, Harrow, Middlesex.

MICHAEL SWASH, MD, FRCP, Senior Lecturer in Neuropathology, The London Hospital Medical College; Consultant Neurologist, The London Hospital, Whitechapel, London E1 1BB, and St Mark's Hospital, London.

I.C. TALBOT, MD, MRCPath, Senior Lecturer, Department of Pathology, University of Leicester Medical School, Leicester; Honorary Consultant, Leicester General Hospital, Gwendolen Road, Leicester, LE5 4PW.

H. WILLIAMS SMITH, DSc, PhD, FRCVS, FRCPath, FRS, Head of the Department of Microbiology, Houghton Poultry Research Station, Houghton, Huntingdon, Cambridgeshire PE17 2DA.

CONTRIBUTORS

D.H. WRIGHT, MD, FRCPath, Professor of Pathology, University of Southampton Medical School; Honorary Consultant Pathologist, Southampton General Hospital, Southampton SO9 4XY.

R. ZEEGEN, MB, MRCP, Recognized Teacher, Westminster Medical School, University of London; Physician in Charge, Department of Gastroenterology, Westminster Hospital, London, and St Stephen's Hospital, Chelsea, London SW10 9TH.

Table of Contents

FOREWORD xi
    Ralph Wright

Part 1 Pathophysiology
1. IMMUNOHISTOCHEMISTRY AND THE GASTROINTESTINAL TRACT 3
    D.Y. Mason and Juan Piris
2. REGULATORY PEPTIDES OF THE GUT: THE ESSENTIAL MECHANISM FOR GUT CONTROL   23
    Julia M. Polak and S.R. Bloom
3. GASTROINTESTINAL MUCUS 47
    John Richard Clamp
4. ANAEMIA AND THE GASTROINTESTINAL TRACT 59
    A.V. Hoffbrand
5. IDIOPATHIC FAECAL INCONTINENCE: HISTOPATHOLOGICAL EVIDENCE ON PATHOGENESIS   71
    Michael Swash

Part 2 Inflammatory Disease
6. IMMUNOLOGICAL MECHANISMS IN THE SMALL INTESTINE 93
    Anne Ferguson and Allan Mowat
7. VIRAL INFECTIONS 105
    C.R. Madeley
8. BACTERIAL INFECTIONS OF THE GASTROINTESTINAL TRACT 125
    H.P. Lambert
9. PLASMID-MEDIATED AND OTHER CHARACTERISTICS OF *ESCHERICHIA COLI* ENTEROPATHOGENIC FOR DOMESTIC MAMMALS: THEIR INFLUENCE ON SMALL INTESTINAL COLONIZATION 135
    H. Williams Smith
10. PSEUDOMEMBRANOUS COLITIS 151
    Ashley B. Price
11. CROHN'S DISEASE: DEFINITION, PATHOGENESIS AND AETIOLOGY 173
    J.E. Lennard-Jones

Part 3 Gastrointestinal Malignancy
12. MALABSORPTION AND INTESTINAL LYMPHOMAS 193
    Peter Isaacson and D.H. Wright
13. NON-HODGKIN'S LYMPHOMAS OF THE GUT 213
    A.J. Blackshaw
14. CYTODIAGNOSIS OF GASTRIC CANCER 241
    O.A.N. Husain, R. Zeegen, R.A. Parkins, K.S. Ibrahim, J. Grainger and R. Basu
15. TUMOUR MARKERS AND THE GASTROINTESTINAL TRACT 255
    A. Munro Neville and Donald J.R. Laurence
16. THE EPIDEMIOLOGY AND PATHOLOGY OF CANCER OF THE OESOPHAGUS 267
    Paula Cook-Mozaffari
17. EPIDEMIOLOGY AND PATHOLOGY OF GASTRIC CANCER 285
    D.W. Day
18. THE AETIOLOGY OF COLORECTAL CANCER 297
    M.J. Hill
19. SCREENING FOR COLORECTAL CANCER 311
    J.D. Hardcastle

20. Dysplasia in the Colorectum	331
B.C. Morson and F. Konishi	
21. Polyposis Syndromes	345
H.J.R. Bussey	
22. Spread of Rectal Cancer Within Veins and Mechanisms of Malignant Embolism	353
I.C. Talbot	
Index	365

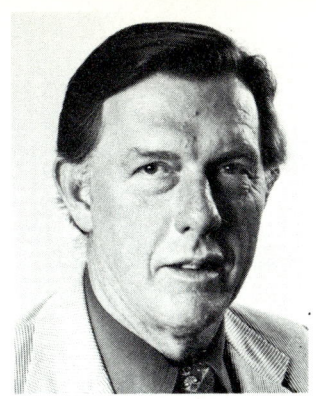

Foreword

During the past decade, there have been major advances in our understanding of gastrointestinal disease. This volume represents the Proceedings of a Symposium on Gastrointestinal Pathology organized by the Royal College of Pathologists and held at the Royal College of Physicians in February 1980. The Symposium covered the pathophysiology of several aspects of gastrointestinal disease, gastrointestinal malignancy and lymphoma. All presentations were highly topical and were by acknowledged experts of international renown in their particular field.

General topics include reviews of new techniques of immunohistochemistry in relation to the gastrointestinal tract, of the measurement and significance of regulatory peptides from the gut, and of the role of gastrointestinal mucus in health and disease.

In the section on inflammatory bowel disease there are up-to-date reviews of immunological mechanisms in the small intestine, viral and bacterial infections in the gut and the most recent clinical and experimental studies on pseudomembranous colitis.

Recent concepts of malabsorption and the intestinal lymphomas were presented by workers from Southampton and St Bartholomew's Hospital, London. There are excellent contributions on the epidemiology of cancer of the oesophagus and of gastric cancer as well as more general papers on tumour markers in the gut and on cytodiagnosis. Papers on colorectal cancer include a review of the aetiology and the difficult problem of screening. The St Mark's Hospital group present their most recent experience of epithelial dysplasia and the polyposis syndromes.

The Symposium, published as a supplement to *Clinics in Gastroenterology*, can equal the best in this highly successful series. Where appropriate, the chapters have been liberally illustrated and the standard of reproduction is extremely high. Since many of the areas covered are growing points in the study of gastrointestinal disease, it is particularly valuable that this volume has appeared within six months of the Symposium being held. Its interdisciplinary nature makes it of value to anyone interested in gastroenterology, whether from an epidemiological, aetiological, pathological or clinical point of view.

RALPH WRIGHT

PART ONE

Pathophysiology

1

Immunohistochemistry and the Gastrointestinal Tract

D.Y. MASON
JUAN PIRIS

The purpose of this paper is to review the immunohistochemical techniques which are currently available to the pathologist for the detection of constituents in human tissues, and to discuss their use in the context of gastrointestinal pathology. This is a field which is likely to expand steadily in the future, both as a result of technical advances (e.g., in ultrastructural immunohistochemistry) and with the increasing availability of antibodies specific for new antigens. In the latter context the production of highly specific monoclonal antibodies by the plasma cell fusion technique (Köhler and Milstein, 1975) is likely to have a major impact. A preliminary indication of the way in which antibodies produced by this technique may be used in the immunohistological analysis of antigenically complex constituents in human tissues has been provided by the studies of Morton and his colleagues (1980) on Mallory bodies.

IMMUNOHISTOLOGICAL TECHNIQUES

Technical aspects of immunohistochemical procedures can conveniently be considered under the two headings of *Tissue Preparation* and *Labelling Techniques*.

Tissue Preparation

Cell suspensions

Although the majority of immunocytochemical investigations of gastrointestinal tissue are performed on tissue sections, in certain circumstances there may be considerable advantages to the use of isolated cell suspensions, since they allow immunocytochemical reactions to be investigated without interference from extraneous factors. This approach has been used for the study of IgA and secretory component (Brandtzaeg, 1978), Ia antigens (Forsum, Klareskog and Peterson, 1979), and apolipoprotein B (Glickman et al, 1979) in isolated human intestinal epithelial cells. Lymphoid cells can

© 1980 W.B. Saunders Company Ltd.

also now be obtained in good yield from human gastrointestinal biopsies (Crofton, Cochrane and McClelland, 1978; Goodacre et al, 1979) in a state suitable for immunocytochemical analysis.

Tissue blocks

The pathologist who elects to work on tissue blocks rather than with cell suspensions faces a choice between unfixed frozen tissue (for cryostat sectioning) and fixed tissues which have been embedded in a medium such as paraffin or resin.

Cryostat sections. Cryostat sections should be used when studying tissue constituents which may lose antigenic reactivity as a result of tissue fixation and embedding. Surface membrane antigens frequently fall into this category, a fact reflected by the use of cryostat sections for the immunohistochemical detection of T and B lymphoid cells in human intestinal and liver biopsies (Strickland et al, 1975; Meuwissen et al, 1976; Fargion et al, 1979). However, the ability of surface membrane antigens to survive tissue processing shows considerable variation, and constituents such as carcinoembryonic antigen (Isaacson and Judd, 1978; Primus et al, 1978), hepatitis B surface antigen (Busachi, Ray and Desmet, 1978; Radaszkiewicz et al, 1979), a recently described epithelial antigen (Heyderman, Steele and Ormerod, 1979) and ABO blood group substances (Heyderman 1979) have all successfully been demonstrated by routine immunohistological techniques on embedded gastrointestinal tissues. In some of these instances the presence of a carbohydrate component to the antigen may be relevant to its survival. Furthermore, if tissues are processed by special techniques designed to maximize antigenic preservation (Brandtzaeg, Surjan and Berdal, 1978) or if the most sensitive immunohistochemical staining procedures are used (Curran and Gregory, 1978; Curran and Jones, 1978) it may be possible to demonstrate surface antigens (i.e., B cell membrane immunoglobulin) which are not conventionally considered to survive tissue fixation and embedding.

Although cryostat sections are optimal for the study of membrane-bound antigens they often allow diffusion of soluble antigens, both extracellular and cytoplasmic. For example, plasma cell staining for immunoglobulin in cryostat sections frequently appears as a diffuse zone of reactivity centred on each cell, and when clusters of plasma cells are present these 'haloes' may merge together so that individual plasma cells are impossible to identify (Curran and Jones, 1978). In contrast, paraffin sections of the same material always show crisp localization of immunoglobulin within the plasma cell cytoplasm.

Embedded tissues. The use of embedded material offers the advantages of good morphological preservation together with the possibility of prolonged storage of tissue samples. Frozen tissue, in contrast, tends to become desiccated on storage unless special precautions are taken, and it is not technically convenient to cut sections from the same block on repeated occasions.

Early immunohistochemical studies of paraffin-embedded gastrointestinal tissues were based upon the use of special fixation procedures, since conventional fixatives such as formol saline were associated with excessive background autofluorescence and were also thought to cause denaturation of tissue constituents. The two processing techniques most widely used in the study of gastrointestinal tissue were the Sainte-Marie (1962) cold ethanol procedure, which formed the basis of the exemplary immunofluorescent studies of immunoglobulin, J chain, secretory component and gastrin by Brandtzaeg and his colleagues (see Korsrud and Brandtzaeg, 1980, for references); and the procedure developed for the study of neuropeptides by Pearce and associates (1974) based upon tissue freeze drying and vapour fixation. Mention may also be made of the paraformaldehyde-lysine-periodate fixative developed by McLean and Nakane (1974) to meet the special requirements of ultrastructural immunohistology. This procedure has been used, principally in Nakane's laboratory, in studies of human gastrointestinal constituents (IgA, secretory component and J chain) at the electron microscopic level (Brown, Isobe and Nakane, 1976; Brown et al, 1977; Isobe et al, 1977; Jos et al, 1979; Nagura, Nakane and Brown, 1979; Nagura et al, 1979).

In the past ten years, however, it has been realized that many more fixatives are compatible with immunohistological staining than were initially appreciated. This came about partly as a result of the introduction of immunoperoxidase staining methods (which obviated the problems of tissue autofluorescence). It was also due, however, to the initiative of pathologists and histochemists such as Taylor and Burns (1974), who ignored conventional wisdom concerning the deleterious effect of formalin fixation on tissue antigens and found their temerity rewarded by excellent immunoperoxidase staining of paraffin sections. When it became apparent that a wide range of human tissue constituents could be demonstrated in conventional histological material, the possibility was opened up of retrospectively analysing tissue samples (including post-mortem material) which had initially been embedded without any realization of their potential value to posterity (Taylor, 1978; DeLellis et al, 1979). It may be added that although the majority of work in this field has been based upon the use of paraffin wax as an embedding medium, it is now apparent that optical microscopic localization of antigens in Araldite- or Epon- embedded sections is also feasible (Erlandsen, Parsons and Rodning, 1979; Heyderman and Monaghan, 1979; Takamiya et al, 1979).

Quite how long tissue antigens remain detectable following conventional histological processing is not clear. Celio (1979) has recently reported the detection of endorphin in Bouin's fixed fetal tissue which had been stored in ethanol for 30 years, whilst Halmi (1978) was able to detect growth hormone and prolactin in seven-year-old conventionally stained and mounted paraffin sections by removal of the cover slips and application of an immunoperoxidase sandwich. Consequently, if the antigenicity of a tissue constituent survives the initial fixation and embedding steps perhaps it may remain detectable virtually indefinitely.

However, it is now apparent that not all tissue constituents can be retrospectively studied with equal facility in conventional histological material. Certain substances (particularly small peptides and carbohydrate antigens) appear to be demonstrable more readily than other constituents (e.g., large protein molecules). An example in the latter category, which is of particular relevance in the field of gastrointestinal pathology, is plasma cell immunoglobulin. In formalin-fixed material immunohistochemical staining for this constituent may be absent or else limited to a small clump of reactivity close to the plasma cell nucleus (Figure 1a). This loss of antigenic reactivity is frequently an unpredictable phenomenon, varying in severity from sample to sample and from laboratory to laboratory.

One approach to this problem is to 'unmask' antigenic reactivity in formalin fixed material by the proteolytic digestion of sections prior to immunohistochemical staining. This procedure has now been widely used (Huang, Minassian and More, 1976; Curran and Gregory, 1977, 1978; Denk, Radaszkiewicz and Weirich, 1977; Mepham, Frater and Mitchell, 1979; Takamiya et al, 1979) and, although the mode of action is still unknown, its effect may be very striking (Figure 1b), allowing antigens which were previously undetectable to be clearly visualized.

Antigenic 'masking' appears to be particularly associated with formalin fixation. The reactivity of plasma cell immunoglobulin in gut biopsies and in other tissues survives much better in mercury-based fixatives such as formol sublimate (Bosman et al, 1979; Piris and Thomas, 1980), or in Bouin's or Zenker's fixatives (Dorsett and Ioachim, 1978; Reitamo and Reitamo, 1978; Bosman et al, 1979; Heyderman, 1979), than in conventional formol saline (Figure 2). Proteolytic digestion is not required following these alternative fixatives.

In consequence, immunohistologists show signs of undergoing a schism into two groups, one of which prefers to use digested formalin-fixed material (Mepham, Frater and Mitchell, 1979), the other insisting on the use of alternative fixatives such as Bouin's, thereby avoiding the need for proteolytic digestion (Heyderman, 1979).

Unfortunately, no studies have been published so far in which the relative merits of these two approaches for any individual antigen have been systematically compared. Proteolytic digestion undoubtedly has a number of disadvantages, including the extra time and care required to obtain consistent results, and the variation which may be found in optimal digestion periods between different sections and between one antigen and another. Furthermore, the digestion time required to reveal an antigen in one site may be excessive and lead to loss of antigenic reactivity at another site. Nevertheless, proteolytic treatment undoubtedly has an important role to play, if only because it may offer the only means of retrospectively studying tissue constituents in formalin-fixed routine histological material. The technique is sometimes accused of causing heavy non-specific background staining. This is commonly attributable to the use of antisera at dilutions which are appropriate for non-digested sections, but which are too concentrated for use on digested material. Unmasking of extracellular protein probably also contributes to background staining. As far as the authors are aware, there is no published evidence, either immunochemical or immunohistolog-

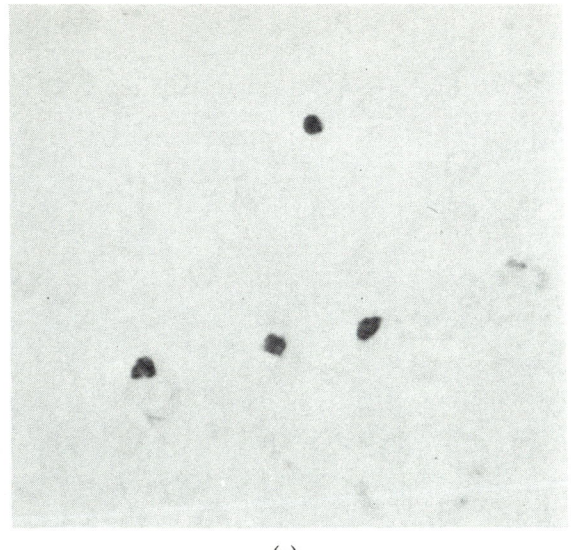

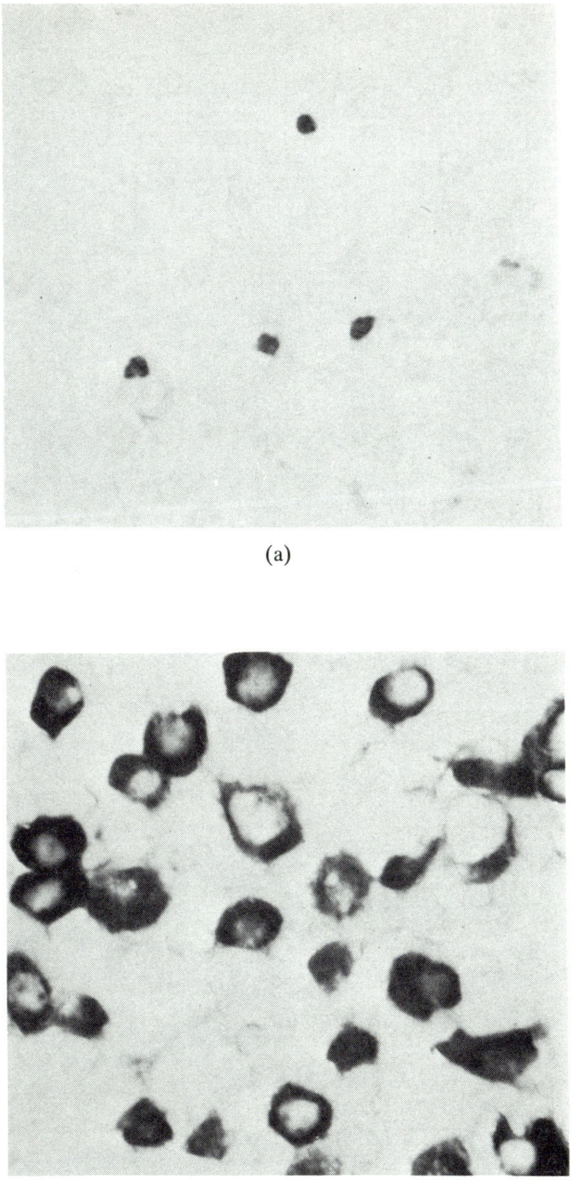

Figure 1. Influence of trypsinization on plasma cell IgG staining by the PAP immunoperoxidase technique. Adjacent paraffin sections from a formalin fixed sample of human reactive lymphoid tissue were stained before (a) and after (b) trypsin digestion. Note that IgG reactivity in the untreated section (a) is restricted to small areas close to the plasma cell nucleus. Following trypsinization (b) many more plasma cells are revealed, and staining is diffusely distributed throughout the cytoplasm.

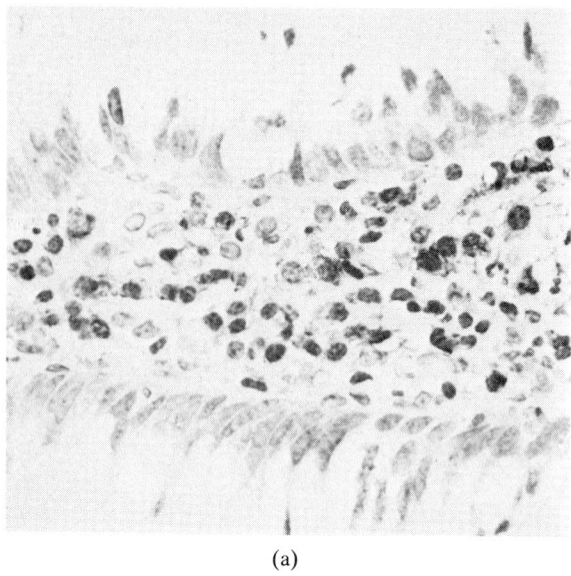

(a)

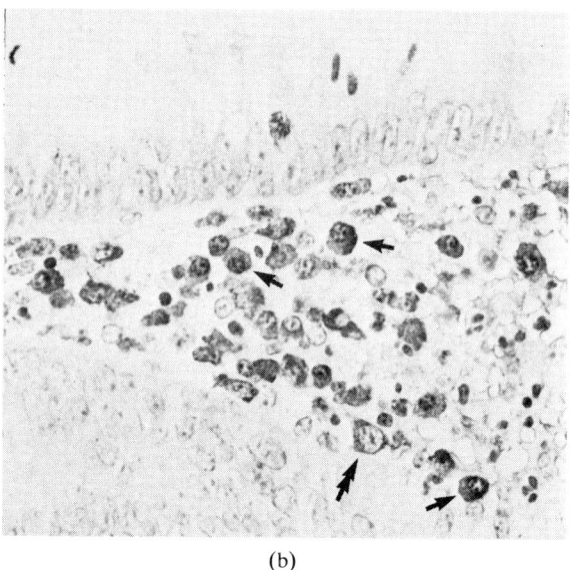

(b)

Figure 2. Immunoperoxidase staining of plasma cell Ig in sections of human rectal biopsies fixed in (a) formol saline and (b) formol sublimate. Note that the latter fixative is associated not only with higher numbers of clearly positive plasma cells (typical examples arrowed) but also with much crisper preservation of nuclear and cytoplasmic detail. (An Ig positive plasma cell precursor with immature nuclear chromatin is indicated by the double arrow.)

From Piris and Thomas (1980), with kind permission of the editor of *Journal of Clinical Pathology*.

ical, to support Heyderman's belief (1979) in a 'very real . . . possibility that the proteolytic cleavage of tissue antigens may yield fragments common to many determinants'. It may be pointed out that if we are ignorant of the mechanism of proteolytic 'unmasking' we are scarcely more knowledgeable concerning the effect of conventional fixatives on tissue antigenic reactivity. The complexity of this field is illustrated by Reitamo's report (1978) that lysozyme in some sites (e.g., gastric mucosa) shows greater susceptibility to denaturation by fixatives than does the same enzyme in other sites (e.g., salivary glands).

The major conclusion which may be drawn from this discussion is that when studying any given constituent of human gastrointestinal tissue it is necessary as a preliminary step to establish an optimal fixation procedure and to explore whether or not proteolytic digestion can improve upon the results obtained with this fixative. Furthermore, the behaviour of the constituent should be studied in the particular cell type under investigation, rather than being inferred by extrapolation from results obtained for other tissue sites.

Immunohistochemical Labelling Techniques

The great majority of immunohistochemical studies of human gastrointestinal tissue are performed using either immunofluorescent or immunoenzymatic labelling methods.

Immunofluorescent methods

There is little new development in this field. Double labelling using FITC (fluorescein) and TRITC (rhodamine) labelled antisera is a well-established technique for the simultaneous detection of two different antigens (Korsrud and Brandtzaeg, 1980). The possibility of triple immunofluorescent labelling has been raised by the development of a new fluorochrome (SITS) emitting a blue fluorescence, but unfortunately tissue autofluorescence makes it unsuitable for staining histological sections (Rothbarth et al, 1978).

Immunoenzymatic methods

The technical development of immunoenzymatic procedures has also reached a halt, which one hopes is temporary. The majority of laboratories now use either the periodate oxidation technique (Nakane and Kawaoi, 1974; Wilson and Nakane, 1978) or glutaraldehyde coupling techniques (Avrameas and Ternynck, 1971) for the preparation of covalent peroxidase-antibody conjugates. Comparative data on the molecular and immunocytochemical characteristics of these two types of conjugates have been published by Boorsma and Streefkerk (1976, 1979). The use of alternative coupling agents such as benzoquinone (Ternynck and Avrameas, 1977) and heterobifunctional reagents (Kitagawa and Aikawa, 1976; Carlsson, Drevin and Axen, 1978; O'Sullivan et al, 1979) has yet to be fully evaluated.

The peroxidase-antiperoxidase (PAP) procedure (Sternberger et al,

1970) is also widely used for immunohistochemical staining of human tissues, although its reputation for high sensitivity may in part be a reflection of the poor quality of many covalent conjugates (in which there is competition between free and conjugated antibody). It should be noted that the preparation of PAP complexes may be speeded up considerably by the use of a chromatographic method (Mason and Sammons, 1978a) or by using a shortened version of the originally published procedure. This method, which we currently use for the preparation of PAP, involves washing the initial immune precipitate briefly in a bench-top centrifuge at room temperature (rather than at 10 000 rpm for 20 minutes at 5 °C) and dialysing the soluble PAP directly against buffered saline after the acid dissociation and neutralization steps (rather than precipitating and washing with ammonium sulphate). PAP complexes prepared in this way offer the theoretical advantages that they will tend to contain high avidity antibody, and that free peroxidase remains at the end of the procedure to stabilize the soluble PAP complexes in antigen excess. The technique can be completed within a few hours and the staining results are indistinguishable from those obtained using PAP prepared by the considerably more laborious conventional procedure.

Double immunoenzymatic-labelling techniques yielding two contrasting reaction products have been reported by several laboratories (Nakane, 1968; Campbell and Bhatnagar, 1976; Erlandsen et al, 1976; Martin-Comin and Robyn, 1976; Tramu, Pillez and Leordanelli, 1978). However, these methods have a number of disadvantages, including the fact that the two 'sandwiches' must be applied sequentially, thereby doubling the time required for immunoenzymatic staining. In consequence, these methods have found very little practical application in the investigation of human disease. A simultaneous double-labelling procedure (using peroxidase and alkaline phosphatase), which takes only a few minutes longer than does conventional single immunoenzymatic labelling, has been recently developed in this laboratory (Mason and Sammons, 1978b). This procedure enables two antigens to be clearly distinguished, even when they are present within the same cell. One use which we have found for this technique in the field of gastrointestinal pathology has been in the analysis of the specificity of anti-Ig antisera. A commercial antiserum, nominally specific for IgE, was found on immunoperoxidase staining to react with an unexpectedly high number of plasma cells in the lamina propria of rectal biopsies. Double labelling for IgE with this antiserum in conjunction with antisera against IgG or IgM revealed in each case two populations of single-stained plasma cells. Double staining for IgE and IgA, on the other hand, revealed a large number of double-stained plasma cells, indicating that the anti-IgE antiserum contained antibodies reacting with IgA. When the anti-IgE antiserum was adequately absorbed this reactivity against mucosal IgA plasma cells was suppressed.

These findings highlight the risks of false positive staining reactions for mucosal IgE (Brandtzaeg and Baklien, 1976) and are relevant to reports (based on inadequately characterized commercial antisera) of increased numbers of IgE plasma cells in inflammatory bowel disease (Heatley et al,

1975; O'Donoghue and Kumar, 1979). It would appear that the double immunoenzymatic-labelling technique provides a valuable means of analysing the immunohistochemical specificity of antisera.

The double-labelling technique has also been used in this laboratory in a study (Bell, Piris and Mason, 1980) of serum protein uptake by gastrointestinal epithelium (see below under *False Positive Staining*).

Choice of immunohistological labelling technique

The conventionally quoted advantages and disadvantages of immunofluorescent versus immunoenzymatic techniques are listed in Table 1. Since

Table 1. *Labelling techniques for immunohistological studies of human tissues*

Technique	Advantages	Disadvantages
Immunofluorescence	Rapidity. Possibility of double labelling.	Fading of label. Incompatibility with conventional fixatives and counterstains, preventing visualization of tissue morphology.
Immunoenzymatic methods	Label visible by conventional microscopy and compatible with conventional histological fixatives and stains. No fading of label. Sensitivity.	Complexity. Carcinogenic substrates.

The characteristics of immunofluorescent and immunoenzymatic labelling techniques listed in this table are those commonly quoted in the immunohistochemical literature. As discussed in the text some of these views are inaccurate.

the limitations of either of these techniques are usually discussed at the greatest length by exponents of the other technique (often on the basis of limited personal experience), more credence should be given to the advantages quoted in this list than to the disadvantages. This is particularly true in the context of immunofluorescent methods. The impermanence of immunofluorescent preparations is frequently exaggerated by partisans of immunoenzymatic-labelling methods. Rhodamine (and to a lesser extent fluorescein) stained sections retain their label virtually undiminished for long periods of storage. Furthermore, if staining fades it may be restored by a second incubation in fluorescent antibody (Weinstein and Lechago, 1977).

Two additional myths which persist concerning immunofluorescence are that counterstaining with conventional histological stains is incompatible with fluorescent labelling, and that routinely fixed paraffin-embedded sections are unsuitable for immunofluorescent staining. Preliminary haematoxylin staining of sections has minimal deleterious effect on subsequent labelling intensity (Weinstein and Lechago, 1977) and, when rhodamine is used, the label survives dehydration and mounting in traditional mounting media. In consequence, the same field can be viewed under optimal morphological conditions by conventional light microscopy and then by immunofluorescence. As far as the unsuitability of conventionally fixed material is concerned, this belief originates from the days of inefficient transmitted-light fluorescent microscopes. Modern narrow-band incident-light filter systems cause minimal autofluorescence in tissues fixed in formalin or Bouin's (Burns, Hambridge and Taylor, 1974; Nayak and Sachdeva, 1975; Dorsett and Ioachim, 1978; Huang, Minassian and More, 1976; Portman et al, 1976; Camelleri et al, 1977; Witting, 1977; McElrath, Galbraith and Allen, 1979; Radaszkiewicz et al, 1979). It may also be noted that if tissue sections are treated with proteolytic enzymes autofluorescence is reduced still further.

A consideration of the relative merits of immunoenzymatic and immunofluorescent methods in the field of gastrointestinal pathology is not of purely academic interest. It is frequently claimed that immunoperoxidase methods will in the future be introduced as routine diagnostic stains for use alongside conventional histochemical methods. However, this prediction has yet to be convincingly fulfilled for want of antigens of obvious diagnostic importance (e.g., malignancy-specific markers). Consequently, immunoperoxidase methods remain principally of value in the context of research rather than routine diagnosis. However, when such antigens of essential diagnostic value are discovered it may well be that many routine histopathologists will prefer the speed and simplicity of immunofluorescent techniques (as they already do when studying skin and renal biopsies) to the complexities of immunoenzymatic-labelling methods, for all their obvious attractions of permanence, sensitivity and preservation of morphological detail.

APPLICATIONS OF IMMUNOHISTOCHEMICAL TECHNIQUES IN GASTROINTESTINAL PATHOLOGY

A wide range of constituents has now been demonstrated in human gastrointestinal tissue (including the liver and pancreas) by immunohistochemical techniques (Table 2) and it is not possible in this paper to review all of these reports adequately. However, a number of comments may be made on some of the problems and pitfalls in this field which have become apparent in recent years.

Table 2. *Antigens studied by immunohistochemical techniques in human gastrointestinal tissues*

Cytoplasmic	Surface membrane
Immunoglobulin	Immunoglobulin
Secretory component	Secretory component
Lysozyme	T and B cell antigens
J chain	Ia antigens
Lactoferrin	Carcinoembryonic antigen
a_1-antitrypsin	
Peptides (e.g., gastrin, somatostatin, substance P, etc.)	

This list is not intended to be an exhaustive survey of all antigens studied in human gastrointestinal tissues, but rather to give some idea of the wide range of substances already investigated.

False Negative Staining

Failure to demonstrate an antigen in a tissue sample by immunocytochemical techniques should never be taken as evidence that the antigen is not present in a tissue. One reason for failure to obtain positive staining is the fact that tissue antigens may be denatured or eluted during tissue processing. As noted previously, antigens in different sites often differ in their susceptibility to tissue preparation procedures; for example, extracellular immunoglobulin appears to be more rapidly denatured or masked by routine histological fixatives than is intracellular plasma cell immunoglobulin. One possible approach to fixation-related problems of this nature may be to raise antisera not against native tissue constituents but against material on which neo-antigens have been created by treatment with the fixative in which the tissue for investigation will be fixed (Eckert and Snyder, 1978). A second cause of negative staining, which is sometimes underestimated, is the fact that antigens may be present at extremely low concentrations in the tissues. The high sensitivity of modern immunoperoxidase techniques is frequently quoted with satisfaction by immunocytochemists. However, the fact that many biologically active substances (e.g., enzymes, growth factors, transmitter substances) are present at very low levels in cells and tissues is much less frequently discussed. If the list of antigens and cell types to which immunocytochemical staining techniques have been applied is considered, it is apparent that the best staining is obtained when the antigen is either packaged within granules (e.g., lysozyme in Paneth's cells, neuropeptides in APUD cells) or endoplasmic reticulum (e.g., immunoglobulin in plasma cells); or forms a structural element in a tissue or cell (e.g., collagen or tubulin); or is present at high density on the surface membrane of a cell (e.g., carcinoembryonic antigen). Many cellular constituents are not locally concentrated in this way, however, and are likely to be difficult if not impossible to detect immunohistochemically. A convenient illustration of this problem is provided by the enzyme lysozyme. This material is readily demonstrated in Paneth's cells, myeloid cells and salivary glandular tissue (Mason and Taylor, 1975), being stored in each of these cell types within granules. In contrast, monocytic cells, despite the fact that they synthesize lysozyme at a high rate (Gordon, Todd and Cohn, 1974), show only weak staining for the enzyme (Mason, Farrell and Taylor, 1975; Mason, 1977). This is attributable to the fact that these cells export lysozyme as soon as it is synthesized and do not allow it to reach high intracellular levels. Presumably, neoplastic histiocytes behave in the same way, since histiocytic tumours of the intestine (Isaacson et al, 1979), despite their ability to synthesize large amounts of lysozyme (Hodges et al, 1979), often stain relatively poorly for this constituent (Isaacson, 1980, personal communication).

False Positive Staining

The problems of establishing the specificity of immunohistochemical staining reactions continue to be hotly debated, and a full discussion of this topic is beyond the scope of this paper. However, it may be worth bringing three aspects of this problem to the reader's attention.

Firstly, on a technical level, the development of novel immunohistochemical methods designed to avoid non-specific labelling may be mentioned. A procedure of this sort (the 'labelled-antigen' technique) has been developed in this laboratory (Mason and Sammons, 1979) and used for immunoperoxidase staining of gastrointestinal tissues (Figure 3). Essentially identical methods (bearing the cheerful acronyms of GLAD and RICH), in which colloidal gold or a radioactive isotope is used as the antibody label, were independently developed in Denmark (Larsson and Schwartz, 1977; Larsson, 1979).

Secondly, it should be recognized that when attempting to prove the specificity of a staining reaction it may be more fruitful to divert resources into a number of different techniques, rather than to increase the information obtained in a single system. Thus if an antiserum appears to demonstrate by immunohistochemical techniques the presence of a constituent

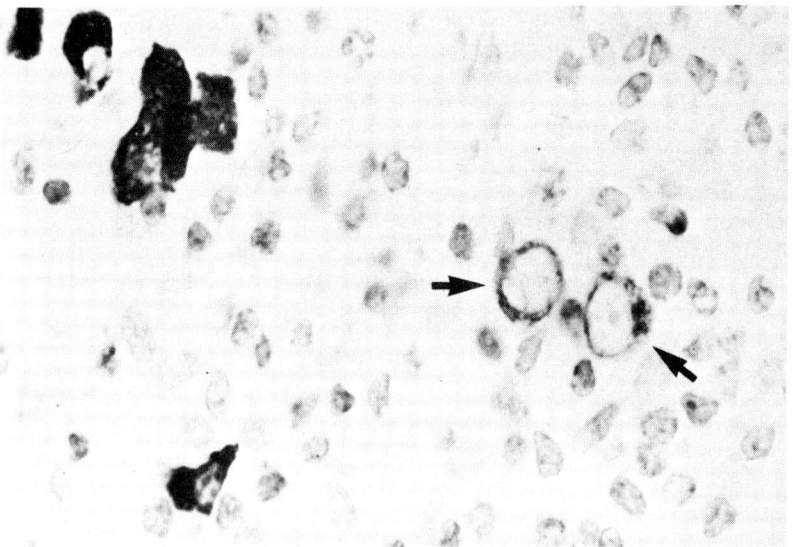

Figure 3. Use of the highly specific low-background 'labelled antigen' immunoperoxidase technique for staining plasma cell Ig in a human rectal biopsy. The edge of a small lymphoid follicle is shown containing two weakly staining primitive cells (arrowed), probably centroblasts, in addition to more heavily stained plasma cells (left).

within a certain cell type, and conventional absorption specificity controls are in agreement, it is more valuable to use an unrelated technique, such as immunoprecipitation of a radiolabelled extract of the cell followed by analysis of the molecular weight (or other characteristic) of the precipitated material, than to continue with ever more exhaustive immunohistochemical absorption controls. This approach was used by Forsum, Klareskog and Peterson (1979) to validate independently their immunocytochemical demonstration of Ia antigens on intestinal epithelial cells. A similar approach has been used by Isaacson and his colleagues (personal communication, 1980) in their study of α-1-antitrypsin in neoplastic human histiocytic cells. A further example of how the localization of a tissue constituent by immunohistochemical means may be independently confirmed by an alternative technique is found in the fact that the demonstration of lysozyme in Paneth's cells by immunoperoxidase staining is in agreement with its distribution as revealed histochemically by chitin hydrolysis (Ghoos and Vantrappen, 1971).

Finally, this paper will conclude with a description of an important cause of misleading immunohistochemical labelling in the gastrointestinal tract which has recently been studied in our laboratory. This phenomenon was first observed in the course of an investigation of transferrin distribution in human tissues (Mason and Taylor, 1978) which revealed (as illustrated in Figure 4) isolated epithelial cells in the small bowel mucosa which stained strongly for this protein. However, it was subsequently found that staining

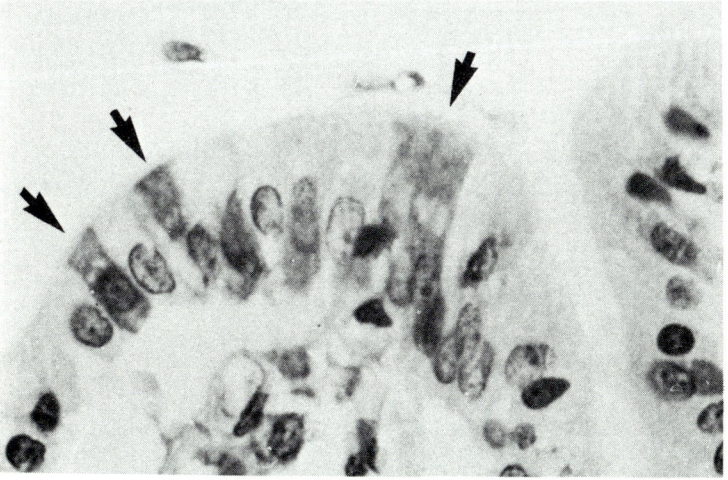

Figure 4. Human duodenal tissue stained by the PAP immunoperoxidase technique for transferrin (using anti-transferrin purified by elution from a Sepharose-transferrin immunoabsorbant). Note the presence of scattered positively staining epithelial cells (arrowed).

for other serum proteins such as albumin and IgG was always present in association with transferrin staining. In consequence, it was postulated that cells with a permeable basal membrane allow protein to leak into their cytoplasm from the lamina propria (Bell, Piris and Mason, 1980), as schematically illustrated in Figure 5. Direct experimental confirmation that a mechanism of this sort could account for transferrin staining in intestinal epithelium comes from the fact that intravenously-injected horseradish peroxidase penetrates very rapidly into scattered duodenal mucosal cells in the mouse, giving a cytochemical staining pattern very similar to that illustrated in Figure 4 (Hugon and Borgers, 1968). An identical staining pattern can be found in the columnar epithelium of the organ of Corti of the guinea pig following perilymphatic injection of horseradish peroxidase (Geyer,

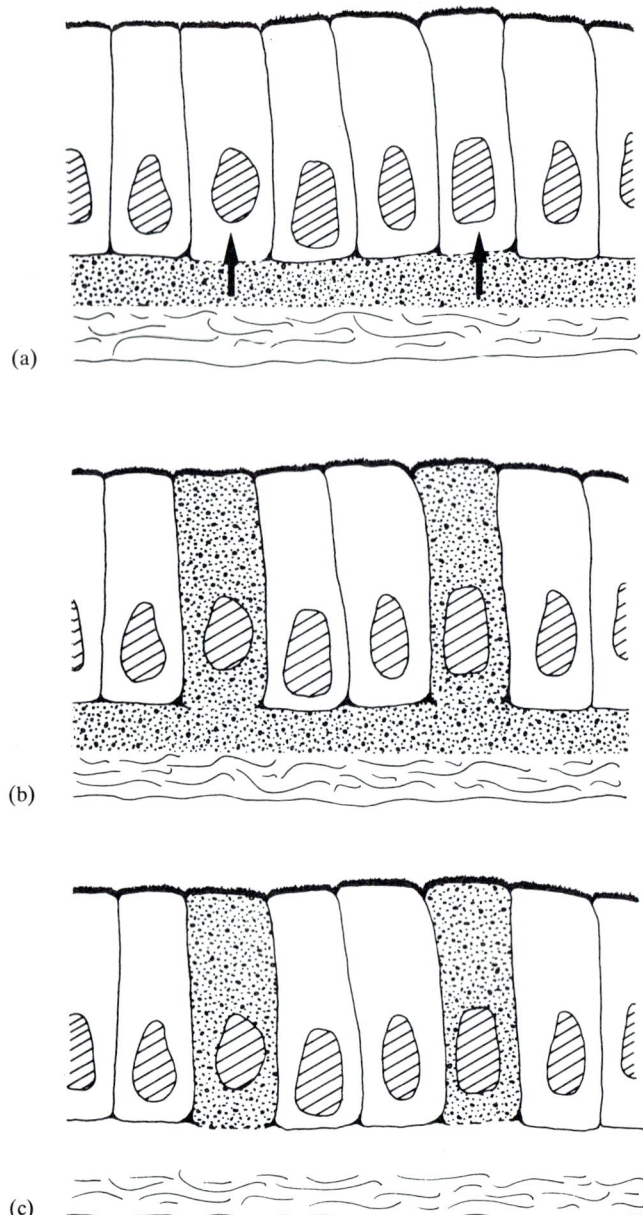

Figure 5. Schematic illustration of the way in which the labelling illustrated in Figure 4 may arise. (a) Extracellular serum protein present in the lamina propria begins to diffuse into two epithelial cells through their permeable basal membranes; (b) the permeable cells are now diffusely filled with serum protein; (c) in the course of tissue processing for immunohistochemical staining the extracellular protein in the lamina propria is denatured or masked, while the intracellular protein in the two epithelial cells remains detectable.

Schmidt and Biedermann, 1979). In the context of human gastrointestinal pathology the staining pattern for lysozyme in epithelial cells in cases of ulcerative colitis closely resembles that illustrated in Figure 4, suggesting that the same phenomenon of intracellular diffusion is responsible (Klockars et al, 1977). To judge from the immunohistochemical staining patterns illustrated in the paper by Buckley and Fox (1979), human chorionic gonadotrophin may also diffuse in a similar way into carcinomatous epithelial cells.

This phenomenon of 'leakage' of proteins into cells is not confined to columnar epithelium. We have observed it in squamous epithelium (Coruh and Mason, 1980), in the central nervous system (Esiri, Taylor and Mason, 1976) and in lymphoid tissue (Mason et al, 1980), and have argued that it accounts for the otherwise inexplicable report by Hartmann and Liacopoulos (1977) of human mucosal lymphoid cells containing both kappa and lambda light chains.

Several characteristic features of the phenomenon may be noted. The intensity of staining for an individual protein is related to its extracellular concentration: for example, albumin staining is stronger than transferrin staining. However, it is important to realize that the extracellular concentration of a protein may rise above the normal serum level if local synthesis occurs; this is relevant to the epithelial cell staining for lysozyme in inflammatory bowel disease referred to above (Klockars et al, 1977). The intensity of staining for an individual protein shows an inverse relationship to its molecular size: for example, IgM diffuses into cells much more readily than does IgG.

CONCLUSIONS

Immunohistochemical procedures clearly have a great deal to offer in the context of gastrointestinal pathology. However, it is necessary for the pathologist who uses these methods to gain experience in their technical aspects if they are to be successfully exploited. In the early days of immunocytochemistry the development of immunofluorescence techniques for cell labelling was held up because, as Pressman pointed out, 'the people who could do the chemistry couldn't do the morphology, and those who could do the morphology couldn't do the chemistry' (Coons, 1978). Fortunately, there are signs today that an increasing number of gastrointestinal pathologists are able to do both.

REFERENCES

Avrameas, S. & Ternynck, T. (1971) Peroxidase labelled antibody and Fab conjugates with enhanced intracellular penetration. *Immunochemistry*, **8**, 1175.

Bell, J.I., Piris, J. & Mason, D.Y. (1980) The exogenous origin of transferrin in human gastrointestinal epithelium. Submitted for publication.

Boorsma, D.M. & Streefkerk, J.G. (1976) Peroxidase conjugate chromatography: isolation of conjugates prepared with glutaraldehyde or periodate using polyacrylamide-agarose gel. *Journal of Histochemistry and Cytochemistry*, **24**, 481.

Boorsma, D.M. & Streefkerk, J.G. (1979) Periodate or glutaraldehyde for preparing peroxidase conjugates. *Journal of Immunological Methods*, **30**, 245.

Bosman, F.T., Lindeman, J., Kuiper, G., Van Der Wall, A. & Kreunig, J. (1979) The influence of fixation on immunoperoxidase staining of plasma cells in paraffin sections of intestinal biopsy specimens. *Histochemistry*, **53**, 57.

Brandtzaeg, P. (1978) Polymeric IgA is complexed with secretory component (SC) on the surface of human intestinal epithelial cells. *Scandinavian Journal of Immunology*, **8**, 39.

Brandtzaeg, P. & Baklien, K. (1976) Inconclusive immunohistochemistry of human IgE in mucosal pathology. *Lancet*, **i**, 1297.

Brandtzaeg, P., Surjan, L. & Berdal, P. (1978) Immunoglobulin system of human tonsils. I. Control subjects of various ages: quantification of Ig-producing cells, tonsillar morphometry and serum Ig concentration. *Clinical and Experimental Immunology*, **31**, 367.

Brown, W.R., Isobe, Y. & Nakane, P.K. (1976) Studies on translocation of immunoglobulins across intestinal epithelium. II. Immunoelectronmicroscopic localization of immunoglobulin and secretory component in human intestinal mucosa. *Gastroenterology*, **71**, 985.

Brown, W.R., Isobe, K., Nakane, P.K. & Pacini, B. (1977) Studies on translocation of immunoglobulin across intestinal epithelium. IV. Evidence for binding of IgA and IgM to secretory component in intestinal epithelium. *Gastroenterology*, **73**, 1333.

Buckley, C.H. & Fox, H. (1979) An immunohistochemical study of the significance of HCG secretion by large bowel adenocarcinoma. *Journal of Clinical Pathology*, **32**, 368.

Burns, J., Hambridge, M. & Taylor, C.R. (1974) Intracellular immunoglobin: a comparative study of three standard tissue processing methods using horseradish peroxidase and fluorochrome conjugates. *Journal of Clinical Pathology*, **27**, 548.

Busachi, C.A., Ray, M.B. & Desmet, V.J. (1978) An immunoperoxidase technique for demonstrating membrane localised HBsAg in paraffin sections of liver biopsies. *Journal of Immunological Methods*, **19**, 95.

Camelleri, J.-P., Amat, C., Chousterman, M., Petite, J.P., Duboust, A., Boddaert, A. & Paraf, A. (1977) Immunohistochemical patterns of hepatitis B surface antigen (HBsAg) in patients with hepatitis, renal homograft recipients and normal carriers. *Virchow's Archives* [*A*], **376**, 329.

Campbell, G.T. & Bhatnagar, A.J. (1976) Simultaneous visualisation by light microscopy of two pituitary hormones in a single tissue section using a combination of indirect immunohistochemical methods. *Journal of Histochemistry and Cytochemistry*, **24**, 448.

Carlsson, J., Drevin, H. & Axen, R. (1978) Protein thiolation and reversible protein-protein conjugation. *Biochemical Journal*, **173**, 723.

Celio, M.R. (1979) Immunohistochemistry on Bouin's fixed fetal tissue stored for thirty years in ethanol. *Histochemistry*, **61**, 347.

Coons, A.H. (1978) Opening remarks. In *Immunofluorescence and Related Staining Procedures* (Ed.) Knapp, W., Holubar, K. & Wick, G. pp. xi-xiii. Amsterdam: Elsevier North Holland.

Coruh, G. & Mason, D.Y. (1980) Serum proteins in human squamous epithelium. *British Journal of Dermatology*, in press.

Crofton, R.W., Cochrane, C. & McClelland, D.B.L. (1978) Preparation of lymphoid cells from small specimens of human gastrointestinal mucosa. *Gut*, **19**, 898.

Curran, R.C. & Gregory, J. (1977) The unmasking of antigens in paraffin sections of tissue by trypsin. *Experientia*, **33**, 1400.

Curran, R.C. & Gregory, J. (1978) Demonstration of immunoglobulin in cryostat and paraffin sections of human tonsil by immunofluorescence and immunoperoxidase techniques. *Journal of Clinical Pathology*, **31**, 947.

Curran, R.C. & Jones, E.L. (1978) The lymphoid follicles of the human palatine tonsil. *Clinical and Experimental Immunology*, **31**, 251.

DeLellis, R.A., Sternberger, L.A., Mann, R.B., Banks, P.M. & Nakane, P.K. (1979) Immunoperoxidase techniques in diagnostic pathology. *American Journal of Clinical Pathology*, **71**, 483.

Denk, H., Radaszkiewicz, T. & Weirich, E. (1977) Pronase pretreatment of tissue sections enhances sensitivity of the unlabelled antibody-enzyme (PAP) technique. *Journal of Immunological Methods*, **15**, 163.

Dorsett, B.H. & Ioachim, H.C. (1978) A method for the use of immunofluorescence on paraffin embedded tissues. *American Journal of Clinical Pathology*, **69**, 66.

Eckert, B.S. & Snyder, J.A. (1978) Combined immunofluorescence and high voltage electron microscopy of cultured mammalian cells, using an antibody that binds to glutaraldehyde treated tubulin. *Proceedings of the National Academy of Sciences of the United States of America*, **75**, 334.

Erlandsen, S.L., Parsons, J.A. & Rodning, C.B. (1979) Technical parameters of immunostaining of osmicated tissue in epoxy sections. *Journal of Histochemistry and Cytochemistry*, **27**, 1286.

Erlandsen, S.L., Hegre, O.D., Parsons, J.A., McEvoy, R.C. & Elde, R.P. (1976) Pancreatic islet cell hormones: distribution of cell types in the islet and evidence for the presence of somatostatin and gastrin within the D cell. *Journal of Histochemistry and Cytochemistry*, **24**, 883.

Esiri, M.M., Taylor, C.R. & Mason, D.Y. (1976) Application of an immunoperoxidase method to the study of the central nervous system; preliminary findings in a study of human formalin fixed material. *Neuropathology and Applied Neurobiology*, **2**, 233.

Fargion, S., Sangalli, G., Ronchi, G. & Fiorelli, G. (1979) Evaluation of T and B lymphocytes in liver infiltrates of patients with chronic active hepatitis. *Journal of Clinical Pathology*, **32**, 344.

Forsum, U., Klareskog, L. & Peterson, P.A. (1979) Distribution of Ia antigen-like molecules on non-lymphoid tissue. *Scandinavian Journal of Immunology*, **9**, 343.

Geyer, G., Schmidt, H.-P. & Biedermann, M. (1979) Horseradish peroxidase as a label of injured cells. *Histochemical Journal*, **11**, 337.

Ghoos, Y. & Vantrappen, G. (1971) The cytochemical localisation of lysozyme in Paneth cell granules. *Histochemical Journal*, **3**, 175.

Glickman, R.M., Green, P.H.R., Lees, R.S., Lux, S.E. & Kilgore, A. (1979) Immunofluorescence studies of apolipoprotein B in intestinal mucosa. *Gastroenterology*, **76**, 288.

Goodacre, R., Davidson, R., Singal, D. & Bienenstock, J. (1979) Morphologic and functional characteristics of human intestinal lymphoid cells isolated by a mechanical technique. *Gastroenterology*, **76**, 300.

Gordon, S., Todd, J. & Cohn, Z.A. (1974) In vitro synthesis and secretion of lysozyme by mononuclear phagocytes. *Journal of Experimental Medicine*, **139**, 1228.

Halmi, N.S. (1978) Immunostaining of growth hormone and prolactin in paraffin-embedded and stored or previously stained materials. *Journal of Histochemistry and Cytochemistry*, **26**, 486.

Hartmann, L. & Liacopoulos, P. (1977) Lymphoid cells of the normal human intestinal mucosa possessing both kappa and lambda light chain specificities. *Biomedicine*, **27**, 123.

Heatley, R.V., Rhodes, J., Calcraft, B.J., Whitehead, R.H., Fifield, R. & Newcombe, R.G. (1975) Immunoglobulin E in rectal mucosa of patients with proctitis. *Lancet*, **ii**, 1010.

Heyderman, E. (1979) Immunoperoxidase techniques in histopathology: applications, methods and controls. *Journal of Clinical Pathology*, **32**, 971.

Heyderman, E. & Monaghan, P. (1979) Immunoperoxidase reactions in resin embedded sections. *Journal of Investigative and Cellular Biology*, **2**, 119.

Heyderman, E., Steele, K. & Ormerod, M.G. (1979) A new antigen on the epithelial membrane: its immunoperoxidase localisation in normal and neoplastic tissue. *Journal of Clinical Pathology*, **32**, 35.

Hodges, J.R., Isaacson, P., Eade, O.E. & Wright, R. (1979) Serum lysozyme levels in malignant histiocytosis of the intestine. *Gut*, **20**, 854.

Huang, S.N., Minassian, H. & More, J.D. (1976) Application of immunofluorescent staining on paraffin sections improved by trypsin digestion. *Laboratory Investigation*, **35**, 383.

Hugon, J.S. & Borgers, M. (1968) Absorption of horseradish peroxidase by the mucosal cells of the duodenum of the mouse. *Journal of Histochemistry and Cytochemistry*, **16**, 229.

Isaacson, P. & Judd, M.A. (1978) Immunohistochemistry of carcinoembryonic antigen in the small intestine. *Cancer*, **42**, 1554.

Isaacson, P., Wright, D.H., Judd, M.A. & Mepham, B.L. (1979) Primary gastrointestinal lymphomas. *Cancer*, **43**, 1805.

Isobe, Y., Chen, S.-T., Nakane, P.K. & Brown, W.R. (1977) Studies on translocation of immunoglobulins across intestinal epithelium. I. Improvement in the peroxidase-labelled method for application to study of human intestinal mucosa. *Acta Histochemica et Cytochemica*, **10**, 161.

Jos, J., Labbe, F., Geny, B. & Griscelli, C. (1979) Immunoelectron-microscopic localisation of immunoglobulin A and secretory component in jejunal mucosa from children with coeliac disease. *Scandinavian Journal of Immunology*, **9**, 441.

Kitagawa, T. & Aikawa, T. (1976) Enzyme coupled immunoassay of insulin using a novel coupling agent. *Journal of Biochemistry*, **79**, 233.

Kitagawa, T., Fujitake, T., Taniyama, H. & Aikawa, T. (1978) Enzyme immunoassay of viomycin. *Journal of Biochemistry*, **12**, 326.

Klockars, M., Reitamo, S., Reitamo, J.J. & Möller, C. (1977) Immunohistochemical identification of lysozyme in intestinal lesions in ulcerative colitis and Crohn's disease. *Gut*, **18**, 377.

Korsrud, F.R. & Brandtzaeg, P. (1980) Quantitative immunohistochemistry of immunoglobulin and J chain producing cells in human parotid and submandibular glands. *Immunology*, **39**, 129.

Köhler, G. & Milstein, C. (1975) Continuous culture of fused cells secreting antibody of defined specificity. *Nature*, **256**, 495.

Larsson, L.-I. (1979) Simultaneous ultrastructural demonstration of multiple peptides in endocrine cells by a novel immunocytochemical method. *Nature*, **282**, 743.

Larsson, L.-I. & Schwartz, T.W. (1977) Radioimmunocytochemistry — a novel immunocytochemical principle. *Journal of Histochemistry and Cytochemistry*, **25**, 1140.

Martin-Comin, J. & Robyn, C. (1976) Comparative immunoenzymatic localisation of prolactin and growth hormone in human and rat pituitaries. *Journal of Histochemistry and Cytochemistry*, **24**, 1012.

Mason, D.Y. (1977) Intracellular lysozyme and lactoferrin in myeloproliferative disorders. *Journal of Clinical Pathology*, **30**, 541.

Mason, D.Y. & Sammons, R.E. (1978a) Rapid preparation of peroxidase:antiperoxidase complexes for immunocytochemical use. *Journal of Immunological Methods*, **20**, 317.

Mason, D.Y. & Sammons, R.E. (1978b) Alkaline phosphatase and peroxidase for double immunoenzymatic labelling of cellular constituents. *Journal of Clinical Pathology*, **31**, 454.

Mason, D.Y. & Sammons, R.E. (1979) The labelled antigen method of immunoenzymatic staining. *Journal of Histochemistry and Cytochemistry*, **27**, 832.

Mason, D.Y. & Taylor, C.R. (1975) The distribution of lysozyme in human tissues. *Journal of Clinical Pathology*, **28**, 124.

Mason, D.Y. & Taylor, C.R. (1978) Distribution of transferrin ferritin and lactoferrin in human tissues. *Journal of Clinical Pathology*, **31**, 316.

Mason, D.Y., Farrell, C. & Taylor, C.R. (1975) The detection of intracellular antigens in human leucocytes by immunoperoxidase staining. *British Journal of Haematology*, **31**, 361.

Mason, D.Y., Bell, J.I., Christensson, B. & Biberfeld, P. (1980) An immunohistological study of human lymphoma. *Clinical and Experimental Immunology*, in press.

McElrath, M.J., Galbraith, R.M. & Allen, R.C. (1979) Demonstration of alpha$_1$-antitrypsin by immunofluorescence on paraffin embedded hepatic and pancreatic tissue. *Journal of Histochemistry and Cytochemistry*, **27**, 794.

McLean, I.W. & Nakane, P.K. (1974) Periodate-lysine-paraformaldehyde fixative. A new fixation for immunoelectron microscopy. *Journal of Histochemistry and Cytochemistry*, **22**, 1077.

Mepham, B.L., Frater, W. & Mitchell, B.S. (1979) The use of proteolytic enzymes to improve immunoglobulin staining by the PAP technique. *Histochemical Journal*, **11**, 345.

Meuwissen, S.G.M., Feltkamp-Vroom, T.M., Brutel de la Riviere, A., Von dem Borne, A.E.G.K. & Tytgat, G.N. (1976) Analysis of lympho-plasmacytic infiltrate in Crohn's disease with special reference to indentification of lymphocyte subpopulations. *Gut*, **17**, 770.

Morton, J.A., Bastin, J., Fleming, K.A., McMichael, A.J., Burns, J. & McGee, J.O'D. (1980) Mallory bodies in alcoholic liver disease; identification of unique and cell membrane/cytoplasmic filament antigens by monoclonal antibodies. Submitted for publication.

Nagura, H., Nakane, P.K. & Brown, W.R. (1979) Translocation of dimeric IgA through neoplastic colon cells *in vitro*. *Journal of Immunology*, **123**, 2359.

Nagura, H., Brandtzaeg, P., Nakane, P.K. & Brown, W.R. (1979) Ultrastructural localisation of J chain in human intestinal mucosa. *Journal of Immunology*, **123**, 1044.

Nakane, P.K. (1968) Simultaneous localisation of multiple tissue antigens using the peroxidase-labelled antibody method: a study on pituitary glands of the rat. *Journal of Histochemistry and Cytochemistry*, **16**, 557.

Nakane, P. K. & Kawaoi, A. (1974) A peroxidase-labelled antibody. A new method of conjugation. *Journal of Histochemistry and Cytochemistry*, **22**, 1084.

Nayak, N.C. & Sachdeva, R. (1975) Localisation of hepatitis B antigen in conventional paraffin sections of the liver. *American Journal of Pathology*, **81**, 479.

O'Donoghue, D.P. & Kumar, P. (1979) Rectal IgE cells in inflammatory bowel disease. *Gut*, **20**, 149.

O'Sullivan, M.J., Gnemmi, E., Simmonds, A.D., Chieregatti, G., Heyderman, E., Bridges, J.W. & Marks, V. (1979) A comparison of the ability of β-galactosidase and horseradish peroxidase enzyme-antibody conjugates to detect specific antibodies. *Journal of Immunological Methods*, **31**, 247.

Pearse, A.G.E., Polak, J.M., Adams, C. & Kendall, P.A. (1974) Diethylpyrocarbonate, a vapour phase fixative for immunofluorescence on polypeptide hormones. *Histochemical Journal*, **6**, 347.

Piris, J. & Thomas, N.D. (1980) A quantitative study of the influence of fixation on immunoperoxidase staining of rectal tissue plasma cells. *Journal of Clinical Pathology*, in press.

Portman, B., Galbraith, R.M., Eddleston, L.W.F., Zuckerman, A.J. & Williams, R. (1976) Detection of HBAg in fixed liver tissue: use of a modified immunofluorescent technique and comparison with histochemical methods. *Gut*, **17**, 1.

Primus, F.J., Sharkey, R.M., Hansen, H.J. & Goldenberg, D.M. (1978) Immunoperoxidase detection of carcinoembryonic antigen. *Cancer*, **42**, 1540.

Radaszkiewicz, T., Dragosics, B., Abdelfattahgad, M. & Denk, H. (1979) Effect of protease pretreatment on immunomorphologic demonstration of hepatitis B surface antigen in conventional paraffin embedded liver biopsy material. *Journal of Immunological Methods*, **29**, 27.

Reitamo, S. (1978) Lysozyme antigenicity and tissue fixation. *Histochemistry*, **55**, 197.

Reitamo, S. & Reitamo, J.J. (1978) Immunoperoxidase identification of intracellular immunoglobulin in human tissues. *American Journal of Clinical Pathology*, **70**, 845.

Rothbarth, P.H., Tanke, H.J., Mul, N.A.J., Ploem, J.S., Vliegenthart, J.F.G. & Ballieux, R.E. (1978) Immunofluorescence studies with 4-acetimido-4'-isothiocyanate stilbene-2,2'-disulphonic acid (SITS). *Journal of Immunological Methods*, **19**, 101.

Sainte-Marie, G. (1962) A paraffin embedding technique for studies employing immunofluorescence. *Journal of Histochemistry and Cytochemistry*, **10**, 250.

Sternberger, L.A., Hardy, P.H., Cuculis, J.J. & Meyer, H.G. (1970) The unlabelled antibody method of immunohistochemistry. Preparation and properties of soluble antigen antibody complex (horseradish peroxidase-antihorseradish peroxidase) and its use in identification of spirochaetes. *Journal of Histochemistry and Cytochemistry*, **22**, 782.

Strickland, R.G., Husby, G., Black, W.C. & Williams, R.C. (1975) Peripheral blood and intestinal lymphocyte sub-populations in Crohn's disease. *Gut*, **16**, 847.

Takamiya, H., Batsford, S.R., Tokunaga, J. & Vogt, A. (1979) Immunohistological staining of antigens on semithin sections of specimens in plastic (QMA-Quetol 523). *Journal of Immunological Methods*, **30**, 277.

Taylor, C.R. (1978) Immunoperoxidase techniques. *Archives of Pathology and Laboratory Medicine*, **102**, 113.

Taylor, C.R. & Burns, J. (1974) The demonstration of plasma cells and other immunoglobulin producing cells in formalin-fixed paraffin embedded tissues using peroxidase labelled antibody. *Journal of Clinical Pathology*, **27**, 14.

Ternynck, T. & Avrameas, S. (1977) Conjugation of p-benzoquinone treated enzymes with antibodies and Fab fragments. *Immunochemistry*, **14**, 767.

Tramu, G., Pillez, A. & Leordanelli, J. (1978) An efficient method of antibody elution for the successive or simultaneous localisation of two antigens by immunocytochemistry. *Journal of Histochemistry and Cytochemistry*, **26**, 322.

Weinstein, W.M. & Lechago, J. (1977) A restaining method to restore fluorescence in faded preparations of tissues treated with the indirect immunofluorescence technique. *Journal of Immunological Methods*, **17**, 375.

Wilson, M.B. & Nakane, P.K. (1978) Recent developments in the periodate method of conjugating horseradish peroxidase (HRPO) to antibodies. In *Immunofluorescence and*

Related Staining Techniques (Ed.) Knapp, W., Holubar, K. & Wick, G. pp. 215–224. Amsterdam: Elsevier North Holland.

Witting, C. (1977) Immunofluorescence studies on formalin-fixed and paraffin-embedded material. *Beitrage für Pathologie*, **161**, 288.

2
Regulatory Peptides of the Gut: the Essential Mechanism for Gut Control

JULIA M. POLAK
S.R. BLOOM

When Bayliss and Starling in 1902 discovered secretin, the first regulatory peptide of the gut, they opened the era of knowledge of hormonal control of the gut by means of 'chemical messengers' acting at a distance. This revolutionary concept rapidly overtook Pavlov's Nobel Prize-winning ideas of neural control of gastrointestinal functions (nervism).

The discovery of secretin was rapidly followed by that of gastrin (Edkins, 1905) and later cholecystokinin-pancreozymin (CCK-PZ). In spite of this early start progress was hampered by technical problems due to the diffuse nature of the endocrine system of the gut which makes it hard to study hormonal effects. Extraction and purification of the gut hormones was originally difficult because they are short-chain peptides likely to be rapidly destroyed by the abundant proteolytic enzymes of the gastrointestinal tract. However, after the discovery that the peptides were heat stable this problem was overcome.

Advances in the technology of protein chemistry such as the use of ion exchange chromatography and high-pressure liquid-gas chromatography led to the rapid discovery, characterization, sequencing and synthesis of a large number of gut regulatory peptides, many of which have also been found in the central and peripheral neural tissue (brain and gut peptides). It is now clear that these peptides may act in a tripartite manner (Polak and Bloom, 1979):

1. as 'circulating hormones', acting on distant target organs;
2. as 'paracrine' or local hormones, acting on the neighbouring tissue;
3. as neurotransmitters/neuromodulators locally released from nerve terminals by axonal depolarization. To date, eight gut peptides are known to act via the circulation (Table 1). One (somatostatin) is a classical paracrine or local hormone and several others, including vasoactive intestinal polypeptide (VIP), the enkephalins, bombesin and substance P, probably act as neurotransmitters or neuromodulators (Table 1).

© 1980 W.B. Saunders Company Ltd.

Table 1. Gut hormones: their chemistry, distribution and actions

Function	Peptide	Stomach Fund.	Stomach Ant.	Upper gut Duod.	Upper gut Jej.	Lower gut Ile.	Lower gut Col.	Pancreas	Mol. wt	Amino-acid no.	Granules nm ± s.d.	Actions
	Gastrin (17)		√	√					2100	17	360 ± 56	Trophism, gastric secretion
	(34) Secretin		√	√√	√√				3800 3073	34 27	175 ± 32 240 ± 32	Pancreatic bicarbonate secretion
Circulating hormone	Motilin CCK			√√	√√				2700 3883	22 34	180 ± 24 250 ± 17	Gut motility Pancreatic enzyme secretion
	GIP			√	√				5105	13	350 ± 24	Insulin release
	Enteroglucagon			√	√	√√	√				210 ± 26	Trophism
	Neurotensin					√√			1673	13	300 ± 39	?
	Pancreatic polypeptide					√	√	√	4273	36	200 ± 22	Inhibition of pancreatic function
Paracrine	Somatostatin	√	√	√	√	√	√	√	1639	14	310 ± 46	Inhibition of gut hormone release
	VIP	√	√	√	√	√	√	√	3326	28		Vasodilation, muscle relaxation and secretion
Neurotransmitter	Substance P	√	√	√	√	√			1347	11		Vasodilation, muscle constriction
	Bombesin	√	√	√	√	√			1620	14		Release of gut hormones
	Enkephalin-Leu Met	√√	√√	√√	√√	√√	√√		556 574	5 5		Opiate effects Opiate effects

TECHNOLOGY

Knowledge of the distribution and cellular localization of these regulatory peptides has been made possible by the availability of pure or synthetic peptides and the use of two immunological methods — radioimmunoassay (RIA) and immunocytochemistry (IC). RIA provides information regarding the precise quantities and molecular forms of the peptide in tissue and its concentration in local fluids and/or the peripheral circulation. IC localizes the peptide in histological tissue sections and shows whether it is produced by the neural elements or by the endocrine cells of the gut mucosa.

Several problems are inherent in both techniques, however, and these must be recognized and taken into account. RIA technique is based on the competitive attachment of unlabelled and radiolabelled hormone to its specific antibody. It has been increasingly recognized that antibodies are raised to only part of the entire amino-acid sequence of hormone and, therefore, radioimmunological measurements may not indicate the biologically active part of the peptide. However, the recent availability of synthetic peptide fragments has allowed the full characterization of the antibodies used in RIA systems and thus the better interpretation of results.

Although IC is an extremely useful technique, several problems must be overcome before it can be used with confidence. These are concerned with:

1. the insolubilizing or fixation of the peptide antigens, which may be readily lost by diffusion from the section, and
2. complete specificity of staining so that the reaction occurs only with the peptide in question.

Fixation

All neuropeptides are water soluble. It is thus essential to prevent their loss from the tissue during processing by rendering them effectively insoluble. This is best achieved by the use of cross-linking agents such as diethylpyrocarbonate and p-benzoquinone, which act by producing insoluble polymerized complexes without undue damage to the antigenic sites or tertiary structure of the peptide (Pearse and Polak, 1975).

Specificity

Antisera for immunocytochemistry usually contain a mixed population of high-affinity specific and low-affinity unspecific antibodies. It is extremely important to ensure that the antigen-antibody reaction is specific for the peptide in question. Two major steps must be taken to control the specificity:

1. Dilution of the primary antibody. The optimal dilution is the greatest possible that is consistent with strong positive staining. The high dilution removes minor populations of unspecific antibodies, and a long (24 to 48 hours) incubation time ensures adequate reaction. Very high dilutions

have recently become possible by use of the extremely sensitive unlabelled antibody enzyme method, known as the 'peroxidase-antiperoxidase' (PAP) technique (Sternberger, 1974).
2. The universally applied and obligatory control is the demonstration that addition of the pure peptide to the antibody before reaction on the section completely quenches all staining by blocking the specific antibody binding site.

In addition, as in the RIA system, the recent use of synthetic peptide fragments has allowed the further characterization of specific antibodies.

GENERAL MORPHOLOGY OF THE ENDOCRINE CELLS OF THE GUT

In conventional histological preparations (haematoxylin and eosin, or toluidine blue) the gut endocrine cells appear as 'clear' elements (Figure 1),

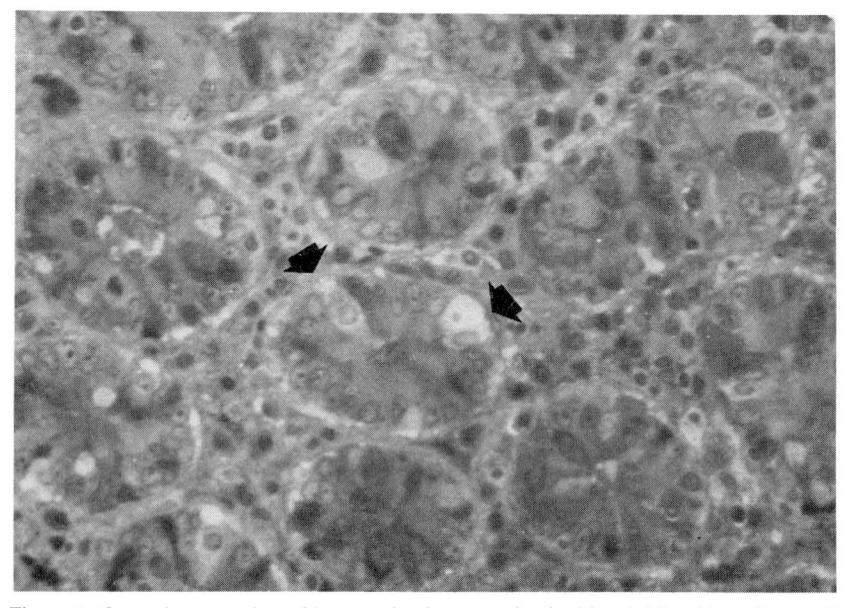

Figure 1. One micron section of human duodenum stained with toluidine blue. Clear cells marked by arrows. × 450.

as they react poorly to routine staining. They are well stained, however, by silver impregnation (Figure 2) which can distinguish two main groups (argyrophil and argentaffin) according to their reactivity. Electron microscopy is, in addition, of considerable diagnostic value, as the gut endocrine cells are well provided with electron-dense secretory granules (Figure 3) whose shape, density and limiting membrane permit their ultrastructural classification (Solcia et al, 1978). The endocrine cells of the gut share a number of cytochemical and functional characteristics with many other peptide-producing cells outside the gut. These have all been grouped together by Pearse as APUD (*A*mine *P*recursor *U*ptake and *D*ecarboxylation) cells.

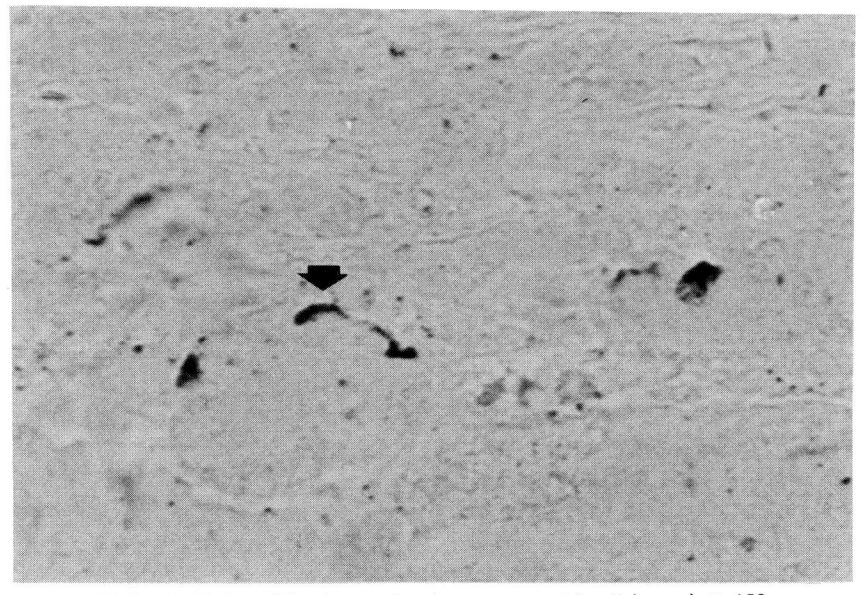

Figure 2. Section of duodenum showing an argyrophil cell (arrow). × 450.

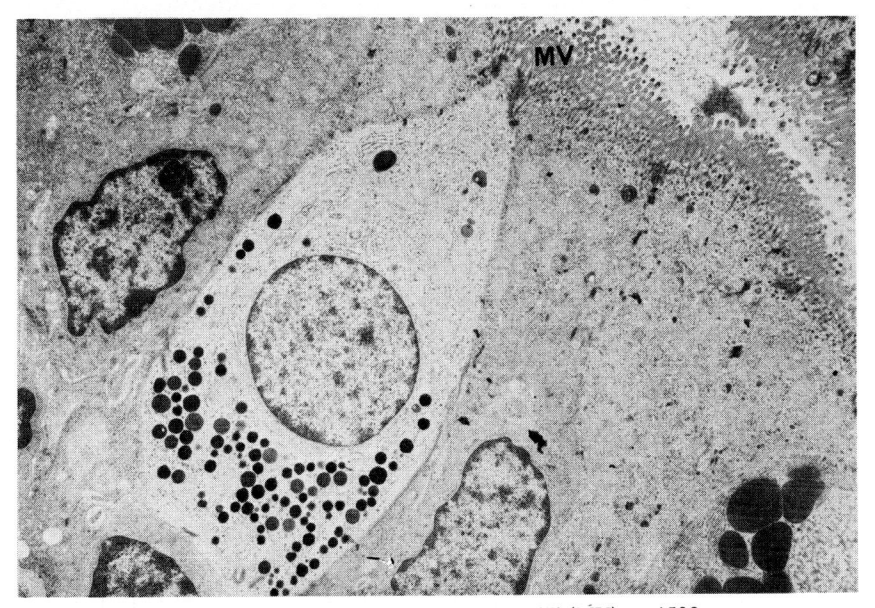

Figure 3. Endocrine cell showing microvilli (MV). × 4500.

INDIVIDUAL PEPTIDES

In this section we shall briefly discuss the chemistry, distribution, cellular origin, physiology and pathology of the peptides which will be grouped according to their mode of action (Table 1).

Hormones Acting via the Circulation

The hormones acting via the circulation have a longer half-life than the peptides acting locally or as neurotransmitters. Basal circulating levels of the hormones are always detectable and a significant rise is seen after a meal, of which particular components can release particular peptides. The distribution of the peptides throughout the gut is quite well circumscribed to specific anatomical areas. The cells of origin are often triangular or pear shaped, with the apex reaching the lumen and ending in a tuft of microvilli (Figure 3). The secretory granules are mostly found in the basal part of the cell in close contact with blood vessels (Figure 3).

Gastrin

Gastrin was discovered in 1905 but was purified and sequenced only in 1964. It was originally thought to be composed of 17 amino-acids. However, larger (34 amino-acids) and smaller (14 and four amino-acids) forms have subsequently been found. The entire biological activity resides in the last four (C-terminal) amino-acids. Apart from its function as the main hormone stimulating the secretion of gastric acid, gastrin is reputed to be a major trophic factor acting particularly on the gut and pancreas (Walsh and Grossman, 1975; Rehfeld and Larsson, 1979).

Gastrin is found predominantly in the antrum, although considerable quantities are also found, especially in man, in the upper small intestine (Figure 4). The gastrin cells of the antrum, which store predominantly gastrin 17 (G17), are characterized at the electron microscopical level by the presence of large (300 nm) electron-lucent granules (Figure 5a), whereas the gastrin cell of the intestine, which stores considerable quantities of the larger form of gastrin, gastrin 34 (G34), contains much smaller and denser secretory granules with an average size of 170 nm (Buchan et al, 1979a) (Figure 5b). Antral gastrin cells are predominantly localized in the midportion of the mucosa. The G cell is one of the most abundant of the endocrine cell types in the antrum where it is present in far greater numbers than are gastrin cells in the intestine. The intestinal gastrin cells, present in the duodenal and jejunal mucosa, display the classical morphology of endocrine cells (see above).

Pathology. Gastrin is the agent responsible for the Zollinger-Ellison syndrome. The majority of gastrinomas are found in the pancreas although some are also found in the small intestine. Since gastrin is not found in adults in the pancreas, the high incidence of pancreatic gastrinomas is difficult to interpret. Small quantities of gastrin and a few very scattered gastrin cells are, however, found in the fetal pancreas and it is therefore possible that remnants of these fetal gastrin cells may give rise to gastrinomas in the adult. Histologically, gastrinomas do not differ from other islet cell tumours.

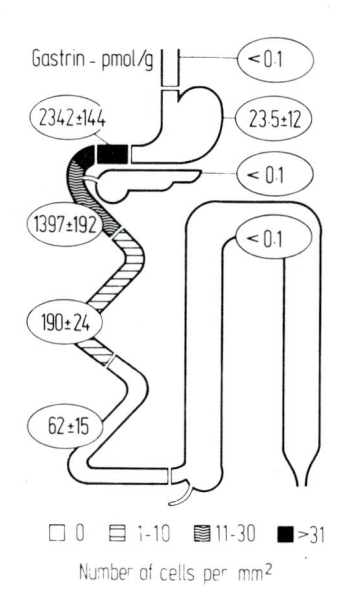

Figure 4. Distribution of gastrin in human gut. Shading indicates cells per mm^2 of mucosa and figures the total extractable hormone per gram of whole bowel.

Benign and malignant tumours occur in approximately equal proportions. A large number of these tumours are multiple and although they are of rather slow growth, metastases are not uncommon, principally in the nearby lymph nodes. Ultrastructurally, both the antral and the intestinal types of granules are found (Figure 6, a and b), corresponding to the proportions of G17 and G34 respectively (Buchan et al, 1979a).

Secretin

Secretin is a 27 amino-acid residue peptide which belongs to the secretin-glucagon family of peptides. Secretin has been so far exclusively found in the small intestine where it is produced by the mucosal S cells (Polak et al, 1971a, 1971b), which contain small to intermediate-sized secretory granules (260 nm). Secretin is a potent stimulant for the release of alkaline juice from the pancreas. Although this hormone is found in the circulation, its level does not rise after a meal. Secretin is released, however, as the classical experiments of Bayliss and Starling suggested, after acid is introduced into the duodenum (Schaffalitzky de Muckadell, Fahrenkrug and Rune, 1979). This release is considerably impaired in patients with coeliac

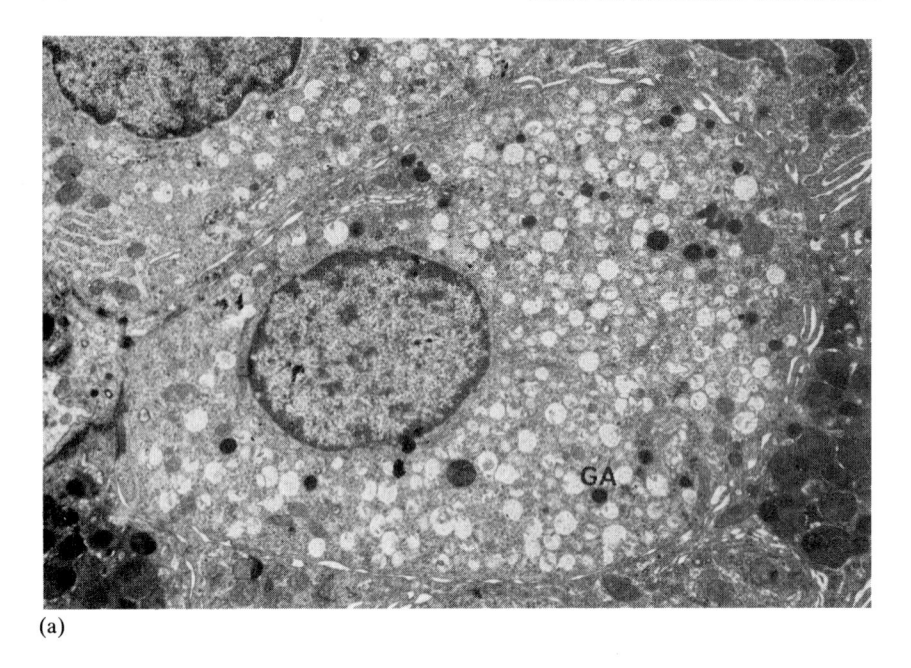

Figure 5. (a) Gastrin-containing cell from human antrum (GA). × 6750. (b) (i) Semithin section of human duodenum showing gastrin-containing cell. Cell identified by arrow is shown in serial thin section. × 450. (ii) Same cell as in (i). × 4800. (iii) High magnification of granules. × 13 500.

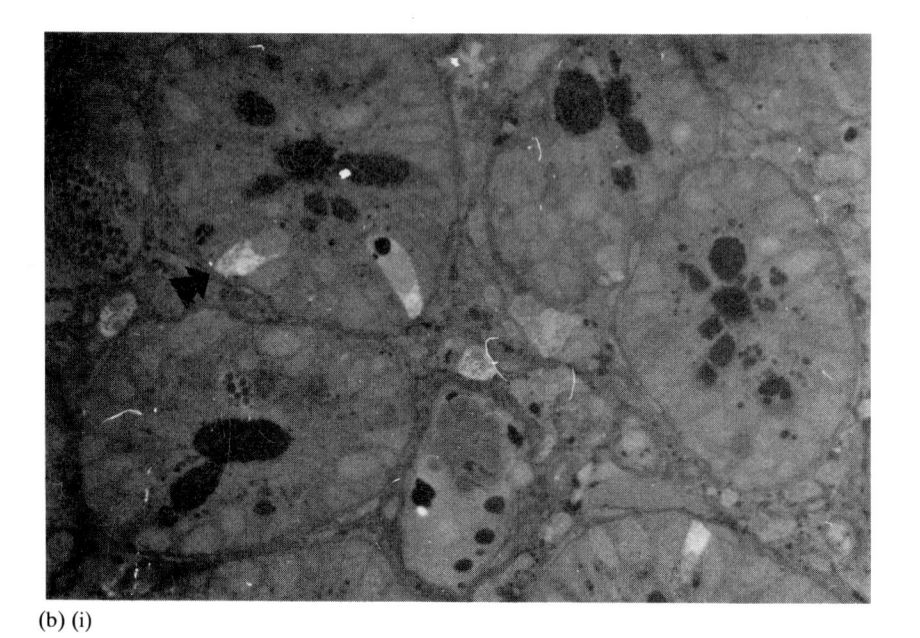

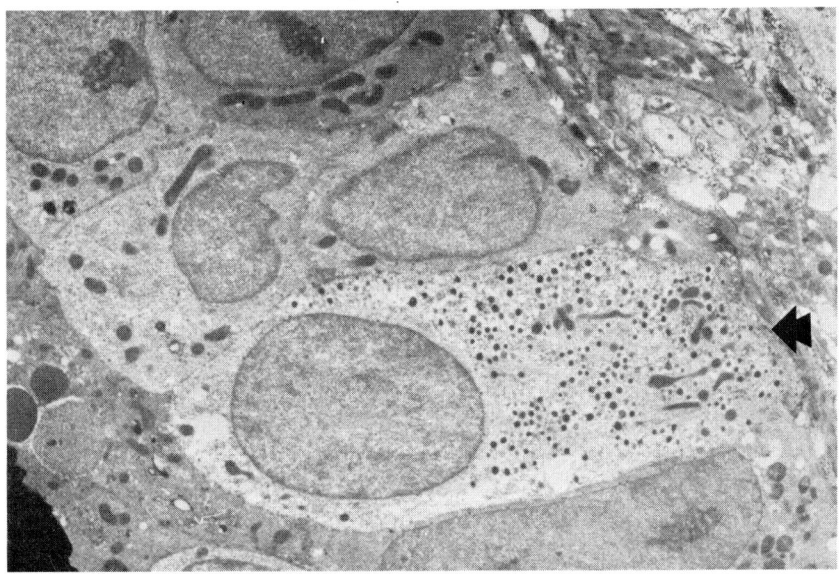

(b) (ii)

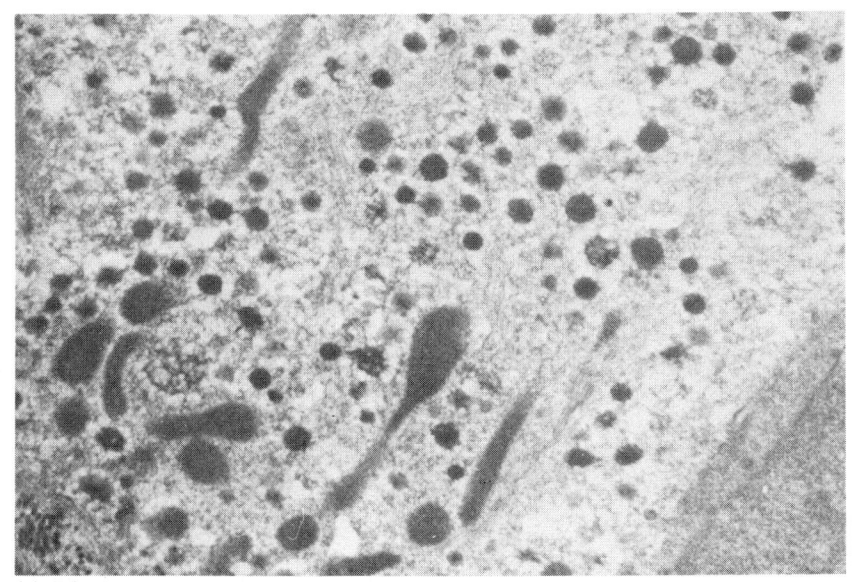

(b) (iii)

disease. This fits well with the finding of increased secretin storage in this disease, manifested by an increase in the strength of immunoreaction and apparent number of secretin cells (Polak et al, 1973b). That the release of secretin and not its target organ (the pancreas) is impaired is shown by the successful pancreatic bicarbonate response of patients after infusion of purified secretin. The abnormalities, probably secondary to mucosal

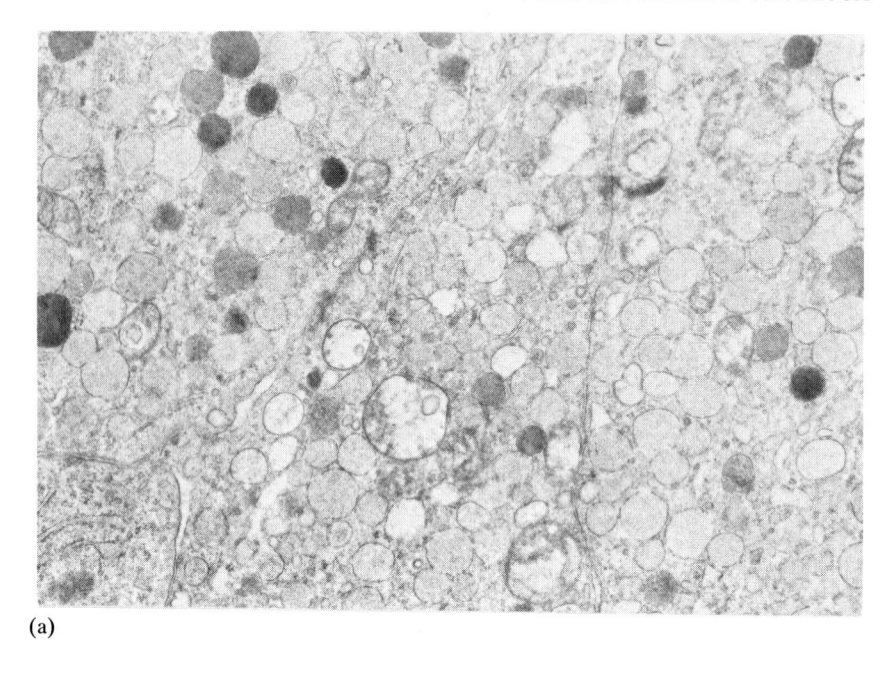

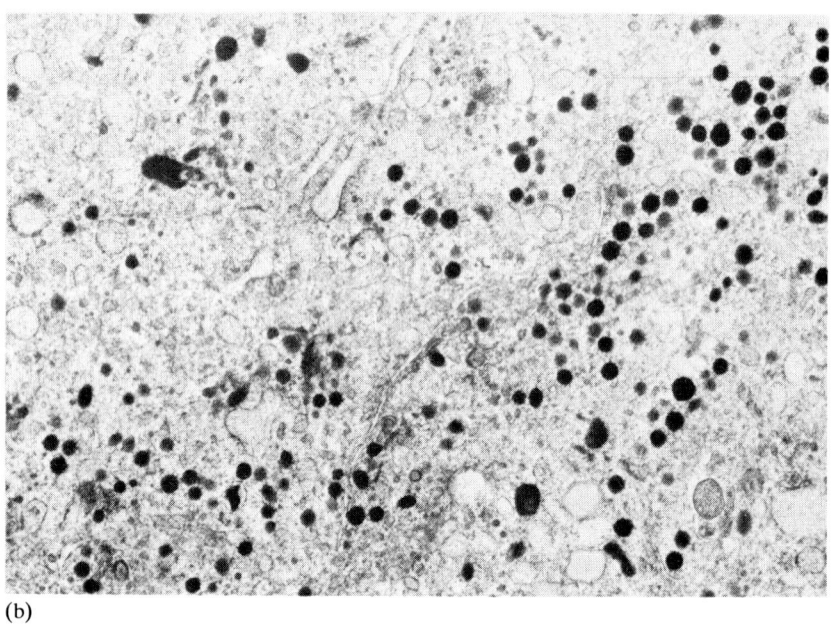

Figure 6. (a) Gastrinoma containing antral-type gastrin granules. × 4500. (b) Gastrinoma containing intestinal-type gastrin granules. × 4500.

inflammation, are reversed after a gluten-free diet has restored the normal appearance of the mucosa.

Cholecystokinin (CCK)

The original 33 amino-acid peptide CCK was found, like gastrin, to be present in both blood and tissues in several molecular forms. Its biologically active part resides in the last eight amino-acids. CCK is found in the small intestine, in typical endocrine cells, the I cells (Buchan et al, 1978), with secretory granules of intermediate size (250 nm), and in the autonomic innervation. CCK, especially its octapeptide, is also found in large quantities in the brain cortex. The main action of CCK appears to be as a stimulant of enzyme secretion from the pancreas and as a gallbladder contractor. It is possible that CCK acts principally as a neurotransmitter in the octapeptide form and as a circulating hormone in the larger forms. The latter are at present difficult to assess as many molecular forms of CCK, with differing biological activity, are known to circulate, and development of accurate and specific assays is difficult (Rehfeld, 1978).

GIP

GIP is a 43 amino-acid peptide which was originally isolated for its inhibitory action on gastric acid production (*G*astric *I*nhibitory *P*olypeptide). However, it was later found to be principally a powerful insulin releaser, though glucose dependent. It was therefore renamed *G*lucose-dependent *I*nsulinotropic *P*eptide, thus retaining its original acronym GIP. GIP is found exclusively in the mucosa of the small intestine, in typical endocrine cells (Polak et al, 1973a) containing large (350 nm) secretory granules with a highly electron-dense core. GIP is a circulating hormone and its blood level rises dramatically after a meal. Like secretin, GIP release is totally obliterated in untreated coeliac disease, possibly due to mucosal inflammation. In addition, GIP is impaired in obese patients who have undergone a by-pass operation, possibly due to the large number of 'by-passed' GIP cells. This consequently leads to abnormalities of glucose metabolism and impairment of insulin release (breakdown of the entero-insular 'incretin' axis) (Bloom and Polak, 1980b).

Motilin

Motilin is a potent motor-stimulating peptide of 22 amino-acids found exclusively in the mucosa of the small intestine. Two major molecular forms of motilin are distinguished in both blood and tissue (Bloom et al, 1979a). One, the smaller, corresponds in gel-permeation chromatographic studies to the original peptide extracted from porcine gut. The nature of the larger form is as yet unclear but it seems to correspond to 'pro-motilin'. Both molecular forms are stored in typical endocrine cells of the small intestine, although some enterochromaffin (EC) cells in addition seem to contain the larger form, detected by N-terminally directed antibodies (Polak and

Buchan, 1979). Basal motilin levels show a skewed distribution and motilin is released by both oral and intravenous fat. The true physiological role of motilin is not known but it would seem that motilin may control gastric emptying and the frequency of the interdigestive myoelectric complexes. Motilin levels are elevated in all kinds of diarrhoeic states, including Crohn's disease, ulcerative colitis and infective diarrhoea (Bloom and Polak, 1980b).

Neurotensin

Neurotensin is a 13 amino-acid peptide originally extracted from the hypothalamus. The hypothalamic content was later found to correspond to only 10 per cent of the total body neurotensin, as the largest bulk, some 85 per cent, is concentrated in the ileum. In this region of the bowel, neurotensin is produced by large granuled cells, the NT cells (Polak et al, 1977). The C-terminal part of neurotensin is the active part. Neurotensin is rapidly released after a meal, the magnitude of this rise being proportional to the size of the meal. Two major molecular forms are found in the circulation, although only the smaller form, which co-elutes in chromatographic studies at the level of synthetic neurotensin, is released after a meal (Blackburn and Bloom, 1979). The physiological role of neurotensin is as yet unknown. However, pharmacological studies seem to indicate that neurotensin releases insulin and glucagon from the pancreas and gastrin from the stomach as well as being a powerful hypotensive-vasodilatory substance. The postprandial neurotensin concentration rises unusually rapidly and reaches an abnormally high level in patients with dumping syndrome.

Enteroglucagon

Enteroglucagon (EG) is a convenient name to denote the glucagon-like immunoreactivity of the intestine. Enteroglucagon is present in significant quantities in the ileum and colon and is produced by the EG cells (Polak et al, 1971b). The large granules of these cells are distinct from those of the other large granuled cells of the same area, the neurotensin (NT) cells. Enteroglucagon has recently been purified from the intestine and named 'glicentin' (Moody, Jacobsen and Sundby, 1978). It was subsequently found to be composed of approximately 100 amino-acids containing within its structure the entire 29 amino-acid sequence of pancreatic glucagon. Glicentin has recently been found also in the pancreas, which raises the possibility that it is a proglucagon which in the pancreas is broken down into true pancreatic glucagon and a larger by-product, the N-terminal remnant. Enteroglucagon is not yet freely available; thus its physiological role can only be deduced from studies of its pathology. In a single enteroglucagon-producing tumour (Bloom, 1972), a significant mucosal villous hypertrophy and increase in intestinal transit time were found. In addition, a markedly raised basal enteroglucagon level is always observed in diseases involving mucosal damage, such as coeliac disease, tropical sprue or after operation such as small intestinal resection or intestinal by-pass for obesity (Bloom and

Polak, 1980a, 1980b). Thus it seems that enteroglucagon is one of the factors regulating intestinal mucosal growth. Correlative studies between enteroglucagon levels and enterocyte turnover rate appear to be warranted.

Pancreatic polypeptide (PP)

PP was discovered by Lin and Chance (1972) while purifying insulin. It is now known as the fourth pancreatic hormone and is composed of 35 amino-acids. PP is almost exclusively found in the pancreas, with greater concentration in the head than in the tail of this organ. The cell of origin is known as the 'small granuled cell of the pancreas' and is present around the islets and as scattered cells in the exocrine pancreas and the pancreatic ducts (Polak and Buchan, 1980). PP is a circulating hormone, and its level rises dramatically after a meal. The role of PP in digestive physiology is little understood, as it exerts actions antagonistic to those of CCK (inhibition of enzyme output from the pancreas and relaxation of the gallbladder). As it is released after a meal to prevent digestion, PP is commonly called the hormone of 'indigestion' (Bloom and Polak, 1980a, 1980b). A very interesting recent finding was the presence of extremely elevated PP levels in both blood and tissue in 50 per cent of patients with islet cell tumours of the pancreas (insulinomas, VIPomas, glucagonomas and gastrinomas) (Polak et al, 1976). A high blood level of PP is thus a very useful diagnostic marker for pancreatic endocrine tumours.

Local (Paracrine) Hormones

Feyrter's postulate of a local or paracrine action for his 'clear cells' (Feyrter, 1938) has recently proved true for at least some of the cells of the 'diffuse endocrine system'. A number of recently discovered regulatory peptides has been shown not to act via the circulation. In addition, their short half-life, extensive distribution and wide spectrum of actions on many organs suggest that they may have a local influence on tissues, within their orbit of diffusion. The most illustrative example is *somatostatin*. Somatostatin is a 14 amino-acid peptide, which exerts a large number of central and peripheral 'inhibitory' actions, hence its name (Table 2).

Table 2. *Pharmacological effects of somatostatin in the gut*

Inhibition of:	
Growth hormone	Gastric acid
TSH	Pepsin
Insulin	Gastric emptying
Glucagon	Pancreatic enzymes
Pancreatic polypeptide	Pancreatic bicarbonate
Gastrin	Choleresis
GIP	Gallbladder contraction
Motilin	Motility
CCK	Xylose absorption
Enteroglucagon	Coeliac blood flow

Somatostatin is found in the brain and also in the periphery. The gut contains large quantities, principally in the antrum and pancreas (Figure 7), although the peptide is widely distributed along its entire length. The cell of origin is the D cell of the gut and pancreas (Polak et al, 1975), described 44

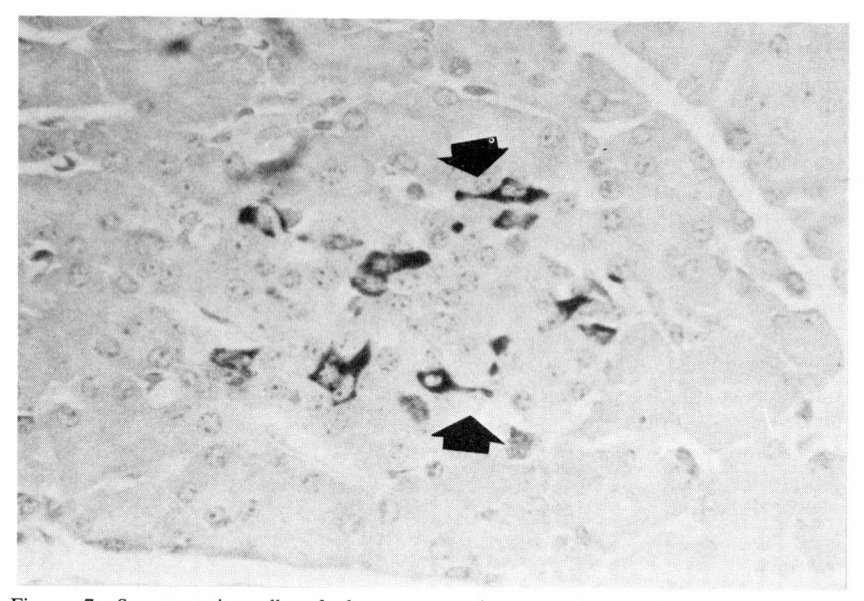

Figure 7. Somatostatin cells of the pancreas immunostained using the peroxidase-antiperoxidase (PAP) technique. Note the cellular processes (arrowed). × 225.

years prior to the discovery of its product, somatostatin. The D (somatostatin) cell is recognized at the ultrastructural level by its characteristic large secretory granules (Figure 8).

Although somatostatin-producing tumours (somatostatinomas) have been described, their incidence is rare. However, scattered somatostatin cells are frequently found in pancreatic endocrine tumours (Bloom, Polak and West, 1978). Their relevance is so far undetermined. Patients with somatostatinomas have been found to have hypochlorhydria, diabetes, gallstones, and steatorrhoea. Somatostatin is one of the main controlling factors for the release of insulin and thus it, or the lack of it, may be responsible for the severe hyperinsulinaemia and intractable hypoglycaemia seen in children with 'nesidioblastosis' of the pancreas as there is a significant decrease in the number and content of somatostatin cells in their pancreases (Polak and Bloom, 1980).

A small proportion of duodenal ulcer patients has less gastric somatostatin than normal (Chayvaille et al, 1978).

Neurotransmitters/Neuromodulators

The principal localization of VIP, the enkephalins, bombesin (mammals) and substance P is in the autonomic innervation of the gut wall. The intrinsic

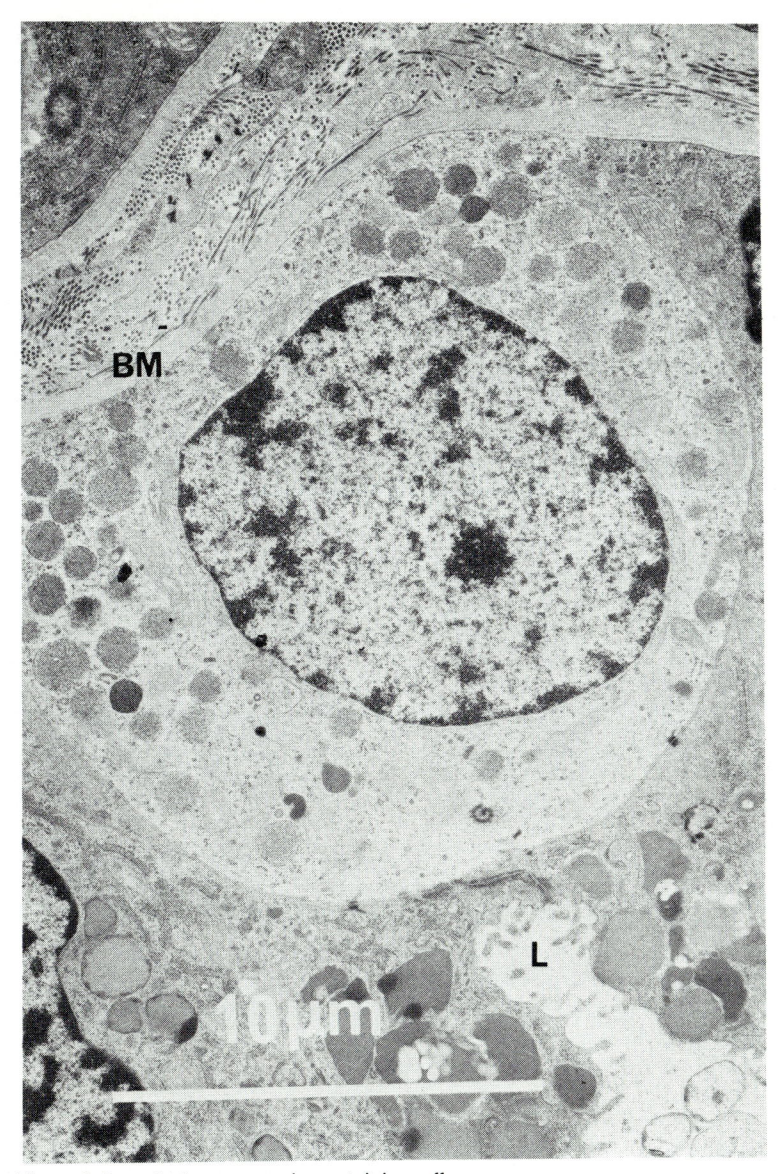

Figure 8. Intestinal somatostatin-containing cell.
BM = Basement membrane;
L = Lumen. × 6000.

neuronal origin of these peptides was suggested in 1976 and has been fully validated by experiments involving immunostaining of myenteric (Auerbach's) and submucous (Meissner's) plexus cultures devoid of extrinsic innervation and inter-plexus nerve connections (Jessen et al, 1980). Confirmation has also been obtained by immunostaining and estimation of peptide content of whole pieces of gut which shows no change after extrinsic denervation (Figure 9) (Jessen et al, 1980).

Substance P

Substance P was discovered when von Euler and Gaddum (1931) recovered, after vagal stimulation, a substance capable of inducing an atropine-resistant gut muscle contraction. Substance P was later purified and characterized as

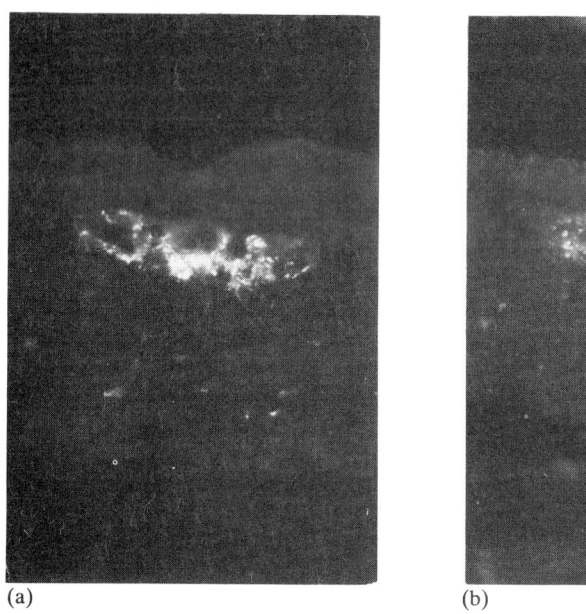

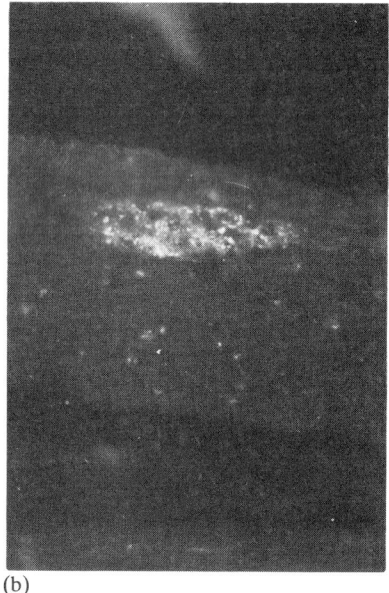

Figure 9. Myenteric plexus of guinea pig immunostained for substance P. (a) Normal colon. (b) Extrinsically denervated colon. × 254. Note there is no apparent alteration in substance P innervation.

an 11 amino-acid peptide identical to Leeman's sialogogic peptide (Leeman and Hammerschlag, 1967). Substance P is found in the brain and in many peripheral areas, including the gut, urogenital tract (Figure 10), heart, skin, lung and carotid body (Polak and Bloom, 1979). In addition, its presence in large quantities in the dorsal horn of the spinal cord (Figure 11), whence it is depleted after section of the dorsal root (substance P is present there in small cells), has indicated that substance P may be a sensory neurotransmitter (Otsuka, Konishi and Takahashi, 1975). This postulate is supported by the finding of numerous substance P-containing fibres in anatomical areas involved with all kinds of sensory transmission (e.g., vagina, skin, bronchial epithelium) (Polak and Bloom, 1978).

Bombesin

Bombesin is a 14 amino-acid peptide first extracted from the skin of the amphibian *Bombina bombina*. Bombesin powerfully influences gastrointes-

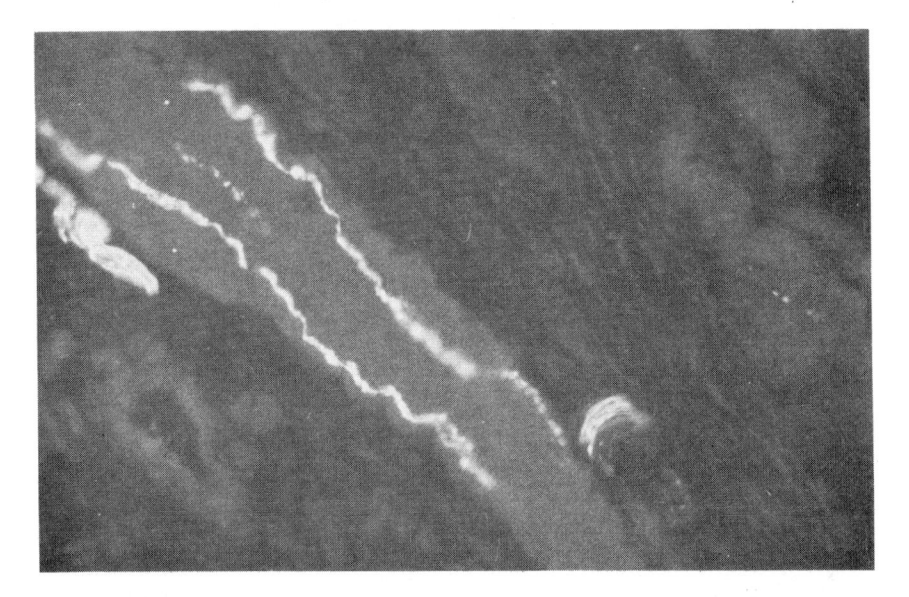

Figure 10. Substance P nerves in muscle of guinea pig ureter immunostained by indirect immunofluorescence. × 282.

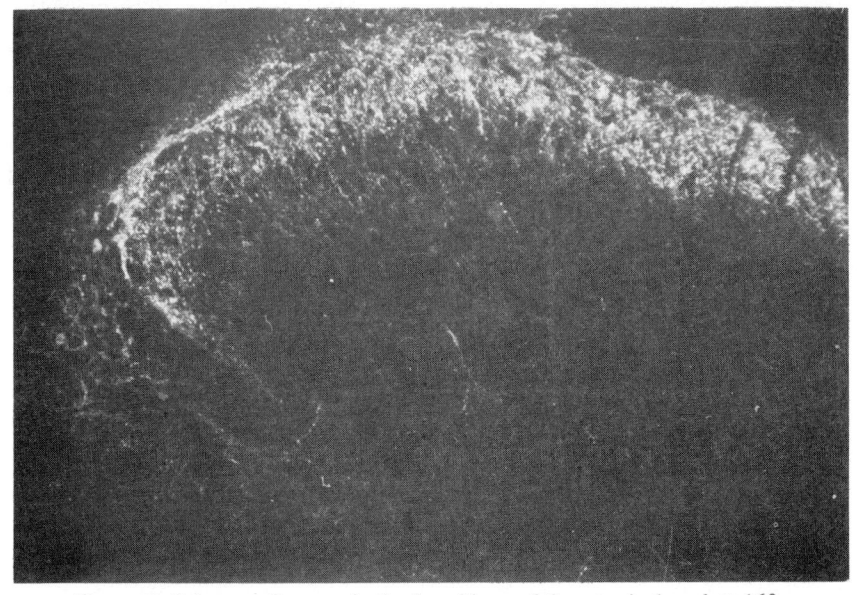

Figure 11. Substance P nerves in the dorsal horn of the rat spinal cord. × 160.

tinal functions as it is a potent gut hormone releaser (Bloom et al, 1979b) (Table 3). It may therefore be considered to be an antagonist of somatostatin, the inhibitory peptide of the gut. Bombesin is found not only in the gut, but also in neurones of the brain and in the lung, where it is present in classical endocrine (Feyrter's) cells (Polak et al, 1978).

Table 3. *Pharmacological effects of bombesin in the gut*

Release of:
  Gastrin
  Neurotensin
  Enteroglucagon
  Pancreatic polypeptide
  Motilin

Stimulation of:
  Gallbladder contraction
  Gastric secretion
  Protein-rich secretion from pancreas

Enkephalins

The enkephalins are a pair of pentapeptides which differ by only one amino-acid (methionine and leucine) at the C-terminal end. The enkephalins exert a wide range of actions in the gut, including the reduction of intestinal motility and secretion, relaxation of gallbladder tone, contraction of the sphincter of Oddi, suppression of pancreatic bicarbonate or enzyme secretion after endogenous or exogenous stimulation and interference with peristaltic reflex (Konturek, 1978). In addition, they inhibit both the release of acetylcholine and the firing of neurones of the myenteric plexus, acting on the processes of the cells rather than their perikarya. The enkephalins may also act as interneurones within a plexus. Sympathetic and chromaffin tissues, as well as the tumours derived from them, also contain the enkephalins (Sullivan, Bloom and Polak, 1978). An interesting recent finding is the presence of enkephalin-like immunoreactivity in the Type I cells of the carotid body (Figure 12) (Wharton et al, 1980), which would account for the modulatory actions of these cells on dopamine release; dopamine is concomitantly stored in the Type I cells.

Vasoactive intestinal polypeptide (VIP)

VIP is a powerful stimulator of vasodilation, muscle relaxation and secretion, composed of 28 amino-acids. It is present in very large quantities in the entire body and its role as a putative neurotransmitter has recently been supported by neurophysiological studies. These have shown that VIP in the gut is responsible for the neurally-mediated atropine-resistant relaxation of gastric muscle, intestinal and salivary gland vasodilation and pancreatic bicarbonate release. Stimulation of the nerves which produce these effects always results in a significant rise of VIP levels in the innervated area (Fahrenkrug et al, 1978). In addition, these atropine-resistant tissue responses can now be mimicked by micro-injections of VIP in the local circulation. VIP in the brain is present in considerable quantities in the cortex, the hypothalamus, the stria terminalis and its bed nucleus and the amygdala (Roberts et al, 1980). In the periphery many VIP nerves are seen not only in the gut and pancreas (Figure 13) but also in the urogenital tract, the upper respiratory tract and nasal mucosa, the skin, the carotid body and

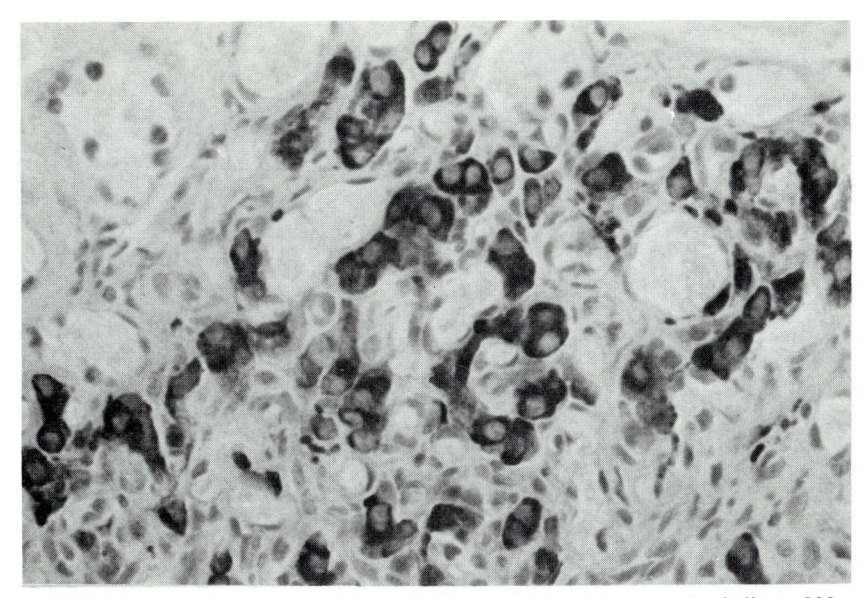

Figure 12. Type I cells of the cat carotid body immunostained for met-enkephalin. × 320.

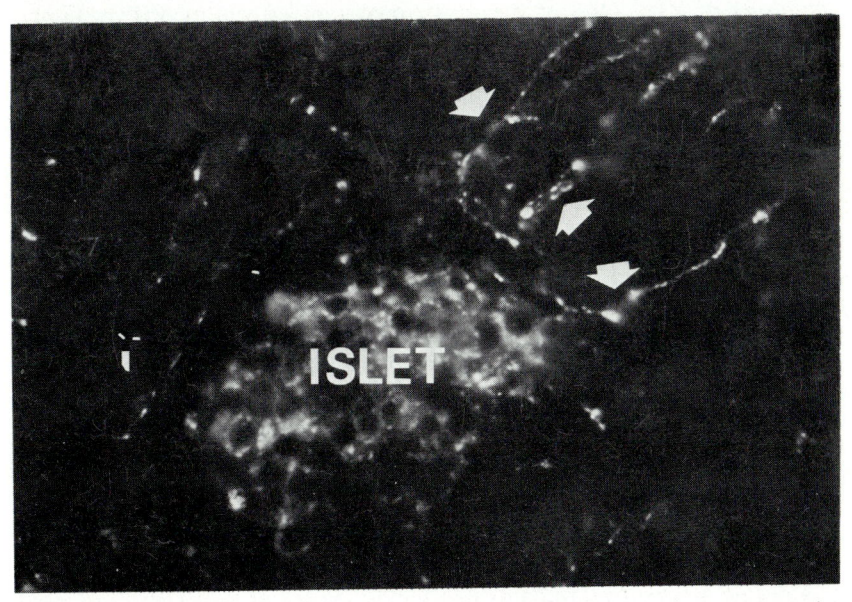

Figure 13. VIP immunoreactive nerves (arrowed) converging on an islet (autofluorescent) in human pancreas. × 225.

the salivary glands (Polak and Bloom, 1978, 1979). In the gut VIP nerves innervate the two muscle layers, the mucosa and submucosa, the two ganglionated plexi and the blood vessels. Most of the VIP neurones are present in the submucous (Meissner's) plexus (Figure 14).

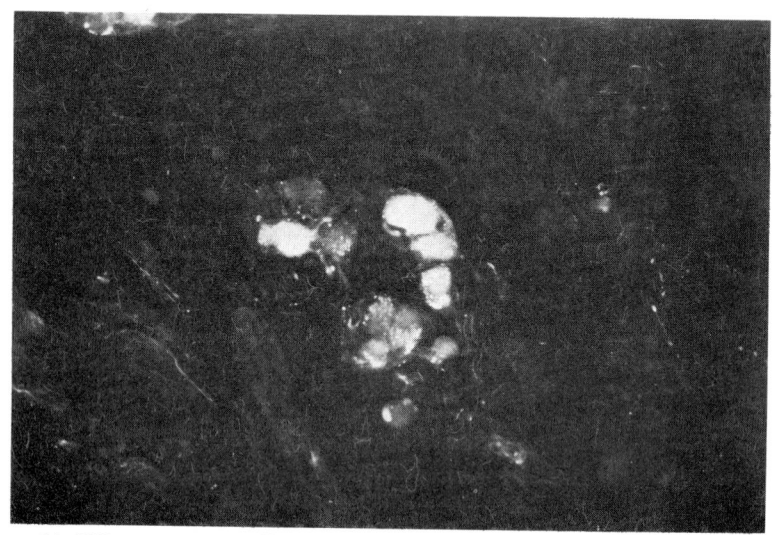

Figure 14. VIP nerves surrounding immunoreactive and non-immunoreactive ganglion cell bodies in Meissner's plexus of human colon. × 225.

Pathology of VIP. One of the most important effects of VIP in human pathology is the production of the Verner-Morrison syndrome, or WDHA (*W*atery *D*iarrhoea *H*ypokalaemia *A*chlorhydria) syndrome or pancreatic cholera or VIPoma syndrome. This syndrome is associated with a VIP-producing tumour of the pancreas or elsewhere (ganglioneuroblastoma). In experimental animals abnormally large quantities of circulating VIP, equivalent to those seen in the VIPoma syndrome, are able to produce a profuse electrolyte-containing watery diarrhoea, leading subsequently to hypokalaemia and other manifestations of electrolytic decompensation.

Many VIP nerves, distorted, hyperplastic and strongly immunostained, are seen in the gut from patients with Crohn's disease. These findings, although widespread in all the layers of the gut wall, are particularly marked in the mucosa and submucosa and constitute an interesting distinctive feature of this disease as they are not seen in the gut from patients with ulcerative colitis (Polak, Bishop and Bloom, 1978) (Figure 15). In addition, both substance P and VIP content and the number of immunostained nerves are markedly reduced in disorders such as Hirschsprung's and Chagas' disease (Figure 16), which affect primarily the intrinsic neuronal cell bodies. Conversely, in generalized autonomic neuropathies which do not specifically affect the gut ganglion cells, such as Shy-Drager syndrome, the peptidergic innervation remains unaffected (Polak et al, 1979; Long et al, 1980).

CONCLUSIONS

Identical peptides are present in neural and endocrine cells. When localized to nerves they may act as neurotransmitters, while those present in endo-

REGULATORY PEPTIDES OF THE GUT 43

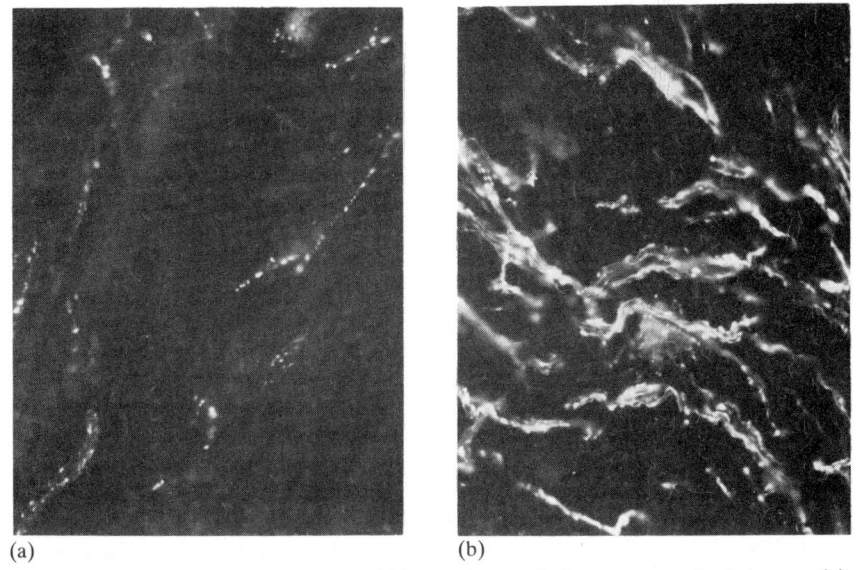

Figure 15. VIP nerves in human colon. (a) Normal muscularis mucosae and submucosa. (b) Hyperplastic nerves in Crohn's disease. × 280.

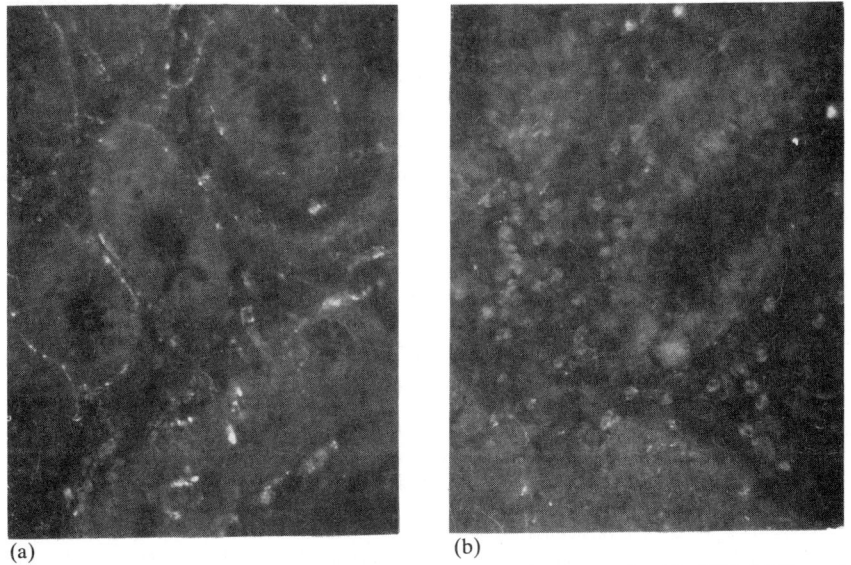

Figure 16. Human colonic mucosa and muscularis mucosae immunostained for VIP. (a) Normal control. (b) Chagas' disease. × 225.

crine cells may act as local or circulating hormones. This not only illustrates the economy of the body's control processes, as a single active peptide may have quite different roles in different places, but also supports the concept suggested by Pearse (1969) that the endocrine system is merely an outpouch of the brain.

Our old ideas of hormones acting via the circulation and the autonomic nervous system being composed of an inhibitory (adrenergic) and excitatory (cholinergic) system must be revised in the light of these new findings. It is therefore necessary to reinvestigate neural and endocrine physiology. The classical experiments of ablation, suppression and hormonal replacement will have to be amplified to take into account the numerous peptides which either act locally or, if circulating, respond to complex stimulation such as lumps of food in a synchronized manner.

The endocrine/paracrine cells of the gut are not confined to a circumscribed, single organ, but are diffusely scattered through the non-endocrine tissue. Pure and synthetic peptides are gradually becoming available. Their infusion into the circulation at doses mimicking those achieved after a meal is progressively providing useful information. The numerous, hitherto inexplicable, atropine-resistant responses to nerve stimulation are being gradually explained by the release from autonomic nerves of these active peptides which, when applied by micro-injection, are capable of reproducing the neurally-mediated responses. The large and complex peptidergic component of the autonomic nervous system is undoubtedly playing an important role in the control of gut functions. We may now look forward to many years of further insight into gut function in health and disease.

ACKNOWLEDGEMENTS

This work was generously supported by the Cancer Research Campaign and Janssen Pharmaceuticals (UK).

REFERENCES

Bayliss, W.M. & Starling, E.H. (1902) The mechanism of pancreatic secretion. *Journal of Physiology*, **28**, 325-353.
Blackburn, A.M. & Bloom, S.R. (1979) A radioimmunoassay for neurotensin in human plasma. *Journal of Endocrinology*, **83**, 175-181.
Bloom, S.R. (1972) An enteroglucagon tumour. *Gut*, **13**, 520-523.
Bloom, S.R. & Polak, J.M. (1980a) Gut hormones. In *Advances in Clinical Chemistry* (Ed.) Bodansky, J. New York: Raven Press.
Bloom, S.R. & Polak, J.M. (1980b) Plasma hormone concentrations in gastrointestinal disease. *Clinics in Gastroenterology*, **9** (3).
Bloom, S.R., Polak, J.M. & West, A.M. (1978) Somatostatin content of pancreatic endocrine tumours. In *Metabolism* (Ed.) Gerich, J.E., Raptis, S. & Rosenthal, J. Vol. 27, No. 9, Suppl. 1, pp. 1235-1238. New York: Grune & Stratton.
Bloom, S.R., Christofides, N.D., Bryant, M.G., Buchan, A.M.J. & Polak, J.M. (1979a) One motilin or several? *Gastroenterology*, **76**, 1102.
Bloom, S.R., Ghatei, M.A., Christofides, N.D., Blackburn, A.M., Adrian, T.E., Lezoche, P., Basso, N., Carlei, F. & Speranzo, F. (1979b) Release of neurotensin, enteroglucagon, motilin and pancreatic polypeptide by bombesin in man. *Gut*, **20**, A912-913.
Buchan, A.M.J., Polak, J.M., Solcia, E., Capella, C., Hudson, D. & Pearse, A.G.E. (1978) Electron immunocytochemical evidence for the human intestinal I cell as the source of CCK. *Gut*, **19**, 403-407.
Buchan, A.M.J., Bryant, M.G., Timson, C.M., Polak, J.M. & Bloom, S.R. (1979a) Intestinal gastrin — ontogeny and tumour distribution. *Gut*, **20** (5), A454.
Buchan, A.M.J., Polak, J.M., Solcia, E. & Pearse, A.G.E. (1979b) Localisation of intestinal gastrin in a distinct endocrine cell type. *Nature*, **277**, 138-140.

Chayvaille, J.A.P., Descos, F., Bernard, C., Martin, A., Barbe, C. & Partensky, C. (1978) Somatostatin in mucosa of stomach and duodenum in gastroduodenal disease. *Gastroenterology*, **75** (1), 13-19.

Edkins, J.S. (1905) On the chemical mechanism of gastric secretion. *Proceedings of the Royal Society, B*, **76**, 376.

Fahrenkrug, J., Galbo, H., Holst, J.J. & Schaffalitzky de Muckadell, O.B. (1978) Influence of the autonomic nervous system on the release of vasoactive intestinal polypeptide from the porcine gastrointestinal tract. *Journal of Physiology (London)*, **280**, 405-422.

Feyrter, F. (1938) *Uber diffuse endokrine Epitheliale Organe*. pp. 6-17. Leipzig: J.A. Barth.

Jessen, K.R., Polak, J.M., Van Noorden, S., Bloom, S.R. & Burnstock, G. (1980) Evidence that peptide-containing neurons connect the two ganglionated plexuses of the enteric nervous system. *Nature*, **283**, 391-393.

Konturek, S.J. (1978) Endogenous opiates and the digestive system. *Scandinavian Journal of Gastroenterology*, **13**, 257-261.

Leeman, S.E. & Hammerschlag, R. (1967) Stimulation of salivary secretion by a factor extracted from hypothalamic tissue. *Endocrinology*, **81**, 803-810.

Lin, T.M. & Chance, R.E. (1972) Spectrum of gastrointestinal actions of a new bovine pancreatic polypeptide (BPP). *Gastroenterology*, **62**, 852.

Long, R.G., Bishop, A.E., Barnes, A.J., Albuquerque, R.H., O'Shaughnessy, D.J., McGregor, G.P., Bannister, R., Polak, J.M. & Bloom, S.R. (1980) Neural and hormonal peptides in rectal biopsies of patients with Chagas' disease and chronic autonomic failure. *Lancet*, **i**, 559-562.

Moody, A.J., Jacobsen, H. & Sundby, F. (1978) Gastric glucagon and gut glucagon-like immunoreactants. In *Gut Hormones* (Ed.) Bloom, S.R. pp. 369-378. Edinburgh: Churchill Livingstone.

Otsuka, M., Konishi, S. & Takahashi, T. (1975) Hypothalamic substance P as a candidate for transmitter of primary afferent neurons. *Federation Proceedings*, **34**, 1922-1928.

Pearse, A.G.E. (1969) The cytochemistry and ultrastructure of polypeptide hormone-producing cells of the APUD series, and the embryologic, physiologic and pathologic implications of the concept. *Journal of Histochemistry and Cytochemistry*, **17**, 303-313.

Pearse, A.G.E. & Polak, J.M. (1975) Bifunctional reagents as vapour- and liquid-phase fixatives for immunohistochemistry. *Histochemie*, **7**, 179-186.

Polak, J.M. & Bloom, S.R. (1978) Peptidergic innervation of the gastrointestinal tract. In *Gastrointestinal Hormones and Pathology of the Digestive System* (Ed.) Grossman, M., Speranza, V., Basso, N. & Lezoche, E. pp. 27-49. New York: Plenum Press.

Polak, J.M. & Bloom, S.R. (1979) The neuroendocrine design of the gut. *Clinics in Endocrinology and Metabolism*,, **8** (2), 313-330.

Polak, J.M. & Bloom, S.R. (1980) Decreased somatostatin content in persistent neonatal hyperinsulinaemic hypoglycaemia. In *Proceedings of Second International Symposium on Hypoglycaemia* (Ed.) Andreani, D. & Marks, V. London and New York: Academic Press.

Polak, J.M. & Buchan, A.M.J. (1979) Motilin immunocytochemical local section indicated possible molecular heterogeneity or the existence of a motilin family. *Gastroenterology*, **76**, 1065-1066.

Polak, J.M. & Buchan, A.M.J. (1980) The D1 cell of the gut and pancreas. In *Cellular Basis of Chemical Messengers* (Ed.) Grossman, M.I. Los Angeles: UCLA Scientific Publications.

Polak, J.M., Bishop, A.E. & Bloom, S.R. (1978) The morphology of VIPergic nerves in Crohn's disease. *Scandinavian Journal of Gastroenterology*, **13** (Suppl. 49), 144.

Polak, J. M., Bloom, S.R., Coulling, I. & Pearse, A.G.E. (1971a) Immunofluorescent localisation of secretin in the canine duodenum. *Gut*, **12**, 605-610.

Polak, J.M., Coulling, I., Bloom, S.R. & Pearse, A.G.E. (1971b) Immunofluorescent localisation of secretin and enteroglucagon in human intestinal mucosa. *Scandinavian Journal of Gastroenterology*, **6**, 739-744.

Polak, J.M., Bloom, S.R., Kuzio, M., Brown, J.C. & Pearse, A.G.E. (1973a) Cellular localisation of gastric inhibitory polypeptide in the duodenum and jejunum. *Gut*, **14**, 284-288.

Polak, J.M., Pearse, A.G.E., Van Noorden, S., Bloom, S.R. & Rossiter, M.A. (1973b) Secretin cells in coeliac disease. *Gut*, **14**, 870-874.

Polak, J.M., Pearse, A.G.E., Grimelius, L. Bloom, S.R. & Arimura, A. (1975) Growth-hormone releasing inhibiting hormone (GH-RIH) in gastrointestinal and pancreatic D cells. *Lancet*, **i**, 1220-1222.

Polak, J.M., Bloom, S.R., Adrian, T.E., Heitz, P., Bryant, M.G. & Pearse, A.G.E. (1976) Pancreatic polypeptide in insulinomas, gastrinomas, VIPomas and glucagonomas. *Lancet*, **i**, 328-330.

Polak, J.M., Sullivan, S.M., Bloom, S.R., Buchan, A.M.J., Facer, P., Brown, M.R. & Pearse, A.G.E. (1977) Specific localisation of neurotensin to the N cell in human intestine by radioimmunoassay and cytochemistry. *Nature*, **270**, 183-184.

Polak, J.M., Ghatei, M.A., Wharton, J., Bishop, A.E., Bloom, S.R., Solcia, E., Brown, M.R. & Pearse, A.G.E. (1978) Bombesin-like immunoreactivity in the gastrointestinal tract, lung and central nervous system. *Scandinavian Journal of Gastroenterology*, **13** (Suppl. 49), 148.

Polak, J.M., Bishop, A.E., Long, R.G., Bryant, M.G., MacGregor, G.P., Albuquerque, R.H. & Bloom, S.R. (1979) Pathology of the gut peptidergic system. *Gut*, **20** (5), A942.

Rehfeld, J.F. (1978) Multiple molecular forms of cholecystokinin. In *Gut Hormones* (Ed.) Bloom, S.R. pp. 213-218. Edinburgh: Churchill Livingstone.

Rehfeld, J.F. & Larsson, L. (1979) The predominating molecular form of gastrin and cholecystokinin in the gut is a small peptide corresponding to their COOH terminal tetrapeptide amide. *Acta Physiologica Scandinavica*, **105**, 117-119.

Roberts, G.W., Woodhams, P.L., Bryant, M.G., Crow, T.J., Bloom, S.R. & Polak, J.M. (1980) VIP in the rat brain. Evidence for a major pathway linking the amygdala and hypothalamus via the stria terminalis. *Histochemistry*, **65**, 103-119.

Schaffalitzky de Muckadell, O.B., Fahrenkrug, J. & Rune, S.J. (1979) Physiological significance of secretin in the pancreatic bicarbonate secretion. I. responsiveness of the secretin releasing system in the upper duodenum. *Scandinavian Journal of Gastroenterology*, **14**, 79-83.

Solcia, E., Polak, J.M., Pearse, A.G.E., Forssmann, W.G., Larsson, L.-I., Sundler, F., Lechago, J., Grimelius, L., Fujita, T., Creutzfeldt, W., Gepts, W., Falkmer, S., Lefranc, G., Heitz, Ph., Hage, E., Buchan, A.M.J., Bloom, S.R. & Grossman, M.I. (1978) Lausanne 1977 classification of gastroenteropancreatic endocrine cells. In *Gut Hormones* (Ed.) Bloom, S.R. pp. 40-48. Edinburgh: Churchill Livingstone.

Sternberger, L. (1974) *The Unlabelled Antibody Enzyme Method*. pp. 142-161. Englewood Cliffs, N.J.: Prentice Hall.

Sullivan, S.N., Bloom, S.R. & Polak, J.M. (1978) Enkephalin in peripheral neuroendocrine tumours. *Lancet*, **i**, 1155.

von Euler, U.S. & Gaddum, J.H. (1931) An unidentified depressor substance in certain tissue extracts. *Journal of Physiology (London)*, **192**, 74-87.

Walsh, J.H. & Grossman, M.I. (1975) Gastrin, chemistry and physiology. *New England Journal of Medicine*, **292**, 1377-1384.

Wharton, J., Polak, J.M., Will, J.A., Biscard, J., Bryant, M.G., MacGregor, G.P., Bloom, S.R. & Emson, P.C. (1980) Enkephalin-, vasoactive intestinal polypeptide- and substance P-like immunoreactivity in the cat carotid body. *Journal of Endocrinology*, in press.

3
Gastrointestinal Mucus

JOHN RICHARD CLAMP

NOMENCLATURE

Mucus is widespread in nature, being present in many species ranging from earthworm to man, and has evolved to fulfil a number of extracellular roles. In humans mucus is of obvious importance in systems as functionally different as the respiratory, gastrointestinal and genito-urinary tracts. In addition to the medical interest, the fascinating chemical and physical properties of mucus have long been an object of interest to biochemists and physical chemists. It is not surprising, therefore, that a subject studied by so many different disciplines should have led to so much confusion in the nomenclature, both of mucus and related materials.

Most nomenclature problems in science are of two kinds: firstly, where the same term is used to mean different entities, and secondly, where several terms are used to describe the same entity. Both kinds of confusion exist in the mucus field. An example of the first type is the term 'mucoid', which has been used by different disciplines with at least four quite separate meanings. These range from the 'non-purulent' sputum of the respiratory physician to the 'neutral' mucin of the histochemist. The second type of confusion can be seen in the many terms used to define the major component of mucus secretions. The list includes mucoprotein, mucosubstance, mucocomplex, mucopolysaccharide, mucin, glycoprotein, and so on.

Fortunately, the nomenclature problem is now recognized and some modest proposals have been made to bring the various disciplines into line (Elstein and Parke, 1977; Clamp, 1978). Imprecise terms such as 'mucoid' or those prefixed by 'muco-' should be abandoned. The total secretion is 'mucus' and the major component of mucus that confers the characteristic physicochemical properties upon the secretion should be called 'mucus glycoprotein'. Degradation products of the glycoprotein are 'glycopolypeptides'. The word 'mucin' should be used only as a histochemical term. These proposals have been accepted by biochemists as part of a more comprehensive classification system. In this system, the term 'glycoconjugate' embraces all those polymeric materials containing covalently-linked carbohydrate, but excluding nucleic acids. For all practical purposes glycoconjugates may be subdivided into carbohydrate linked to either lipid or protein and may be further subdivided as follows:

GLYCOCONJUGATE

CARBOHYDRATE — LIPID		CARBOHYDRATE — PROTEIN	
GLYCOLIPIDS (e.g., sphingolipids)	LIPOPOLYSACCHARIDES (e.g., certain bacterial cell walls)	PROTEOGLYCANS (e.g., chondroitin sulphate)	GLYCOPROTEINS (e.g., plasma globulins, mucus glycoprotein)

Although proteoglycans and glycoproteins both consist of carbohydrate linked to protein, they are quite different materials. They occur in different parts of the body and fulfil different roles. In addition, the two substances are chemically different, particularly with regard to the carbohydrate portion (Reid and Clamp, 1978).

CHEMISTRY OF MUCUS GLYCOPROTEIN

As mentioned above, the principal constituent of mucus and the component that gives the secretion its characteristic properties is a glycoprotein. The glycoproteins are a diverse group of proteins possessing covalently-linked carbohydrate and they include the plasma globulins, structural glycoproteins (for example collagen and histocompatibility antigens), mucus glycoproteins, and so on. The principal property that glycoproteins have in common is that the carbohydrate is present in relatively small oligosaccharide units which have little or no repeating structure. Mucus glycoproteins form a distinct subgroup with a number of characteristic features. They are extremely large molecules; the glycoprotein from gastric mucus, for example, has a molecular weight of about 2×10^6. Mucus glycoproteins exhibit polydispersity and carbohydrate heterogeneity. These are probably features of the biosynthetic mechanism and therefore when found in isolated material are not entirely due to bacterial degradation in the gastrointestinal tract, since they are seen in mucus from germ-free rats (Wold, Khan and Midtvedt, 1971).

Over half of the mass of mucus glycoprotein consists of carbohydrate. This very large amount of carbohydrate is nevertheless present in relatively small oligosaccharide units, containing on average only about eight monosaccharide residues. A typical mucus glycoprotein therefore possesses many hundreds of such units and indeed every third or fourth amino-acid carries an oligosaccharide unit. Thus the molecule consists of an extended polypeptide chain surrounded and shielded by tightly packed carbohydrate. This structure partly explains an important property of gastrointestinal mucus, namely its relative resistance to proteolytic attack and its survival in the intestines for a sufficient period of time to carry out its function of lubrication and protection of mucosal surfaces.

The mucus glycoprotein molecule does have short stretches of polypeptide chain which are carbohydrate-free, and these so-called 'naked' peptide regions enable neighbouring chains to come together and to be linked through disulphide bonds. These linkages between chains are important in maintaining the physicochemical properties of mucus.

The oligosaccharide units are attached to the polypeptide chain through N-acetylgalactosamine to the hydroxyamino-acids, serine and threonine, and these two amino-acids, together with proline, account for almost half of the total amino-acid content. The oligosaccharide units may contain up to four different types of monosaccharide, namely a deoxyhexose (fucose), a neutral hexose (galactose), N-acetylhexosamine (N-acetylglucosamine and N-acetylgalactosamine) and sialic acid. 'Sialic acid' is the name given to any substituted neuraminic acid. The most important sialic acid in humans is N-acetylneuraminic acid, although O-acylated derivatives have been described in human colonic mucus (Reid et al, 1978; Rogers, Cooke and Filipe, 1978). The role of these different monosaccharides in the function of mucus is by no means clear. Fucose (6-deoxy-L-galactose) and N-acetylhexosamine possess hydrophobic groups which may contribute to the conformation of the oligosaccharide unit or to non-covalent interactions between units. Galactose has two kinds of hydroxyl groups, depending on their orientation to the plane of the pyranose ring (axial and equatorial). Attachment of other monosaccharides to these would give rise to oligosaccharides differing in structure and possibly function. Sialic acid confers negative charge upon the molecule and this is supplemented in some types of mucus by ester sulphate groups.

The above remarks are a general description of mucus glycoproteins and are substantially correct for mucus from any site, whether bronchial, cervical or gastrointestinal. There is indeed little evidence that the structure of human mucus differs in any fundamental way between these systems, despite their widely varying functions. This may, in part, be because there have been few detailed studies, performed in the same laboratory, of mucus isolated from these different sites. Such studies need to be carried out on undegraded mucus and should establish the overall molecular weight, the degree of cross-linkage and the number, size and nature of the oligosaccharide units. Most investigations have been confined to estimations of carbohydrate content, although these have shown analytical differences between mucus samples from various sites, particularly in the peripheral monosaccharide residues. Thus histochemical techniques indicate that gastric mucus contains only neutral glycoprotein whereas colonic mucus is largely acidic glycoprotein, being particularly rich in sulphate ester groups. The staining reaction appears to show quite clear-cut differences between neutral, sialic acid-containing and sulphated glycoproteins. These distinct types of mucus glycoproteins are not found during biochemical studies. Gastric mucus, for example, always contains small amounts of sialic acid and careful fractionation of bronchial mucus (Roberts, 1974) indicates that the glycoprotein components show a continuous variation rather than separating into distinct clear-cut types. One of the major problems in the mucus field is therefore the precise correlation of histochemical findings with the biochemical results.

The techniques for isolating mucus glycoprotein vary from laboratory to laboratory probably because the usual biochemical criteria for purity do not apply to these samples. Attempts to achieve homogeneity have often led to quite elaborate isolation procedures. These usually include gel-permeation chromatography on columns of Sepharose 2B or similar resin in which the mucus glycoprotein is eluted in the high molecular weight fraction. An important technique in this field is density-gradient ultracentrifugation in 1.4 M caesium bromide solution (Creeth et al, 1977). Many isolation procedures also include an exhaustive proteolysis step which converts the mucus glycoprotein into a glycopolypeptide which is still of relatively high molecular weight. Thus it can be easily separated from any contaminating proteins which would have undergone more extensive degradation.

When mucus glycoproteins are isolated from stomach and colon, the analyses (Table 1) show differences in the content of a number of monosaccharides, but particularly sialic acid. Gastric mucus contains only 0.5 residues of sialic acid relative to six residues of galactose whereas colonic mucus contains seven residues. Suphate estimation was carried out only on the gastric mucus glycoprotein and showed an absence of this acidic radical.

Table 1. *The proportions of monosaccharide residues in gastric and colonic mucus glycoproteins*

	Gastric mucus	Colonic mucus
Fucose	2.9	2.3
Mannose	0.3	0.5
Galactose	6.0	6.0
N-Acetylglucosamine	3.8	7.4
N-Acetylgalactosamine	2.3	6.8
Sialic acid	0.5	7.0

The monosaccharide content is given relative to a galactose content of six residues.

Interestingly, both gastric and colonic mucus glycoprotein contain significant amounts of mannose. The absence of this monosaccharide has been used as a criterion of purity for mucus glycoprotein material. However, we have always found small but consistent amounts of mannose in the undegraded mucus glycoprotein preparations, as have other workers (Andre and Descos, 1975). It is true, however, that when a proteolysis step is included in the procedure the resultant glycopolypeptide is mannose-free (Table 2). Possibly a mannose-containing oligosaccharide unit is located on a stretch of polypeptide chain that is susceptible to proteolysis.

Table 2. *Comparison of the carbohydrate content of mucus glycoprotein and glycopolypeptide from meconium*

	Mucus glycoprotein	Mucus glycopolypeptide
Fucose	2.3	2.2
Mannose	0.7	0
Galactose	6.0	6.0
N-Acetylglucosamine	4.8	4.5
N-Acetylgalactosamine	2.5	3.2
Sialic acid	1.5	1.9

The monosaccharide content is given relative to a galactose content of six residues.

Most of the work on gastrointestinal mucus has tended to concentrate on gastric mucus because it is the most easily obtained. These studies have been carried out either on resting juice or the secretion obtained after a variety of stimuli. We therefore decided to compare the nature of the mucus released under basal (resting) conditions and after stimulation by insulin and pentagastrin in the same subject (Table 3). The mucus glycoproteins that are

Table 3. *The amount and composition of gastric mucus glycoproteins collected under basal resting conditions and after stimulation by insulin and pentagastrin*

	Basal	Insulin	Pentagastrin
Duration of collection (hr)	1	2	1
Volume of gastric secretions (ml)	74(45)	252(52)	198(65)
Total mucus glycoprotein (mg)	48(34)	85(17)	50(19)
Monosaccharide content (nmols/mg)			
Fucose	346(110)	369(140)	361(148)
Mannose	28(14)	40(30)	45(43)
Galactose	678(139)	780(165)	757(261)
N-Acetylglucosamine	435(160)	506(175)	460(250)
N-Acetylgalactosamine	257(131)	307(151)	297(163)
Sialic acid	64(35)	95(81)	40(35)

The results are given as the mean (standard deviation) of values from nine normal subjects. The monosaccharide content is expressed as nmols/mg.

released under the three sets of conditions do not differ significantly in their carbohydrate composition although, when adjusted for duration of collection, there is a marginally greater release of total glycoprotein after stimulation by pentagastrin.

The linkage between carbohydrate and polypeptide in mucus glycoprotein is readily cleaved by alkali. If this reaction is carried out in the presence of excess reducing agent, the linkage N-acetylgalactosamine after release from the protein is converted to the corresponding glycitol, N-acetylgalactosaminitol. Thus the linkage monosaccharide is identified and the equivalent weight of the oligosaccharide established. After the oligosaccharides are released, they are fractionated according to size and are found to range from just the linkage N-acetylgalactosamine to units containing over 20 monosaccharide residues. The oligosaccharide unit that was present in all the meconium samples studied (Clamp and Gough, 1979) contained one residue of fucose, three residues of galactose, two of N-acetylglucosamine and one residue of sialic acid, together with the linkage N-acetylgalactosamine. The majority of the units in colonic mucus glycoprotein tend to be smaller than this, containing one residue of fucose, two residues of galactose and one residue each of N-acetylglucosamine and sialic acid, together with the linkage N-acetylgalactosamine.

A convenient method for establishing the carbohydrate content of mucus glycoproteins from precise areas of the gastrointestinal tract is the analysis of endoscopic biopsies. Such biopsies are limited to the superficial layers of the mucosal surface and the carbohydrate content is contributed almost exclusively by mucus glycoprotein either within cells or adherent to the epithelial surface (Barton, Brown and Clamp, 1972; Brown, Clamp and Salmon, 1972). The results obtained with biopsies (Table 4) are similar to those obtained with isolated mucus glycoprotein (see Table 1).

Table 4. *The proportions of monosaccharide residues in gastric and colonic biopsies*

	Gastric biopsies	Colonic biopsies
Fucose	3.1	1.9
Mannose	1.1	2.2
Galactose	6.0	6.0
N-Acetylglucosamine	4.5	7.0
N-Acetylgalactosamine	3.9	5.1
Sialic acid	0.5	6.4

The monosaccharide content is given relative to a galactose content of six residues.

MUCUS CHANGES IN DISEASE

Mucus is a complex secretion containing many different substances contributed by several cell types. Obviously, disease could affect the secretion in many ways, for example by causing the appearance of some new constituent or by changing the concentration of a normal constituent. Secretion of mucus glycoprotein in abnormal amounts or change of epithelial type with secretion from an unusual site may cause problems. Thus our laboratory has analysed material from the middle ear ('glue ear'), the bladder ('colloid urine') and from the submandibular glands, all of which proved to be typical mucus glycoproteins. The patients in each case initially presented with problems associated with the mucus secretion.

The idea that the 'quality' of mucus might be deficient in peptic ulcer has been supported by the association between non-secretor status and duodenal ulcer (Clarke et al, 1956). The ABO (ABH) blood groups are determined by certain terminal monosaccharide residues on cell surface membrane glycolipids. The same blood groups are also expressed on mucus glycoproteins but only if the individual possesses the 'secretor' gene. There is no doubt that there is a marked chemical difference between secretor mucus and non-secretor mucus. The secretor mucus glycoprotein contains approximately twice as much fucose as the non-secretor material (Machado, Clamp and Read, 1977; Clamp and Gough, 1979). There are no significant differences in the other monosaccharide residues between the groups (Table 5). Unfortunately, this attractive hypothesis is not supported by other blood group data. For example, there is an association between blood group O and duodenal ulcer (Clarke et al, 1955) but this is not dependent on secretor status. The terminal monosaccharide residues of blood group A (α-N-acetylgalactosaminyl) and blood group B (α-galactosyl) would not be present to any significant extent in non-secretor mucus glycoprotein. The 'pro-

Table 5. *The carbohydrate content of mucus from secretors and non-secretors*

	Gastric Sec.	Gastric Non.	Meconium Sec.	Meconium Non.
Numbers in sample	25	12	35	14
Fucose	4.1	1.2	2.2	1.0
Galactose	6.0	6.0	6.0	6.0
N-Acetylglucosamine	4.6	4.3	4.5	4.6
N-Acetylgalactosamine	4.0	3.8	3.2	2.4
Sialic acid	0.5	0.4	1.9	2.7

The monosaccharide content is given relative to a galactose content of six residues. Abbreviations are as follows: Sec. = secretors; Non. = non-secretors.

tective' effect of these blood groups must therefore be expressed by some other mechanism, a list of which is given by McConnell (1966). An additional possibility is that the monosaccharides are exercising a protective role at the cell surface where the blood groups would of course be expressed in the glycolipids irrespective of secretor status. Blood group activity in mucus does, however, provide a simple and precise method for determining mucus glycoprotein changes in disease. Thus Hakkinen and Virtanen (1967) and Schrager and Oates (1973) found that gastric secretions often developed anomalous blood group activity in carcinoma of the stomach, in that the secretions were converted to blood group A. This is of interest because of the known correlation of blood group A (but not secretor status) with gastric carcinoma (Aird, Bentall and Roberts, 1953). This activity could be due to modification of mucus glycoprotein as a result of activation of additional glycosyltransferases, and changes in carbohydrate content of mucus have been reported in this condition (Richmond, Caputto and Wolf, 1955; Schrager and Oates, 1973; Machado, Clamp and Read, 1977). Alternatively, the anomalous blood group activity could be present in some new substance appearing in the mucus and a sulphoglycoprotein has been detected in gastric carcinoma (Hakkinen, Jarvi and Gronroos, 1968; Lambert and Andre, 1972).

Other changes in mucus glycoproteins have been observed in a number of gastrointestinal diseases, although all these changes are probably secondary to the disease and are not involved in the aetiology. These mucus changes have usually been detected by histochemical techniques (Lev, 1970), particularly where there has been a change in the acidic groups (sialic acid or sulphate). Thus intestinal metaplasia can be detected in the stomach by the appearance of goblet cells rich in acidic glycoprotein. The decrease or absence of sulphated glycoproteins has been postulated as a sign of a premalignant mucosa (transitional mucosa) for carcinoma of the rectum and lower sigmoid (Filipe, 1972). Even if this change is not specific and only secondary to the carcinoma (Isaacson and Attwood, 1979) it is important from the point of view of mucus glycoproteins. This and other work (Filipe and Cooke, 1970; Machado, Clamp and Read, 1977) indicate that mucus not directly involved by the malignant tissue shows significant differences in carbohydrate content from normal mucus. The mechanism whereby the malignant process affects mucus biosynthesis in the goblet cells is not known.

The above studies depend upon either histochemical findings or changes in carbohydrate content found during analyses of total mucus or glycoprotein. Very few investigations have been carried out on the distribution and nature of the oligosaccharides in mucus glycoprotein. However, work in this laboratory has shown a significant difference between the fucose contents of oligosaccharides isolated from cystic fibrosis meconium and normal meconium (Clamp and Gough, 1979). A selection of the oligosaccharides found in the two types of material is shown in Table 6, but these changes did

Table 6. *The carbohydrate content of oligosaccharides from cystic fibrosis meconium and normal meconium*

	\multicolumn{4}{c}{Monosaccharide ratio to one residue of N-acetylgalactosaminitol}
	Fucose	Galactose	N-Acetyl glucosamine	Sialic acid
Normal	2	2	1	0-1
Cystic fibrosis	2	2	1	0-1
Normal	2	4	3	1
Cystic fibrosis	3	4	3	1
Normal	2	5	4	1-2
Cystic fibrosis	3	5	4	1
Normal	3	6	5	2-3
Cystic fibrosis	4	6	5	2
Normal	3	8	7	2-3
Cystic fibrosis	5	8	7	2
Normal	3	11	8	6
Cystic fibrosis	8	11	8	2

The mucus glycopolypeptides were isolated from meconium and used for the preparation of oligosaccharides. These were cleaved from the glycopolypeptide and separated by gel-permeation chromatography. The selected results from the two types of material are compared on the basis of similar contents of galactose and N-acetylglucosamine and are related to one residue of N-acetylgalactosaminitol.

not become apparent until the oligosaccharide units had been cleaved from the glycoprotein, fractionated and analysed.

Similar studies have been carried out on glycoproteins from colonic mucus in ulcerative colitis. One of the features of ulcerative colitis is epithelial destruction (Morson and Dawson, 1972) with an accompanying reduction in the amount of mucus (Filipe and Dawson, 1970). An indication that there is a qualitative change in mucus from ulcerative colitis came when differences were found (Teague, Fraser and Clamp, 1973) in the carbohydrate content of mucus, particularly in the levels of mannose. Mucus has now been isolated from diseased colons resected at operation and compared with similar normal material obtained at post-mortem (Clamp, Fraser and Read, 1976, unpublished findings). Colonic mucus can be separated into two molecular weight fractions, namely a high molecular weight fraction which is a typical mucus glycoprotein and a fraction with a molecular weight of about 150 000 with a high content of mannose. This latter fraction was shown by immunological techniques to be a product of the colonic mucosa and was not derived from plasma. The changes affecting the high molecular weight fraction (mucus glycoprotein) in ulcerative colitis are twofold. Firstly, there is a reduction in the amount of mucus glycoprotein in mucus, with a corresponding increase in the low molecular weight high-mannose fraction. This, presumably, is the explanation for the findings of Teague, Fraser and Clamp (1973). Secondly, there is a reduction in the total amount of carbohydrate in both fractions. These changes, summarized in Table 7, appear at first sight to

Table 7. *The carbohydrate content of fractions from normal and ulcerative colitis colons*

	Normal		Ulcerative colitis	
	High	Low	High	Low
Amount in original mucus (%)	43	57	23	77
Total carbohydrate content (%)	36	8	17	4
Fucose	2.3	2.7	2.6	2.3
Mannose	0.5	3.3	0.8	5.7
Galactose	6.0	6.0	6.0	6.0
N-Acetylglucosamine	7.4	6.6	7.4	7.0
N-Acetylgalactosamine	6.8	3.7	6.5	4.2
Sialic acid	7.0	3.6	5.4	2.7

The monosaccharide content is given relative to six residues of galactose. Abbreviations are given as follows: High = high molecular weight fraction (mucus glycoprotein); Low = low molecular weight fraction.

be at variance with the observation (Bleiberg et al, 1970; MacDermott, Donaldson and Trier, 1974) that the rate of biosynthesis of mucus glycoproteins is increased in ulcerative colitis. However, both these findings are compatible with the changes found in the oligosaccharide units. When the oligosaccharide units are released from the glycoprotein and fractionated, a further difference between normal and colitic mucus becomes manifest. Normal colonic mucus glycoprotein possesses oligosaccharides with a mean size of 8 monosaccharide residues whereas the corresponding figure for ulcerative colitis is 5 residues. We postulate that the increased production of mucus glycoprotein results in incomplete biosynthesis of the oligosaccharide units. There is support for this idea in the observation (J. R. Clamp and C. F. Phelps, 1974, unpublished observations) that prolonged stimulation of mucus secretion leads to a reduction in the numbers of peripheral monosaccharide residues.

MUCUS: THE FUTURE

The study of mucus secretions from the gastrointestinal tract is still at a very preliminary stage. The early workers carried out broad analyses of relatively crude material but nevertheless provided valuable background information for later studies. Present and future investigations should determine the total secretion from known areas of the gastrointestinal tract and establish the precise composition of those secretions in terms of defined constituents. The most important constituent is, of course, mucus glycoprotein. This should be isolated, as far as possible, in an undegraded state free from contaminating protein or non-mucus glycoprotein material. The size, shape, degree and type of cross-linkage, composition and 'monomer' size should be established. The size and distribution of the oligosaccharide units should be determined, together with their composition and structure. In addition, the sequence and structure of the polypeptide chain will have an important bearing on the biosynthesis and conformation of the glycoprotein molecule. When all these points have been established for normal mucus one will then be in a strong position to assess the significance of changes seen in various gastrointestinal diseases.

Of no less importance, of course, are the mucus 'environment' and the interaction of mucus glycoproteins with both surfaces and molecules. For example, interaction with the mucosal surface may play a part in the protection of the gastrointestinal tract and possibly with the process of digestion and absorption. Interaction with the surface of pathogenic organisms may prevent the specific attachment of these organisms to the intestinal epithelium, which is probably an essential feature of the pathogenic process. The interaction of mucus glycoproteins with molecules may be exemplified by lysozyme. The interaction between these two molecules has been established (Creeth, Bridge and Horton, 1979), and it is of interest, therefore, that they both appear in the same intestinal epithelial cell (Montero and Erlandsen, 1978). The importance of such interaction in the protection of the mucosa from susceptible organisms is self-evident. Mucous membranes are also protected by secretory IgA antibodies. The major subclass, IgA_1, contains a sequence in the hinge region of the heavy chain which is rich in proline and hydroxyamino-acids and which possesses O-glycosidically-linked oligosaccharide units. It cannot be a coincidence, therefore, that the IgA_1 antibody present in mucus secretions itself possesses a 'mucus-like' stretch. Interaction of secretory IgA_1 with mucus glycoprotein or mucosal surfaces has been postulated (Clamp, 1975; 1977) to explain this similarity. The above are perhaps examples of 'positive' interactions but there is also the possibility of 'negative' interactions where the mucus layer excludes other macromolecules such as enzymes (Edwards, 1978). This hypothesis suggests that the intact mucus layer exploits the phenomenon of phase separation and is immiscible with solutions of most other macromolecules. This would fit in with the idea of mucus as a protective layer, keeping enzymes, toxins and other potentially harmful macromolecules away from the mucosa, but allowing free diffusion to small molecules. The reason for the mucus-like stretch in secretory IgA_1 would then be explained in a different way. This stretch would be miscible with the mucus layer and would cause the IgA_1 to sit at the interface between the two phases forming a monolayer of antibodies at the mucus surface. The other subclass of IgA, namely IgA_2, has a deletion of the heavy chain which includes the mucus-like stretch. In both hypotheses, therefore, the secretory IgA$_2$ would be present in the fluid overlying the mucus layer, acting, as it were, as a first line of defence.

Gastrointestinal mucus has usually been assigned rather general functions, vaguely described as 'protective' and 'lubricatory'. Hopefully, we are now entering a period when these general functions can be interpreted in terms of known structure and when specific functions and interactions can be related to some of the many processes that go on in the intestinal tract.

REFERENCES

Aird, I., Bentall, H.H. & Roberts, J.A.F. (1953) A relationship between cancer of the stomach and the ABO blood groups. *British Medical Journal*, i, 799-801.

Andre, F. & Descos, F. (1975) Purification d'une glycoprotéine gastrique humaine et étude de ses composants glucosidiques. *Biochimica Biophysica Acta*, 386, 129-137.

Barton, W., Brown, P. & Clamp, J.R. (1972) The carbohydrate content of mucosal biopsies. *Clinica Chimica Acta*, 36, 262-263.

Bleiberg, H., Mainguet, P., Galand, P., Chretien, J. & Dupont-Mairesse, N. (1970) Cell renewal in the human rectum. *In vitro* autoradiographic study on active ulcerative colitis. *Gastroenterology*, 58, 851-855.

Brown, P., Clamp, J.R. & Salmon, P.R. (1972) The carbohydrate-containing component of gastric mucosal biopsies. *Gut*, 13, 1026.

Clamp, J.R. (1975). Structure and function of glycoproteins. In *The Plasma Proteins* (Ed.) Putnam, F.W. pp. 163-211. New York: Academic Press.

Clamp, J.R. (1977) The relationship between secretory immunoglobulin A and mucus. *Biochemical Society Transactions*, 5, 1579-1581.

Clamp, J.R. (1978) Mucus. *British Medical Bulletin*, 34 (1).

Clamp, J.R. & Gough, M. (1979) Study of the oligosaccharide units from mucus glycoproteins of meconium from normal infants and from cases of cystic fibrosis with meconium ileus. *Clinical Science*, 57, 445-451.

Clarke, C.A., Cowan, W.K., Edwards, J.W., Howel-Evans, A.W., McConnel, R.B., Woodrow, J.C. & Sheppard, P.M. (1955) The relationship of the blood groups to duodenal and gastric ulceration. *British Medical Journal*, ii, 643-646.

Clarke, C.A., Edwards, J.W., Haddock, D.R.W., Howel-Evans, A.W., McConnell, R.B. & Sheppard, P.M. (1956) ABO blood groups and secretor character in duodenal ulcer. Population and sibship studies. *British Medical Journal*, ii, 725-731.

Creeth, J.M., Bridge, J.L. & Horton, J.R. (1979) An interaction between lysozyme and mucus glycoproteins. Implications for density-gradient separations. *Biochemical Journal*, 181, 717-724.

Creeth, J.M., Ramakrishnan Bhaskar, K., Horton, J.R., Das, I., Lopez-Vidriero, M.-T. & Reid, L. (1977) The separation and characterization of bronchial glycoproteins by density-gradient methods. *Biochemical Journal*, 167, 557-569.

Edwards, P.A.W. (1978) Is mucus a selective barrier to macromolecules? *British Medical Bulletin*, 34 (1), 55-56.

Elstein, M. & Parke, D.V. (1977) *Mucus In Health And Disease. Advances In Experimental Medicine And Biology*. Vol. 89, 558 pp. New York: Plenum Press.

Filipe, M.I. (1972) The value of a study of the mucosubstances in rectal biopsies from patients with carcinoma of the rectum and lower sigmoid in the diagnosis of premalignant mucosa. *Journal of Clinical Pathology*, 25, 123-128.

Filipe, M.I. & Cooke, K.B. (1970) Changes in epithelial mucosubstances in mucus immediately adjacent to carcinoma of the large intestine: a histochemical autoradiographic and biochemical study. *Proceedings of the 4th World Congress of Gastroenterology, Copenhagen, 1970*. p. 281.

Filipe, M.I. & Dawson, I. (1970) The diagnostic value of mucosubstances in rectal biopsies from patients with ulcerative colitis and Crohn's disease. *Gut*, 11, 229-234.

Hakkinen, I.P.T. & Virtanen, S. (1967) The blood group activity of human gastric sulphoglycoproteins in patients with gastric cancer and normal controls. *Clinical and Experimental Immunology*, **2**, 669-675.

Hakkinen, I., Jarvi, O. & Gronroos, J. (1968) Sulphoglycoprotein antigens in the human alimentary canal and gastric cancer. An immunological study. *International Journal of Cancer*, **3**, 572-581.

Isaacson, P. & Attwood, P.R.A. (1979) Failure to demonstrate specificity of the morphological and histochemical changes in mucosa adjacent to colonic carcinoma (transitional mucosa). *Journal of Clinical Pathology*, **32**, 214-218.

Lambert, R. & Andre, C. (1972) Sulfated mucosubstances and gastric diseases. *Digestion*, **5**, 116-122.

Lev, R. (1970) The histochemistry of mucus-producing cells in the normal and diseased gastrointestinal mucosa. *Progress in Gastroenterology*, **2**, 13-41.

MacDermott, R.P., Donaldson, R.M. & Trier, J.S. (1974) Glycoprotein synthesis and secretion by mucosal biopsies of rabbit colon and human rectum. *Journal of Clinical Investigation*, **54**, 545-554.

Machado, G., Clamp, J.R. & Read, A.E. (1977) Carbohydrate content of endoscopic gastric biopsies in carcinoma of the stomach. *Gut*, **18**, 670-672.

McConnell, R.B. (1966) *The Genetics of Gastrointestinal Disorders.* 282 pp. London: Oxford University Press.

Montero, C. & Erlandsen, S.L. (1978) Immunocytochemical and histochemical studies on intestinal epithelial cells producing both lysozyme and mucosubstance. *Anatomical Record*, **190**, 127-141.

Morson, B.C. & Dawson, I.M.P. (1972) *Gastrointestinal Pathology.* 676 pp. Oxford: Blackwell Scientific Publications.

Reid, L. & Clamp, J.R. (1978) The biochemical and histochemical nomenclature of mucus. *British Medical Bulletin*, **34** (1), 5-8.

Reid, P.E., Culling, C.F.A., Dunn, W.L., Clay, M.G. & Ramey, C.W. (1978) A correlative chemical and histochemical study of the O-acetylated sialic acids of human colonic epithelial glycoproteins in formalin fixed paraffin embedded tissues. *Journal of Histochemistry and Cytochemistry*, **26**, 1033-1041.

Richmond, V., Caputto, R. & Wolf, S. (1955) Biochemical study of the large molecular constituents of gastric juice. *Gastroenterology*, **29**, 1017-1021.

Roberts, G. (1974) Isolation and characterisation of glycoproteins from sputum. *European Journal of Biochemistry*, **50**, 265-280.

Rogers, C.M., Cooke, K.B. & Filipe, M.I. (1978) Sialic acids of human large bowel mucosa: O-acylated variants in normal and malignant states. *Gut*, **19**, 587-592.

Schrager, J. & Oates, M.D.G. (1973) A comparative study of the major glycoproteins isolated from normal and neoplastic gastric mucosa. *Gut*, **14**, 324-329.

Teague, R.H., Fraser, D. & Clamp, J.R. (1973) Changes in monosaccharide content of mucous glycoproteins in ulcerative colitis. *British Medical Journal*, **i**, 645-646.

Wold, J.K., Khan, R. & Midtvedt, T. (1971) Intestinal glycoproteins of germ-free rats. *Acta Pathologica et Microbiologica Scandinavica, Section B*, **79**, 525-530.

4

Anaemia and the Gastrointestinal Tract

A.V. HOFFBRAND

Although many different types of anaemia may occur in association with gastrointestinal disease, the most common are due to deficiencies of one or other of the three haematinics— iron, vitamin B_{12} or folate. In all countries, iron deficiency is by far the commonest cause of anaemia. Whereas vitamin B_{12} deficiency most commonly results from malabsorption, iron deficiency is usually due to excess loss (as haemorrhage from the gastrointestinal tract or in females the genital tract) and folate deficiency is most often due to a poor diet. Malabsorption can play a role in deficiency of all three haematinics, however, and this review will concentrate on recent advances in knowledge of the mechanisms of normal absorption of vitamin B_{12}, folate and iron, and how malabsorption of these compounds may arise because of disease of the gastrointestinal tract.

VITAMIN B_{12}

The major role of gastric intrinsic factor (IF) in vitamin B_{12} absorption has long been established (see Donaldson, 1975; Chanarin, 1979). The receptor for IF and vitamin B_{12} (on the surface of the microvillus membranes of the ileal mucosa) appears to be a macromolecule, probably a lipoprotein, with a molecular weight of over a million (Katz and Cooper, 1974; Marcoullis and Gräsbeck, 1977). There are approximately 10^{12} receptors per gram of human ileal mucosa (Hooper et al, 1973). IF does not enter portal blood where B_{12} appears in humans after a delay of several hours attached to transcobalamin II (TCII) (see below). The importance of proteins other than IF in gastrointestinal secretions has only recently become apparent. Gastric juice contains, in addition to IF, a glycoprotein, the so-called 'R' binder, which is closely related to similar proteins in saliva, plasma transcobalamin I) (TCI) and other body fluids. The name 'R' refers to the rapid mobility of these proteins on electrophoresis.

Pancreatic secretion also plays an important role and more recently transcobalamin II has been shown to be involved. The effect of these proteins, other than IF, on vitamin B_{12} absorption are reviewed next.

EFFECT OF NON-INTRINSIC FACTOR GASTRIC 'R' TYPE VITAMIN B_{12} BINDING PROTEIN

The saliva and gastric juice 'R' glycoprotein binders for vitamin B_{12} have an even greater affinity for the vitamin than IF. Thus, Kolhouse and Allen (1977) have shown that the affinity of these proteins for vitamin B_{12} is three times greater than that of IF at neutral pH and 50 times greater at pH 2. Not only do these R binding proteins bind vitamin B_{12} but they also bind a variety of analogues of vitamin B_{12} which may be contained in a normal diet. Strictly, vitamin B_{12} refers to cyanocobalamin, the form of the vitamin which was first crystallized in 1948. Cyanocobalamin itself occurs only in traces in nature, and the main forms of the vitamin (the cobalamins) are methylcobalamin (which is the main form in human plasma), deoxyadenosylcobalamin (the main form in human tissues) and hydroxocobalamin which is rapidly formed when light shines on methyl- or deoxyadenosylcobalamin and is probably the main form ingested in food. All these four cobalamins bind well to IF, which then facilitates their absorption across the ileum. However, several vitamin B_{12} analogues are thought to exist in nature, which differ from these compounds either in the nucleotide portion of the molecule or by substitutions around the corrin ring (Lester-Smith, 1965). Some of these analogues are also bound by IF and are taken up by ileal mucosa in vitro and absorbed, while others are taken up by IF even though the ileum appears to have mechanisms for preventing their subsequent rapid absorption, while still others are bound with only low affinity by IF and are not then taken up by the ileum (Kolhouse and Allen, 1977). On the other hand, the R proteins tend to bind with high affinity most of these vitamin B_{12} analogues. Since cobalamins bound to R proteins are not absorbed unless released and bound to IF these proteins may provide a mechanism for preventing the absorption of some of the unwanted analogues (Kolhouse and Allen, 1977).

Analogues may also be produced by bacterial synthesis within the small intestine (Brandt, Bernstein and Wagle, 1977) and these may be absorbed into the body. TCI is a plasma-binding glycoprotein for vitamin B_{12} of similar structure to the R binders of gastric juice and saliva. Vitamin B_{12} or its analogues bound to this protein is selectively carried to hepatocytes since TCI has a higher affinity than TCII (which carries vitamin B_{12} preferentially to bone marrow) for the analogues as well as for vitamin B_{12} itself. Thus, the R proteins may provide a mechanism for reducing the absorption of, and accelerating the excretion of, unwanted, potentially toxic, vitamin B_{12} analogues.

Albert, Mathan and Baker (1980) have recently suggested that bacteria in the small intestine may also produce true vitamin B_{12} compounds which may become attached to intrinsic factor and contribute to the subject's vitamin B_{12} stores. This source of vitamin B_{12}, they postulate, may help to protect against vitamin B_{12} deficiency in normal subjects in Southern India, who take a vegan diet lacking in vitamin B_{12} but often have colonic bacteria in the small intestine and in most cases do not develop severe vitamin B_{12} deficiency.

The presence of analogues of vitamin B_{12} in plasma, whether derived from food or bacterial synthesis in the intestine, which are capable of binding to R proteins, has been postulated as a possible explanation for a discrepancy that exists between the microbiological and radioactive assays for vitamin B_{12} in serum. It has been clear for many years that radioassays give higher results for serum vitamin B_{12} than microbiological (*Euglena gracilis* or *Lactobacillus leichmannii*) assays, and this is particularly marked in some patients following partial gastrectomy (Raven et al, 1972). Indeed, if most radioassays are used, the steadily falling serum vitamin B_{12} and increasing incidence of subnormal serum vitamin B_{12} levels with time, found post-partial gastrectomy using microbiological assay, are not observed. Cooper and Whitehead (1978) have reported that this discrepancy may also lead to a failure to diagnose pernicious anaemia in as many as 10 per cent of cases. Kolhouse et al (1978) suggest that the discrepancy arises because cobalamin analogues in plasma compete with true vitamin B_{12} for protein binders other than pure intrinsic factor, which are used in the radioassays, whereas these analogues are not active for the microbiological organisms, or indeed, active in human vitamin B_{12} metabolism. This attractive explanation awaits full confirmation but preliminary results from a number of laboratories, including our own (Ahmed, Luck and Hoffbrand, 1980, unpublished observations), demonstrate that addition of a vitamin B_{12} analogue to 'block' non-intrinsic factor binder present in impure IF preparations used in the radioassay does lower the serum vitamin B_{12} measured by radioassay to that of the microbiological assay in many sera.

ROLE OF THE PANCREAS

The observation of malabsorption of vitamin B_{12} in chronic pancreatic disease, whether chronic pancreatitis or cystic fibrosis (see review, Chanarin, 1979), has led to a search for the role of pancreatic secretion in vitamin B_{12} absorption. Bicarbonate as well as trypsin has been found to improve absorption in these patients. Previous suggested mechanisms for the malabsorption of vitamin B_{12} in chronic pancreatitis have been lack of an optimum pH (approximately neutral) and of optimal calcium ion concentration in the ileum or lack of release of vitamin B_{12} from binding proteins other than intrinsic factor in the small intestine. More recently, Allen et al (1978) have shown that trypsin and, to a lesser extent, chymotrypsin and elastase are needed to digest gastric and saliva R proteins which bind vitamin B_{12} in the stomach, otherwise vitamin B_{12} bound to these proteins is not available for absorption. Incubation of R protein with pancreatic proteases led to a 150-fold reduction in the affinity of the R protein for vitamin B_{12}. The pancreatic proteases do not degrade IF-B_{12} complex. Presumably, in patients with a reduced IF secretion (e.g., with atrophic gastritis), the R protein binding of dietary vitamin B_{12} becomes a major factor and in such patients malabsorption of dietary vitamin B_{12} is more likely if chronic pancreatitis occurs. The explanation for the beneficial effect of bicarbonate proposed was that this neutralized gastric acid and so favoured binding of dietary vitamin B_{12} to intrinsic factor, rather than to R protein which competes with IF for vitamin B_{12} more effectively the lower the pH (Allen et al, 1978).

As yet no patients with chronic pancreatitis have been described who have developed megaloblastic anaemia due to vitamin B_{12} deficiency, presumably because malabsorption of the vitamin in chronic pancreatic disease is neither sufficiently severe nor prolonged to deplete body stores of the vitamin to the level at which megaloblastic anaemia (or vitamin B_{12} neuropathy) occurs.

ROLE OF TRANSCOBALAMIN II (TCII)

Vitamin B_{12} in plasma is largely bound to the R-Type of glycoprotein, TCI. Vitamin B_{12} bound to TCI is functionally 'dead' and does not enter these cells more readily than the free vitamin. TCI-B_{12} is taken up almost exclusively by hepatocytes which contain receptors with specificity for a variety of asialo-glycoproteins (Ashwell and Morell, 1974). A minor fraction (5 to 10 per cent) of plasma B_{12}, however, is bound to the separate polypeptide protein TCII which plays the vital role of facilitating vitamin B_{12} entry to the haemopoietic cells in the bone marrow, to the placenta, and probably to the brain and other organs. Newly absorbed vitamin B_{12} is found mainly on TCII. It had been assumed that this is largely because the free vitamin leaving the enterocyte and entering the portal blood attaches mainly to the most unsaturated of the plasma transcobalamins, TCII. Several more recent observations suggest that this entirely passive role for TCII in vitamin B_{12} absorption may not be true. Children born with the rare inherited defect, TCII deficiency, show severe malabsorption of vitamin B_{12} (Hakami et al, 1971: Gimpert, Jacob and Hitzig, 1975; Burman et al, 1979). Moreover, newly-absorbed vitamin B_{12} appears on TCII even after this protein has been completely saturated with large amounts of injected vitamin B_{12}, suggesting that TCII is synthesized in the ileum during the passage of the vitamin through the absorptive cell (Chanarin et al, 1978). In vitro studies have also suggested that the ileal cell, in the guinea pig at least, is capable of TCII synthesis (Rothenberg, Weiss and Cotter, 1978). Whether this synthesis occurs during the known delay in vitamin B_{12} transport across the ileal cell is unclear. Peters and Hoffbrand (1970) found vitamin B_{12} to be localized to the mitochondria of the guinea pig ileal enterocyte during the delay period, and Rothenberg, Weisberg and Ficarra (1972) confirmed this and also demonstrated immunoreactive IF in the mitochondria, and postulated that the delay in vitamin B_{12} absorption occurs during intramitochondrial digestion of IF or of that portion of IF that has been passed through the brush border of the enterocyte in combination with vitamin B_{12}. IF has not been found in portal blood.

A more recent study suggests that vitamin B_{12} is localized to lysosomes rather than mitochondria during the delay period, suggesting a pinocytic absorptive mechanism, with possible digestion of IF or portions of it by acid hydrolases in the ileal enterocyte (Empson et al, 1980). Certainly, transport of protein-bound vitamin B_{12} into liver cells and across renal tubules occurs by pinocytic mechanisms (Pletsch and Coffey, 1971). The concept of vitamin B_{12} absorption through the ileal cell by a pinocytotic mechanism is consistent with the concept that renal and ileal cells share a common defect in the syndrome of congenital specific malabsorption of vitamin B_{12} (Imerslund-Gräsbeck's disease) in which benign proteinuria also occurs. It may be that a lysosomal defect is present in both the ileal enterocyte and the renal tubular absorptive cell.

VITAMIN B_{12} ABSORPTION TESTS AND MALABSORPTION OF VITAMIN B_{12}

Traditionally, tests of vitamin B_{12} absorption are performed using crystalline radioactively-labelled cyanocobalamin in aqueous solution alone or with commercial intrinsic factor given to fasting subjects. In patients following partial gastrectomy, however, the amount absorbed may be improved if the labelled vitamin B_{12} is given with food. The mechanism is probably stimulation of gastric secretion of IF by food. A similar effect can be obtained by injecting histamine. On the other hand, Doscherholmen, McMahon and Ripley (1976) suggest that some subjects may be able to absorb crystalline vitamin B_{12} from an aqueous solution but may not be able to absorb normal dietary (protein-bound) vitamin B_{12}. They have described a vitamin B_{12} absorption test using egg ovalbumin with radioactive vitamin B_{12} to simulate better dietary vitamin B_{12} absorption. The ovalbumin reduces vitamin B_{12} absorption in normal subjects and even more so in some patients with atrophic gastritis or following partial gastrectomy, and the authors claim that this is a better test of dietary vitamin B_{12} malabsorption (Doscherholmen, McMahon and Ripley, 1976, 1978). However, since the crystalline test has proved so excellent in separating pernicious anaemia from normal and is more convenient, most workers still employ this test (whether using whole body counting or the urine excretion method) as routine.

The causes of malabsorption of vitamin B_{12} are listed in Table 1. Relatively few conditions cause sufficient lack of IF, or abnormality in the small intestine with malabsorption of vitamin B_{12} of sufficient severity, for sufficient length of time to cause megaloblastic anaemia or vitamin B_{12} neuropathy. The frequency of vitamin B_{12} deficiency following partial gastrectomy and with small intestinal diseases has diminished in recent years. Pernicious anaemia is by far the major cause in Great Britain. Although several drugs cause malabsorption of vitamin B_{12} (Table 1), megaloblastic anaemia caused solely by these has not yet been described.

A recent study has shown increased loss of body vitamin B_{12} in pernicious anaemia the most common cause of malabsorption of vitamin B_{12}, compared with that in vegans (Amin et al, 1980). The authors suggest that malabsorption of vitamin B_{12} breaks the enterohepatic circulation for vitamin B_{12}, whereas this is intact in vegans, and this might explain why so many vegans do not develop severe vitamin B_{12} deficiency even after many years.

Table 1. *Malabsorption of vitamin B_{12}*

1. *Associated with megaloblastic anaemia or neuropathy due to vitamin B_{12} deficiency*

    Gastric causes
        Addisonian pernicious anaemia
        total and partial gastrectomy
        congenital lack of (or abnormality of) intrinsic factor

    Small intestinal causes
        intestinal stagnant-loop syndrome
            jejunal diverticulosis
            ileo-colic fistula
            anatomical blind-loop
            stricture, etc.
        ileal resection
        chronic tropical sprue
        congenital specific malabsorption of vitamin B_{12} with proteinuria (Imerslund-Gräsbeck syndrome)
        fish tapeworm
        transcobalamin II deficiency

2. *Not usually associated with vitamin B_{12} deficiency sufficiently severe to cause megaloblastic anaemia or neuropathy*

    chronic pancreatitis and cystic fibrosis
    drugs
        metformin, phenformin, PAS,
        colchicine, cholestyramine,
        potassium supplements, neomycin
    alcohol
    severe deficiencies of vitamin B_{12}, folate, iron or protein
    gluten-induced enteropathy
    Crohn's disease (without resection or fistula)
    ileal by-pass
    giardiasis
    Zollinger-Ellison syndrome
    scleroderma, Whipple's disease

FOLATE

The normal Western diet contains between 500 and 1000 µg of folate daily. The dietary folates consist largely of reduced (dihydro- or tetrahydro-) polyglutamate forms of formyl and methyl derivatives of folic (pteroyl-glutamic) acid (PteGlu). During absorption through the duodenal and jejunal mucosae, these folates are converted to a single compound, 5-methyltetrahydrofolate (methyl-H₄PteGlu) which enters portal blood (Perry and Chanarin, 1970). Although full reduction and conversion to the methyl form occurs within the absorptive cell, the exact site of hydrolysis of the polyglutamate derivatives to the monoglutamate form is less certain. Foodstuffs themselves contain a hydrolase (folate conjugase, pteroylpoly-glutamate hydrolase) capable of this conversion once the cells have been disrupted and before heat has destroyed the enzyme. Intestinal and pancreatic juices also contain folate conjugase, but the enzyme is present at far higher concentration in the intestinal cell (where it is localized to lysosomes) and in plasma (Hoffbrand and Peters, 1970). Halsted et al (1978), on the basis of double-lumen perfusion studies, suggest that hydrolysis of the heptaglutamate, at least, occurs by contact with a mucosal enzyme and not from a reaction with free intraluminal enzyme. Although most previous studies have failed to demonstrate folate conjugase on the brush border of the enterocyte, a brush border enzyme with a pH optimum of 6.5 has been detected recently by Halsted (1979). He has suggested that some deconjugation occurs at the brush border and this may be subsequently completed inside the enterocyte, or via the plasma enzyme. Di- and tri-glutamate derivatives are capable of entering mammalian cells (Hoffbrand et al, 1973) but there is no evidence that higher polyglutamates can do this.

Between 50 and 80 per cent of dietary folates are absorbed, depending on their exact composition (the larger polyglutamates being less well absorbed) and on the presence of other dietary components, for example fibre or conjugase inhibitors which may reduce the absorption. Unreduced folic acid, the pharmacological compound used for treating folate deficiency, largely by-passes the reducing mechanism of the small intestine and enters portal blood mainly unchanged if given in large (mg) doses. It then enters the liver and other cells from which methyltetrahydrofolate is displaced into plasma, the folic acid being converted inside cells to reduced and polyglutamate derivatives. About 80 per cent of a dose of folic acid, whatever its size, is absorbed in normal human subjects, the excess being excreted in the urine or bile unchanged or as breakdown products.

Folate binding proteins have recently been characterized in mammalian tissues and fluids, including milk. Their exact role is uncertain. One protein is present on brush borders and may facilitate folate absorption. As these proteins bind oxidized folates more avidly than reduced folates, however, it may also be that they help to prevent absorption of unwanted oxidized folate derivatives or breakdown products of folate. The folate binder present in milk may protect folate from breakdown in the infant's stomach before it can be absorbed. The plasma binders of folate may provide a route by which unwanted folates and their breakdown derivatives, probably particularly acetamidobenzoylglutamate and pteridines (Murphy et al, 1976), are excreted in the bile after being transported preferentially to the liver instead of the bone marrow (Fernandez-Costa and Metz, 1979; Rubinoff et al, 1980).

ENTEROHEPATIC CIRCULATION

Folate is present in bile and the daily excretion by this route has been estimated to be 60 to 90 μg. Most is presumably reabsorbed in normal subjects. Folate also enters the intestine in sloughing intestinal mucosal cells and this may be an important source of loss in conditions of severe malabsorption.

MALABSORPTION OF FOLATE

The small intestine has a large reserve capacity for folate absorption. Malabsorption of the vitamin sufficient to cause megaloblastic anaemia occurs most typically in gluten-induced enteropathy (whether in adults or children) (Table 2). Since folate deficiency follows rapidly when dietary intake or

Table 2. *Malabsorption of folate*

1. *Associated with megaloblastic anaemia due to folate deficiency*

   gluten-induced enteropathy — child, adult or associated with dermatitis herpetiformis
   tropical sprue
   congenital specific malabsorption of folate (very rare)

2. *Not usually associated with megaloblastic anaemia unless associated with reduced dietary intake of folate*

   following partial or total gastrectomy
   inflammatory bowel disease
   systemic bacterial infections
   drugs
     salazopyrine, cholestyramine, methotrexate,
     doubtfully with oral contraceptives,
     anticonvulsants
   bromsulphthalein
   alcohol
   severe folate deficiency
   congestive heart failure

absorption is cut off, folate deficiency assessed by sensitive tests such as serum and red cell folate assays is detected in virtually all untreated cases with this disease (Hoffbrand, 1974). In children, iron deficiency is the main cause of anaemia and may persist after many years of a gluten-free diet. In adults, on the other hand, approximately half have a megaloblastic marrow and almost an equal proportion mixed megaloblastosis and iron deficiency, a pure iron deficiency picture occurring only in a few teenagers or young adults. The cause of the megaloblastic anaemia is folate rather than vitamin B_{12} deficiency although vitamin B_{12} deficiency may also be present and perhaps contribute in some cases. Splenic atrophy sufficient to cause blood film changes (presence of Howell-Jolly bodies, target cells, Pappenheimer bodies and crenated and fragmented cells) occurs in 10 to 15 per cent of adult cases and most of the others show impaired splenic function on sensitive testing. The mechanism remains uncertain; damage by gluten products or by immune complexes containing gluten and loss of lymphocytes via the damaged intestinal mucosa are some of the possible mechanisms. The demonstration of splenic atrophy in some cases of ulcerative colitis (Ryan et al, 1974) and of impaired RE function in rheumatoid arthritis (Williams et al, 1979) shows that immunological mechanisms may underly the atrophy.

The only other conditions in which malabsorption of folate is frequent are dermatitis herpetiformis (a condition closely related to adult coeliac disease), tropical sprue and the very rare congenital specific malabsorption of folate. When severe folate deficiency occurs in other gastrointestinal diseases (e.g., Crohn's disease, ulcerative colitis, intestinal resection and following gastrectomy) it is likely that poor dietary intake is the major factor. The cause of malabsorption of folate in coeliac disease and all these syndromes may be damage to the mucosa with loss of absorptive surface. Lucas et al (1978) have also postulated that alteration in the microclimate of the intestinal villi is also important. In contrast to the situation for vitamin B_{12}, folate excess rather than deficiency is the characteristic finding in the intestinal stagnant-loop syndrome (Hoffbrand et al, 1971).

As in the case for vitamin B_{12}, a number of drugs have been reported to cause malabsorption of folate (Table 2). Because tests for folate absorption are more difficult to carry out than for vitamin B_{12}, these are less well documented, but it is doubtful if any are sole or even major causes of severe malabsorption of the vitamin, and when megaloblastic anaemia due to folate deficiency occurs in patients receiving them, poor diet can usually be identified as the major precipitating factor.

IRON

The importance of iron absorption in regulating body iron balance is well recognized. The mechanism by which this is achieved remains uncertain. The role of intraluminal factors in presenting dietary iron to the duodenal and jejunal mucosae in a soluble form, either as inorganic iron attached to low molecular weight chelates or as organic iron, has been well reviewed (Jacobs and Worwood, 1975). Several regulatory steps seem to control the amount of iron that subsequently enters portal blood. Cox and Peters (1980) have recently shown that the initial uptake by the mucosal cell has the characteristics of an active, carrier-mediated process and that iron deficiency, known to enhance iron absorption, reversibly induces brush-border iron carriers. They suggest that in man, initial entry to the enterocyte rather than cellular retention of iron is a major regulatory step in the control of iron absorption. Crosby (1966) suggested that temporary mucosal retention of unwanted iron in ferritin with subsequent shedding into the intestinal lumen formed a major site of regulation, while Fletcher and Huehns (1968) and Cavill, Worwood and Jacobs (1975) have postulated that much of the regulation depends on the rate at which transferrin in portal blood takes up and transfers iron to other tissues. A full discussion of all these theories and of the differences between inorganic and organic iron absorption is beyond the scope of this review.

MALABSORPTION OF IRON

Despite the importance of the intestine in regulating iron absorption, malabsorption is rarely the sole cause of iron deficiency. This is partly because of the long time needed for depletion of body iron to occur because of the malabsorption alone. It is also becoming increasingly well recognized that in some conditions in which malabsorption has been thought to be a major factor, for example gluten-induced enteropathy, following gastrectomy, in atrophic gastritis or in infants with milk intolerance, it is excessive iron loss, usually as chronic haemorrhage, that is the major factor causing the deficiency. For instance, Kosnai, Kuitunen and Siimes (1979) recently showed that iron loss in the stools was greater than normal in coeliac children receiving a gluten-free diet if the mucosa was still abnormal, even though iron absorption had returned to normal. Anand, Callender and Warner (1977) have indeed shown that iron absorption is usually normal in such treated patients. This iron loss accounted for the high incidence of iron deficiency in the children. Haemorrhage or increased turnover of epithelial cells could both account for the increased iron loss, but the authors concluded on the basis of labelled ^{51}Cr red cell loss studies that haemorrhage was the major factor. Similarly, iron loss due to haemorrhage and possibly in shedding mucosal cells is probably important in the iron deficiency of atrophic gastritis and following partial gastrectomy.

REFERENCES

Albert, M.J., Mathan, V.I. & Baker, S.J. (1980) Vitamin B_{12} synthesis by human small intestinal bacteria. *Nature*, **283**, 781.

Allen, R.H., Seetharam, B., Podell, E. & Alpers, D.H. (1978) Effect of proteolytic enzymes on the binding of cobalamin to R protein and intrinsic factor. In vitro evidence that a failure to degrade R protein is responsible for cobalamin malabsorption in pancreatic insufficiency. *Journal of Clinical Investigation*, **61**, 47-54.

Amin, S., Spinks, T., Ranicar, A., Short, M.D. & Hoffbrand, A.V. (1980) Long-term clearance of ^{57}Co-cyano-cobalamin in vegans and pernicious anaemia. *Clinical Science*, **58**, 101-103.

Anand, B.S., Callender, S.T. & Warner, G.T. (1977) Absorption of inorganic and haemoglobin iron in coeliac disease. *British Journal of Haematology*, **37**, 409-414.

Ashwell, G. & Morell, A.G. (1974) The role of surface carbohydrates in the hepatic recognition and transport of circulating glycoproteins. *Advances in Enzymology*, **41**, 99-128.

Brandt, L.J., Bernstein, L.H. & Wagle, A. (1977) Production of vitamin B_{12} analogues in patients with small bowel bacterial overgrowth. *Annals of Internal Medicine*, **87**, 546-551.

Burman, J.F., Mollin, D.L., Sourial, N.A. & Sladden, R.A. (1979) Inherited lack of transcobalamin II in serum and megaloblastic anaemia: a further patient. *British Journal of Haematology*, **43**, 27-28.

Cavill, I., Worwood, M. & Jacobs, A. (1975) Internal regulation of iron absorption. *Nature*, **256**, 328-329.

Chanarin, I. (1979) *The megaloblastic anaemias*. 2nd edn. Oxford: Blackwell Scientific Publications.

Chanarin, I., Muir, M., Hughes, A. & Hoffbrand, A.V. (1978) Evidence for intestinal origin of transcobalamin II during vitamin B_{12} absorption. *British Medical Journal*, **i**, 1453-1455.

Cooper, B.A. & Whitehead, V.M. (1978) Evidence that some patients with pernicious anaemia are not recognized by radio dilution assay for cobalamin in serum. *New England Journal of Medicine*, **299**, 816-818.

Cox, T.M. & Peters, T.J. (1980) Cellular mechanisms in the regulation of iron absorption by the human intestine: studies in patients with iron deficiency before and after treatment. *British Journal of Haematology*, **44**, 75-86.

Crosby, W.H. (1966) Mucosal block. An evaluation of concepts relating to control of iron absorption. *Seminars in Hematology*, **3**, 299-313.

Donaldson, R.M. (1975) Mechanism of malabsorption of colabamin. In *Colabalamin: Biochemistry and Pathophysiology* (Ed.) Babior, B.M. pp. 335-368. New York: John Wiley & Sons.

Doscherholmen, A., McMahon, J. & Ripley, D. (1976) Inhibitory effect of eggs on vitamin B_{12} absorption: description of a simple ovalbumin ^{57}Co-vitamin absorption test. *British Journal of Haematology*, 33, 261-272.

Doscherholmen, A., McMahon, J. & Ripley, D. (1978) Vitamin B_{12} assimilation from chicken meat. *American Journal of Clinical Nutrition*, 31, 825-830.

Empson, R., Jenkins, E.J., Jewell, D.P. & Taylor, K.B. (1980) Absorption of vitamin B_{12} in the guinea-pig ileum. *Clinical Science*, 58, 13p.

Fernandez-Costa, F. & Metz, J. (1979) Role of serum folate binders in the delivery of folate to tissues and to the fetus. *British Journal of Haematology*, 41, 335-342.

Fletcher, J. & Huehns, E.R. (1968) Function of transferrin. *Nature*, 218, 1211-1214.

Gimpert, E., Jacob, M. & Hitzig, W.H. (1975) Vitamin B_{12} transport in blood. I. Congenital deficiency of transcobalamin II. *Blood*, 45, 71-82.

Hakami, N., Neiman, P.E., Cannellos, G.P. & Lazerson, J. (1971) Neonatal megaloblastic anaemia due to inherited transcobalamin II deficiency in two siblings. *New England Journal of Medicine*, 285, 1163-1170.

Halsted, C.H. (1979) The intestinal absorption of folates. *American Journal of Clinical Nutrition*, 32, 846-855.

Halsted, C.H., Reisenauer, A.M., Shane, B. & Tamura, T. (1978) Availability of monoglutamyl and polyglutamyl folates in normal subjects and in patients with coeliac sprue. *Gut*, 19, 886.

Hoffbrand, A.V. (1974) Anaemia in adult coeliac disease. *Clinics in Gastroenterology*, 3, 71-89.

Hoffbrand, A.V. & Peters, T.J. (1970) Recent advances in clinical and biochemical aspects of folate. *Schweizer Medizine Wochenschrifte*, 100, 1954.

Hoffbrand, A.V., Tabaqchali, S., Booth, C.C. & Mollin, D.L. (1971) Small intestine bacterial flora and folate status in gastrointestinal disease. *Gut*, 12, 27-33.

Hoffbrand, A.V., Tripp, E., Houlihan, C. & Scott, J.M. (1973) Studies on the uptake of synthetic conjugated folates by human marrow cells. *Blood*, 42, 141.

Hooper, D.C., Alpers, D.H., Burger, R.L., Mehlman, C.S. & Allen, R.H. (1973) Characterization of ileal vitamin B_{12} binding using homogenous human and hog intrinsic factors. *Journal of Clinical Investigation*, 52, 3074-3083.

Jacobs, A. & Worwood, M. (1975). Iron absorption: present state of the art. *British Journal of Haematology*, 31, 89-101.

Katz, M. & Cooper, B.A. (1974) Solubilized receptor for vitamin B_{12} — intrinsic factor complex from human intestine. *British Journal of Haematology*, 26, 569-579.

Kolhouse, J.I. & Allen, R.H. (1977) Absorption, plasma transport, and cellular retention of cobalamin analogues in the rabbit. *Journal of Clinical Investigation*, 60, 1381-1392.

Kolhouse, J.I., Kondo, H., Allen, N.C., Podell, E. & Allen, R.H. (1978) Cobalamin analogues are present in human plasma and can mask cobalamin deficiency because current radioisotope dilution assays are not specific for true cobalamin. *New England Journal of Medicine*, 299, 785-792.

Kosnai, I., Kuitunen P. & Siimes, M.A. (1979) Iron deficiency in children with coeliac disease on treatment with gluten-free diet. Role of intestinal blood loss. *Archives of Disease in Childhood*, 54, 375-378.

Lester-Smith, E. (1965) *Vitamin B_{12}*. London: Methuen.

Lucas, M.L., Cooper, B.T., Lei, F.H., Johnson, I.T., Holmes, G.K.T., Blair, J.A. & Cooke, W.T. (1978) Acid microclimate in coeliac and Crohn's disease: a model for folate malabsorption. *Gut*, 19, 735-742.

Marcoullis, G. & Gräsbeck, R. (1977) Solubilised intrinsic factor receptor from pig ileum and its characteristics. *Biochimica* et *Biophysica Acta*, 36, 496.

Murphy, M., Keating, M., Boyle, P., Weir, D.G. & Scott, J.M. (1976) The elucidation of the mechanism of folate catabolism in the rat. *Biochemical and Biophysical Research Communications*, 71, 1017-1024.

Perry, I. & Chanarin, I. (1970) Intestinal absorption of reduced folate compounds in man. *British Journal of Haematology*, 18, 329-339.

Peters, T.J. & Hoffbrand, A.V. (1970) Absorption of vitamin B_{12} by the guinea pig: subcellular localisation of vitamin B_{12} in the ileal cell during absorption. *British Journal of Haematology*, **19**, 369.

Pletsch, Q.A. & Coffey, J.W. (1971) Intracellular distribution of radioactive vitamin B_{12} in rat liver. *Journal of Biological Chemistry*, **246**, 4619-4629.

Raven, J.L., Robson, M.B., Morgan, J.O. & Hoffbrand, A.V. (1972) Comparison of three methods for measuring vitamin B_{12} in serum: radioisotopic, *Euglena gracilis*, and *Lactobacillus leichmannii*. *British Journal of Haematology*, **22**, 21-31.

Rothenberg, S.P., Weisberg, H. & Ficarra, A. (1972) Evidence for the absorption of immunoreactive intrinsic factor into the intestinal epithelial cell during vitamin B_{12} absorption. *Journal of Laboratory and Clinical Medicine*, **79**, 587-597.

Rothenberg, S.P., Weiss, J.P. & Cotter R. (1978) Formation of transcobalamin II-vitamin B_{12} complex by guinea pig ileal mucosa in organ culture after in vivo incubation with intrinsic factor-vitamin B_{12}. *British Journal of Haematology*, **40**, 401-414.

Rubinoff, M., Abramson R., Schreiber, C. & Waxman, S. (1980) The effect of a folate binding protein on the plasma transport and tissue distribution of folic acid. *British Journal of Haematology*, in press.

Ryan, F.P., Smart, R.C., Preston, F.E. & Holdsworth, C.D. (1974) Hyposplenism in ulcerative colitis. *Lancet*, **ii**, 318-320.

Williams, B.D., Pussell, B.A., Lockwood, C.M. & Cotton, C. (1979) Defective reticuloendothelial system function in rheumatoid arthritis. *Lancet*, **i**, 1311-1313.

5
Idiopathic Faecal Incontinence: Histopathological Evidence on Pathogenesis

MICHAEL SWASH

INTRODUCTION

Anal continence depends on the interaction of several factors (Duthie, 1971). These include the anorectal angulation (Parks, 1975) and resting tonic contraction of the internal and external anal sphincter muscles. Of these three factors, the maintenance of the normal anorectal angulation is the most important (Parks, Porter and Melzack, 1962; Parks, Porter and Hardcastle, 1966; Parks, 1975). This angulation is maintained by the pull of the muscular sling formed in this region by the puborectalis muscles (Thompson, 1899; Kerremans, 1969; Duthie, 1971). The puborectalis muscles are situated at the apex of the funnel-like muscular floor of the pelvis formed by the paired levator ani muscles, but the histological similarity of the puborectalis and external anal sphincter muscles (Kerremans, 1969; Beersiek, Parks and Swash, 1979) suggests that the latter two muscles form a functional unit separate from the levator ani itself. Indeed, the circular external anal sphincter muscle, consisting of deep, superficial and cutaneous parts, is also important in faecal continence although it has often been regarded as playing only a minor role (Kerremans, 1969; Duthie, 1971; Schuster, 1975). The internal anal sphincter is important in controlling continence to flatus, but is of little importance in faecal continence itself (Bennett and Duthie, 1964).

The factors leading to defaecation in normal subjects include pressure and tension changes in the lower rectum and the presence of faecal matter in the anal canal itself, indicating that the internal and external anal sphincters have relaxed slightly. Abnormalities of the control of these muscles occur in patients with spinal cord disease and in other disorders of the central nervous system, and these may lead to released reflex defaecation, and so to incontinence, as in multiple sclerosis. Faecal incontinence may also occur when there is damage to the lumbosacral nerve roots (Butler, 1954), and after trauma to the anal sphincter musculature. In another and larger group of patients, however, faecal incontinence occurs without evidence of neurological disease, or of other anorectal abnormalities; this is termed

© 1980 W.B. Saunders Company Ltd.

idiopathic anorectal (faecal) incontinence. In this paper evidence suggesting that this form of faecal incontinence is due to abnormalities in the anal sphincter musculature resulting from damage to its nerve supply will be reviewed. This evidence derives from clinical, pathological and physiological studies carried out at St Mark's Hospital, and at the London Hospital.

Clinical features of idiopathic faecal incontinence

Idiopathic faecal incontinence occurs almost exclusively in women. The disorder develops gradually during a period of years. There is usually a history of constipation and of repeated and often prolonged straining during defaecation. At first incontinence may be noticed only when there is diarrhoea and the stools are more liquid than normal but later it occurs in response to minor stresses, as during a bout of coughing. In severe cases incontinence of faeces may occur even when sitting or standing, and such patients are depressed and housebound. Examination reveals a patulous external anal sphincter, so that a finger or two may be inserted into the anal canal without resistance. The anal canal itself contains faeces although the patient is unaware of it. Indeed, patients with anorectal incontinence are invariably unable to distinguish flatus from faeces in the lower rectum and in the anal canal. Sometimes examination will reveal impaired sensation to touch, and less commonly to pin-prick, in the skin at the anal margin. This zone is innervated by sensory branches of the pudendal nerves. The anal reflex is often absent.

The pelvic floor has usually dropped in relation to surrounding structures so that the anal orifice may appear slightly everted, and if the patient is asked to strain or 'bear down' by increasing her intra-abdominal pressure during a forced expiration against a closed glottis the perineum descends still further (perineal descent).

Perineal descent also occurs in these patients during a sudden cough; the normal response is for the pelvic floor to contract and for the perineum to rise slightly during straining or coughing (Parks, Porter and Hardcastle, 1966). Perineal descent occurs because of weakness of the puborectalis muscles (Parks, Porter and Hardcastle, 1966; Parks, 1975). Rectal prolapse is a feature of about 60 per cent of patients with idiopathic anorectal incontinence. In patients with rectal prolapse, on the other hand, incontinence is a feature only when the prolapse has been symptomatic for many months, or several years (Porter, 1962).

Studies of the pressure in the anal canal in patients with anorectal incontinence show a relatively normal resting pressure, but only a slight rise in pressure during voluntary or reflex contraction of the external anal sphincter muscle (see Parks, 1975). In a series of 25 patients with anorectal incontinence referred for surgery (Parks, Swash and Urich, 1977) faecal incontinence began after a difficult or precipitate labour, or after obstetric trauma, in eight of the 24 women (33 per cent), but seven women (30 per cent) had never been pregnant. Surgical trauma to the sphincter musculature, associated with haemorrhoidectomy, was implicated in one case. In 65 per cent of the patients excessive straining during defaecation was a prominent feature of the history, and rectal prolapse was present in 60 per cent. Only three patients (12 per cent) had urinary incontinence and none showed evidence of a primary neurological cause, although perineal sensation was absent in one patient in whom a third-degree perineal tear had occurred during childbirth, and most could not distinguish flatus from faeces. These patients' ages ranged from 24 to 80 years (mean 58 years).

The anorectal angle

The major anatomical factor in the maintenance of faecal continence (Parks, Porter and Melzack, 1962; Parks, Porter and Hardcastle, 1966; Parks, 1975) is the flap-valve mechanism at the anorectal junction formed by the right-angle between the longitudinal axes of the lower rectum and the anal canal (Figure 1). The mucosa of the lowest part of the anterior rectal wall

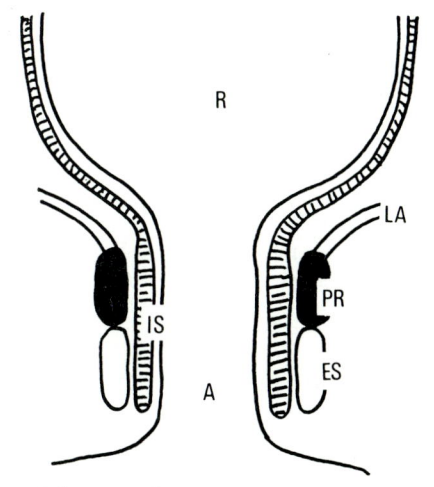

Figure 1. The muscles of the pelvic floor responsible for faecal continence. IS = internal sphincter; ES = external sphincter; PR = puborectalis; LA = levator ani; R = rectum; A = anal canal.

thus closes off the upper end of the anal canal. The higher the intra-abdominal pressure the more securely is continence maintained, provided that the anorectal angulation remains intact. The anorectal angle is itself maintained by the pull of the muscular sling formed in this region by the puborectalis muscles (Thompson, 1899; Kerremans, 1969; Duthie, 1971). Although there has been some controversy as to the anatomical separation of the puborectalis and external anal sphincter muscles (Thompson, 1899; Goligher, Leacock and Brossy, 1953; Kerremans, 1969) our own studies have clearly shown differences. Nonetheless, the close similarity of these two muscles suggests that they have a similar function (Beersiek, Parks and Swash, 1979). The levator ani, which forms the funnel-like muscular base of the pelvic floor, is anatomically discrete from the puborectalis muscles, although its lowermost fibres are apposed to the latter muscle (Figure 2).

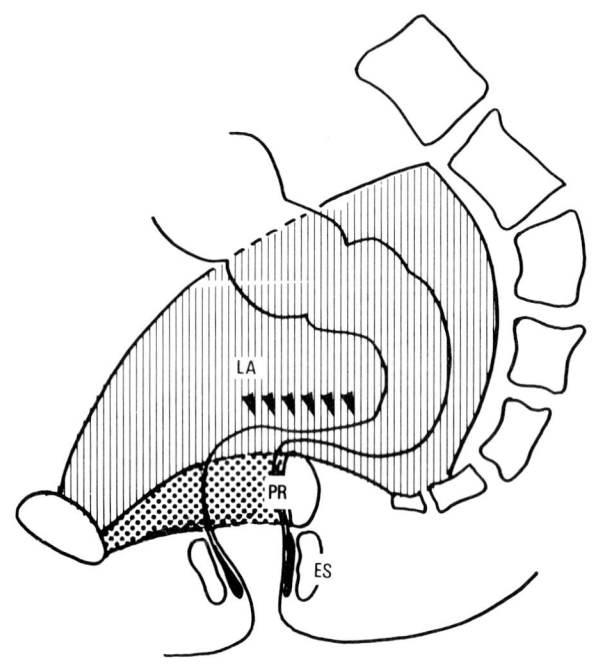

Figure 2. The flap valve mechanism of the anorectal angle. The valve is closed by the intra-abdominal pressure (arrowheads) and by the pull of the puborectalis (PR) muscles. ES = external sphincter; LA = levator ani.

In patients with anorectal incontinence the normally sharp anorectal angle is lost (Parks, 1975). When there is perineal descent the anal canal is drawn downward and the anorectal angle is further compromised, leading to incontinence of faeces during coughing or sneezing. This, therefore, indicates weakness of the puborectalis muscles and, to a lesser degree, of the uppermost fibres of the levator ani funnel. Correction of the incontinence can be accomplished by surgical correction of the anorectal angle, by reconstructing this muscular sling. This can be carried out by a post-anal approach to the puborectalis and levator ani muscles (Parks, 1975) or by an autogeneous muscle graft procedure (Hakelius, 1975).

External anal sphincter, puborectalis and levator ani muscles

The clinical features of idiopathic anorectal incontinence suggest that the anal sphincter and pelvic floor musculature is abnormal. An opportunity to examine these muscles histologically arose during surgical correction of incontinence. The post-anal approach to this operation introduced by Parks (1975) was used and during the operation biopsies of the external anal sphincter, puborectalis and levator ani muscles were taken. Biopsies of these three muscles have been studied in 53 patients. The histological features of these muscles have been described, in previous publications, in 34 of these patients (Parks, Swash and Urich, 1977; Beersiek, Parks and Swash, 1979; Parks and Swash, 1979), and histometric analysis has been carried out in 16 cases (Beersiek, Parks and Swash, 1979).

METHODS

Small pieces of each biopsy were snap-frozen in isopentane-liquid nitrogen, and a consecutive series of transverse sections was cut from blocks of each muscle. These sections were prepared for light microscopy using haematoxylin and eosin, and modified Gomori trichrome stains, and a standard series of enzyme histochemical techniques, including nicotine adenine dinucleotide tetrazolium reductase (NADHtr) and myosin adenosine triphosphatase (ATPase), preincubated at pH 9.5 and 4.3 (Dubowitz and Brooke, 1973). Histochemical fibre typing of the muscle fibres in the biopsies was performed using the ATPase preparations, and the proportions of Type 1 and Type 2 fibres, calculated as a percentage of the total numbers of fibres in each biopsy, were expressed as the dominant fibre type (*fibre type predominance*: see Dubowitz and Brooke, 1973). In addition, the presence of groups of fibres of similar histochemical type and size, and changes in morphology of individual fibres, or other abnormalities, were noted.

In a second study (Beersiek, Parks and Swash, 1979) the same histological methods were used to study biopsies of these three muscles in 16 patients aged 19 to 69 years (mean 48 years) with anorectal incontinence and in 15 normal subjects aged 17 to 76 (mean 47 years). The latter were studied at autopsy; there was no anorectal disorder in these patients and death had occurred from a variety of causes; none was cachectic (Beersiek, Parks and Swash, 1979). The muscle samples were obtained seven to 70 hours after death (mean 32 hours) and satisfactory histological preparations were obtained in 41 of the 51 muscle samples in this group of normal subjects.

In these 33 normal and incontinent subjects the lesser diameters of all the muscle fibres, of both histochemical types, were measured in at least five separate microscope fields, at a magnification of 100 dioptres, using an eye-piece micrometer. Eighty-two muscle biopsies, containing 19 564 muscle fibres, were studied in this way and the mean muscle fibre diameters of Type 1 and Type 2 fibres were determined in each muscle. These diameters, with their standard deviation, in the grouped data of normal and incontinent subjects, were compared using Student's t test (see Beersiek, Parks and Swash, 1979).

RESULTS

In longitudinal sections of the anal canal in control subjects the puborectalis and external anal sphincter muscles were usually separated by a thick layer of connective tissue. This plane of separation could not be recognized in the patients with incontinence, but it is clear that these two muscles are separate and not part of a single larger muscle.

Histological observations

Similar histological abnormalities were found in all the incontinent patients, although they varied in degree from case to case. The external anal sphincter was always the most abnormal of the three muscles and the levator ani was usually the least affected; in some cases the levator ani appeared normal. The abnormalities found in the external anal sphincter differed slightly from those found in the puborectalis; in particular, muscle fibre hypertrophy was much more marked in the puborectalis muscles than in the external anal sphincter muscles, or the levator ani muscles (Table 1).

Table 1

Muscle	Muscle fibre type	% increase in diameter in incontinent patients	% Type 1 fibre predominance Control	% Type 1 fibre predominance Incontinence
External anal sphincter	Type 1	36	78	85
	Type 2	54		
Puborectalis	Type 1	132	75	82
	Type 2	135		
Levator ani	Type 1	21	69	68
	Type 2	61		

External anal sphincter muscle

The most abnormal of the external sphincter biopsies consisted of a few scattered striated muscle fibres embedded in fibrous and adipose tissue, situated adjacent to the smooth muscle fibres of the internal anal sphincter muscle. In other, less abnormal biopsies the muscle fibres were arranged in groups of 10 to 60 fibres separated from each other by bands of fibrous or adipose tissue (Figure 3). The fibres within each group were of approximately uniform size. Some of these fibres contained central sarcolemmal nuclei (Figure 3). In some cases myopathic changes were very prominent so that in haematoxylin and eosin preparations there were apparently random variations in fibre size, individual fibres being widely separated from each other by collagenous connective tissue. However, even in these cases, the ATPase and NADHtr stains revealed fibre-type grouping consistent with reinnervation (Figure 4). Fibre-type grouping was found in 75 per cent of the biopsies.

Scattered necrotic fibres, some undergoing phagocytosis (Figure 5), were sometimes found, usually close to the larger fibres in the biopsy. Splitting or fragmentation of individual muscle fibres was also present in most of these biopsies (see Figure 8) and rare basophilic regenerating fibres were seen.

The Gomori trichrome stain sometimes showed fibres with a granular red margin and with a densely stippled interior: these regions also stained intensely with NADHtr reaction, but they were unstained with the ATPase

(a)

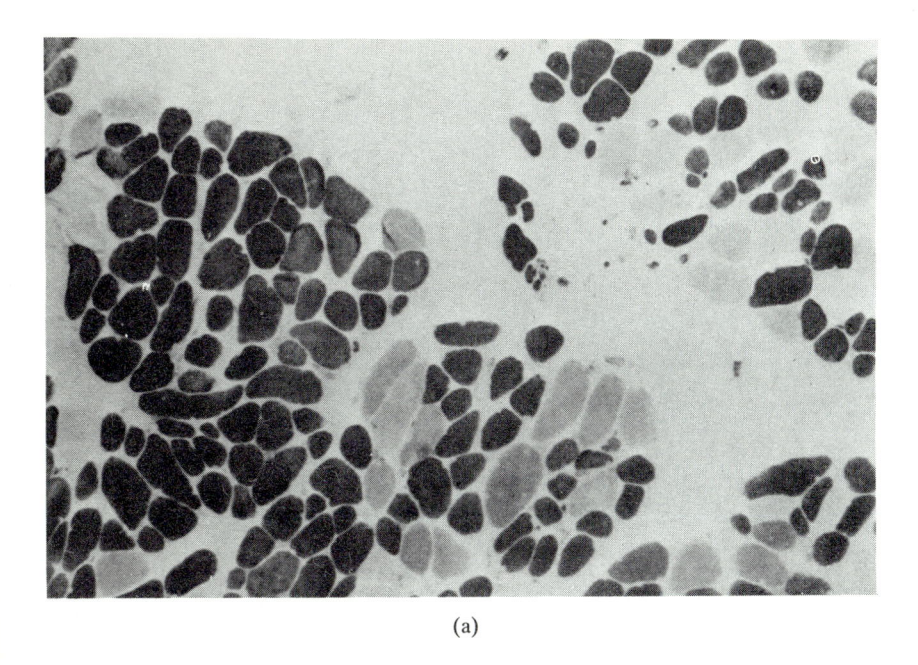

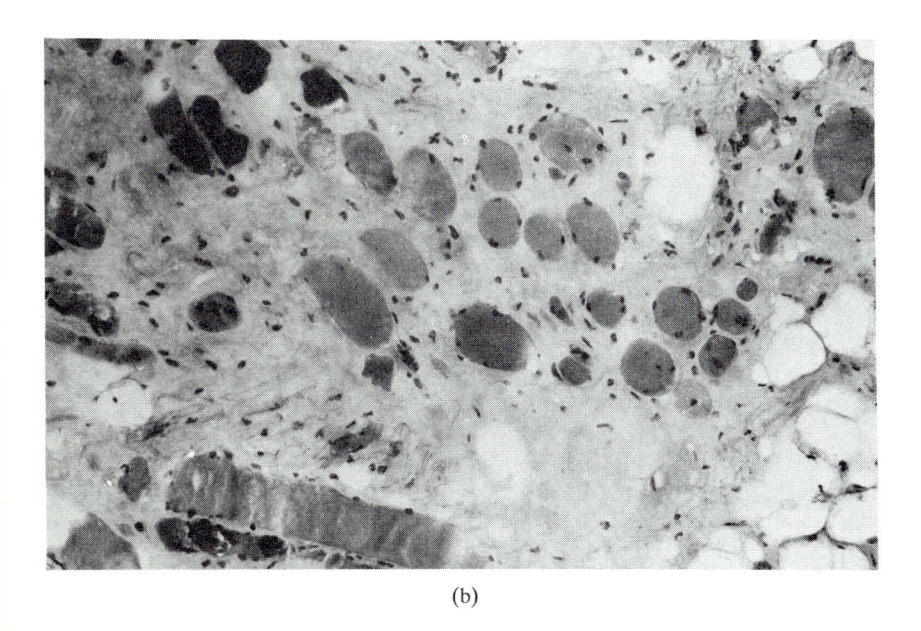

(b)

Figure 3. External anal sphincter in patients with incontinence. (A) Fibre-type grouping and slight fibre hypertrophy; fibre splitting is also present. There are several unstained zones of fat and fibrous tissue replacement. Compare with Figure 10. ATPase, pH 4.3, × 140. (b) Fibrosis, fat replacement and gross loss of muscle fibres are evident. Haematoxylin and eosin, × 140.

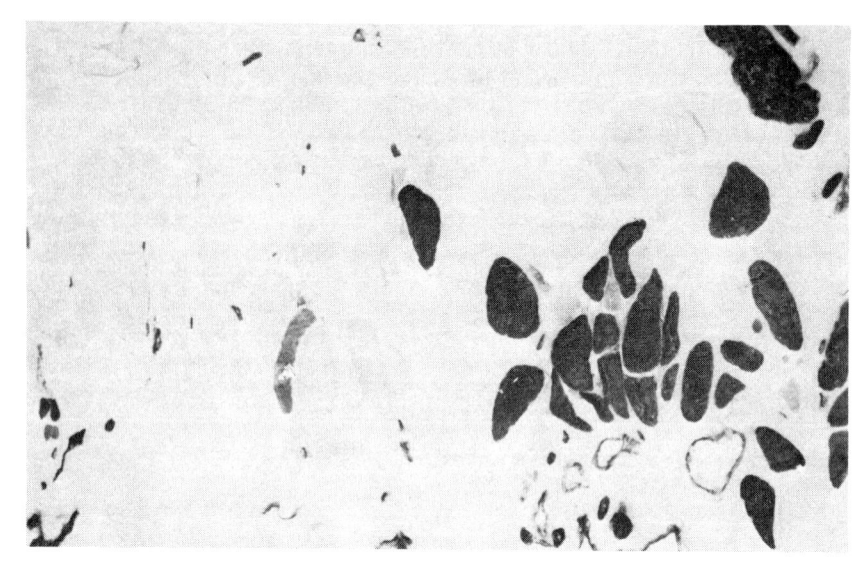

Figure 4. External anal sphincter in a patient with incontinence. Fibre type grouping of both Type 1 (dark) and Type 2 (pale) fibres, with grouped denervation atrophy. ATPase, pH 4.3, × 140.

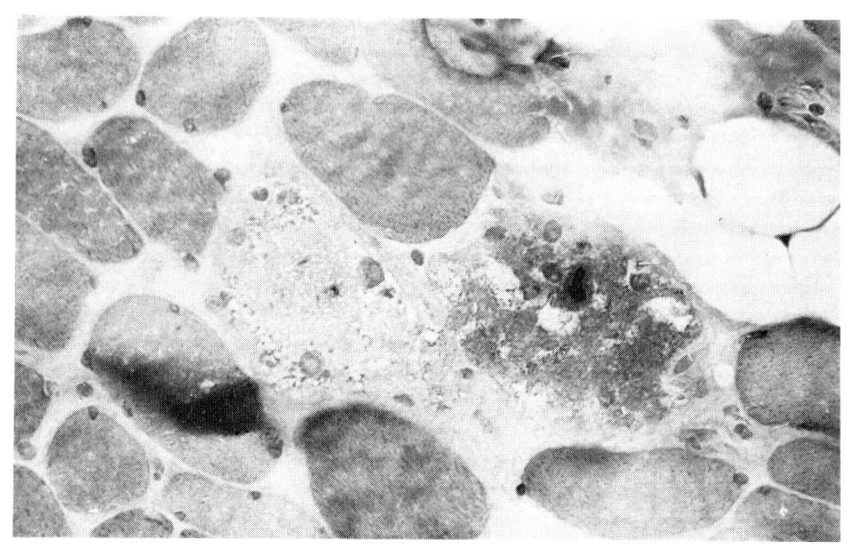

Figure 5. Puborectalis in an incontinent patient. Two vacuolated necrotic fibres: one contains a macrophage. Gomori trichrome, × 350.

technique. These changes are characteristic of 'ragged-red' fibres (Engel, 1971). In the same sections other fibres contained scattered rod-like (nemaline) bodies (Figure 6). Ultrastructural studies confirmed that these rod-bodies were derived from the Z band material (Figure 7). They were located in clusters in regions of focal myofibrillar degeneration and were often associated with collections of lipid droplets.

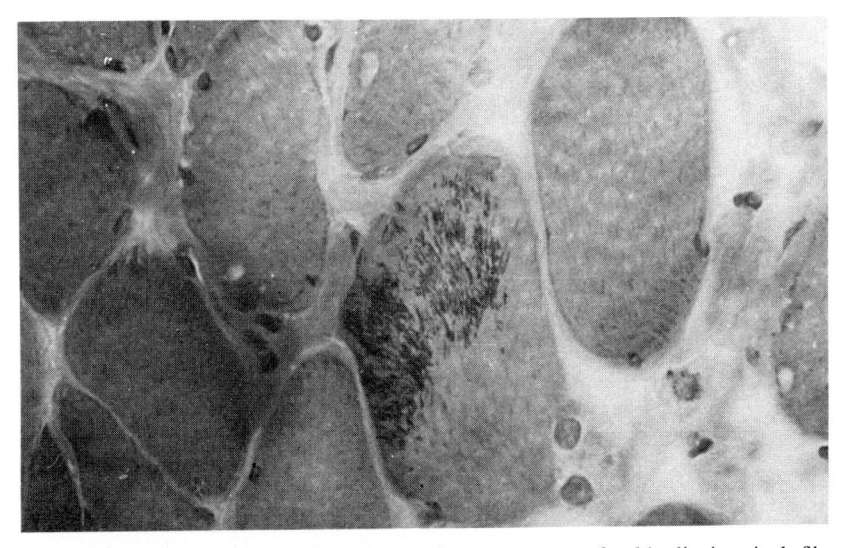

Figure 6. Puborectalis in an incontinent patient. Dense aggregate of rod-bodies in a single fibre. Gomori trichrome, × 560.

Puborectalis muscle

The abnormalities found in the puborectalis muscle biopsies (Figure 8) were similar to those found in the external sphincter muscles. Fibre-type grouping was clearly evident in ATPase preparations, but myopathic changes, such as fibre splitting or fragmentation, necrosis, phagocytosis, or regeneration of single fibres with increased variation in fibre size and central nucleation, were usually far less evident. Accumulations of rod-bodies were found in several cases but they were less prominent than in the external anal sphincter muscles.

Levator ani muscle

The levator ani muscle biopsies usually showed only mild abnormalities such as disseminated neurogenic atrophy. Grouped denervation atrophy was found in some cases. Type 1 fibre preponderance was common in this muscle. Myopathic abnormalities were rarely found and accumulations of rod-bodies were rare.

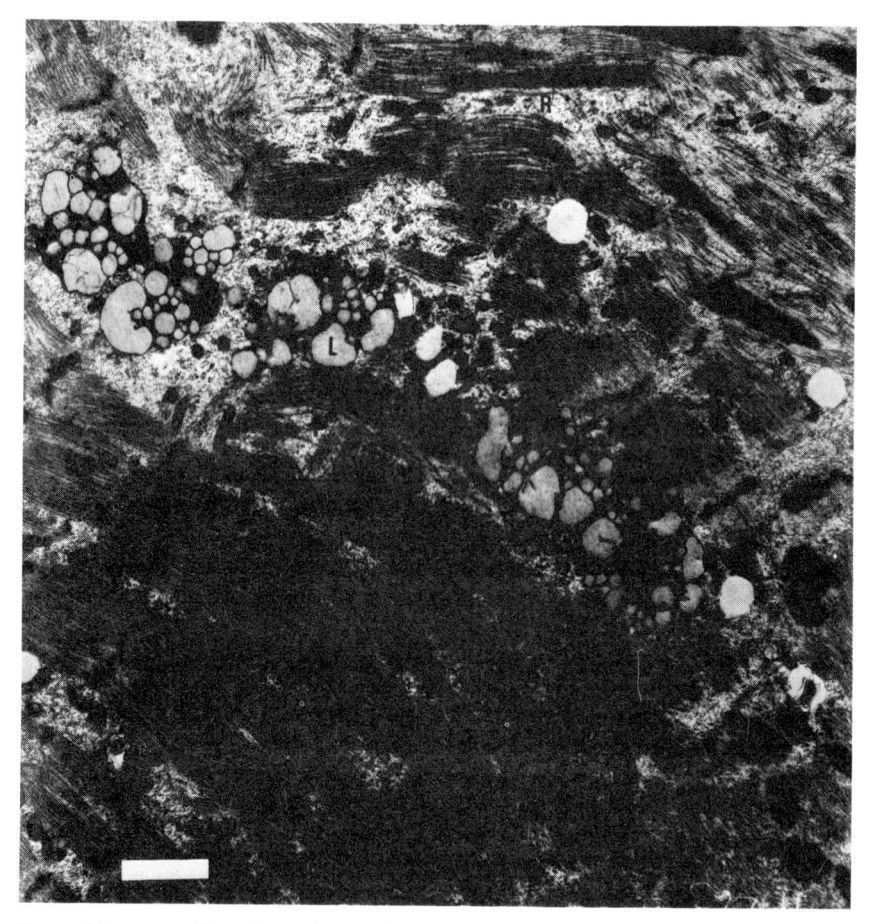

Figure 7. Levator ani in an incontinent patient. Longitudinal section. Lipid droplets (L) and rod bodies (R) in a region of focal myofibrillar disruption. Electron micrograph. Bar = 1 μm.

Other features

Muscle spindles were found occasionally in each of the three muscles examined. They usually appeared normal, but in the external anal sphincter muscles there was some fibrosis of their periaxial spaces and capsules (see Swash and Fox, 1974).

Innervation

Small intramuscular nerve bundles, examined both by light and electron microscopy in the external anal sphincter biopsies, contained few nerve fibres, and were fibrosed. Intramuscular nerve bundles were less affected in the puborectalis muscles of these cases, and were normal in the levator ani biopsies. In the three biopsies of nerves supplying the external anal sphincter

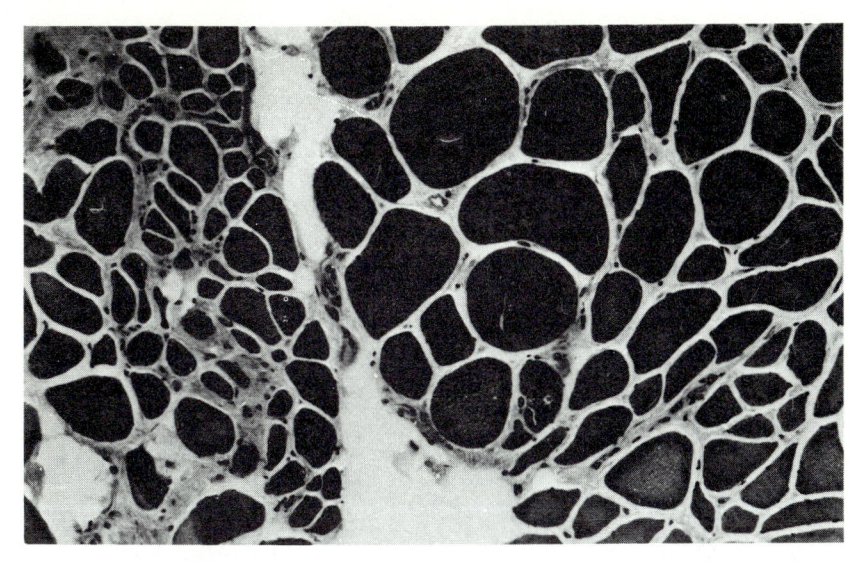

Figure 8. Puborectalis in an incontinent patient. Fibre hypertrophy with fibre splitting and central nucleation is prominent. There is marked fibrosis and there are groups of fibres of differing size. Compare with Fig 12. Haematoxylin and eosin, × 140.

muscles (Figure 9) there was a pronounced reduction in the number of myelinated nerve fibres, with some proliferation of Schwann cells. Segmental or paranodal demyelination was not found, and the unmyelinated nerve fibres were normal. The interstitial collagen was unusually prominent.

Control Cases

As in other human muscles, the normal external anal sphincter, puborectalis and levator ani muscles consist of a mosaic of Type 1 and Type 2 fibres. In the six control cases there was a preponderance of Type 1 fibres in each of these three muscles. The external anal sphincter muscles contained scattered smaller fibres (Figure 10) which were histochemically Type 1 fibres (Figure 11). Some similar smaller fibres were also found in the puborectalis muscles (Figure 12). In some of these normal muscles, particularly in the external anal sphincter muscles, rare necrotic fibres were found.

Quantitative observations

The external anal sphincter, puborectalis and levator ani muscle samples taken from normal subjects all showed Type 1 fibre predominance, but this was slightly more marked in the biopsies from the external anal sphincter and puborectalis muscles of the incontinent patients (see Table 1). No change in Type 1 fibre predominance was observed in the levator ani muscles of the incontinent patients.

The mean diameters of Type 1 and Type 2 muscle fibres in the three muscles in the incontinent patients and in the normal subjects are shown in

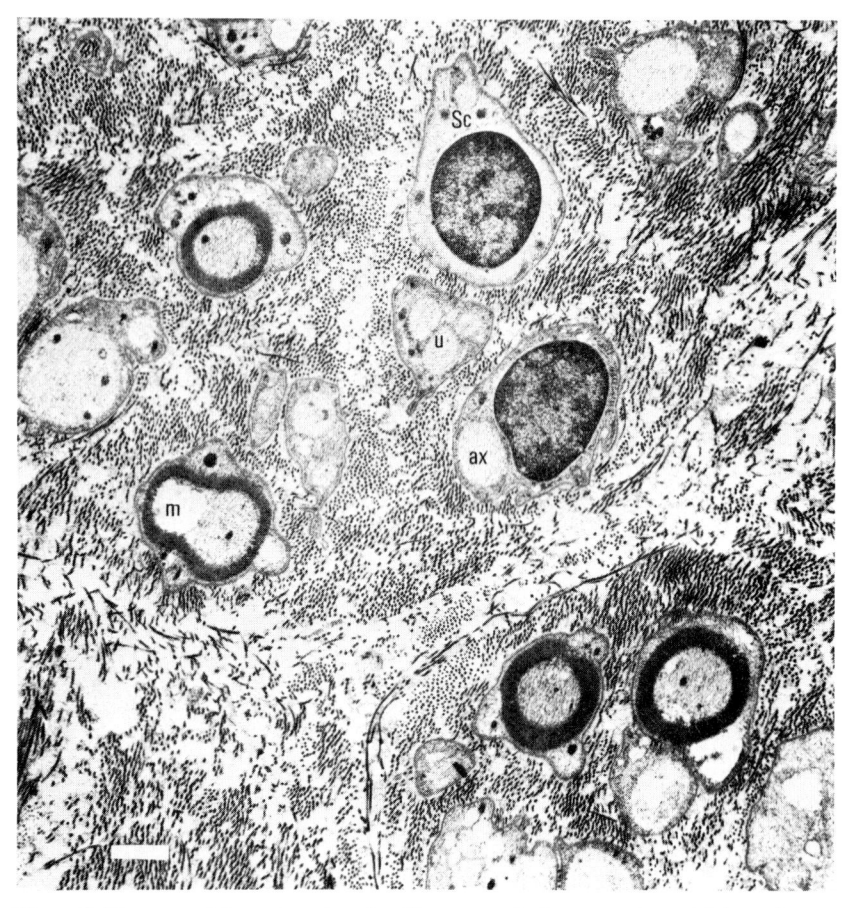

Figure 9. Nerve supplying external anal sphincter muscle from a patient with incontinence. Transverse section. There is an increase in interstitial collagen and a reduction in number of myelinated (m) and unmyelinated (u) nerve fibres. ax = axon; Sc = Schwann cell. Electron micrograph. Bar = μm.

Figure 13. In the external anal sphincter and puborectalis muscles of control subjects Type 2 fibres were slightly larger than Type 1 fibres. Type 2 fibres were generally larger in men than in women, as in other human skeletal muscles (Dubowitz and Brooke, 1973), but fibres of both histochemical type were much smaller in these two muscles than in other striated muscles (see Johnson et al, 1973). However, in the levator ani of adult female control subjects Type 1 fibres were markedly larger than Type 2 fibres. This observation is difficult to explain, but it is possible that the difference in diameter of Type 1 and Type 2 fibres in this muscle in women might be a hormone-dependent phenomenon. In the female rat the levator ani muscles, homologous to the external anal sphincter of primates, undergo involution during puberty (Cihak, Guttmann and Hanzlikova, 1970). Other possible factors, such as work-induced hypertrophy, partial denervation or other

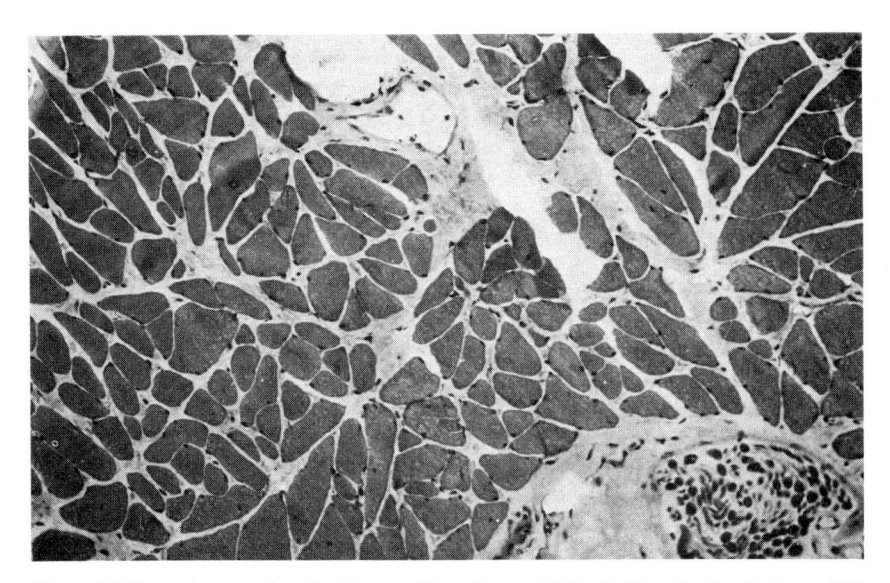

Figure 10. Normal external anal sphincter. Note that variability in fibre size is a feature of this muscle in normal subjects. Haematoxylin and eosin, × 140.

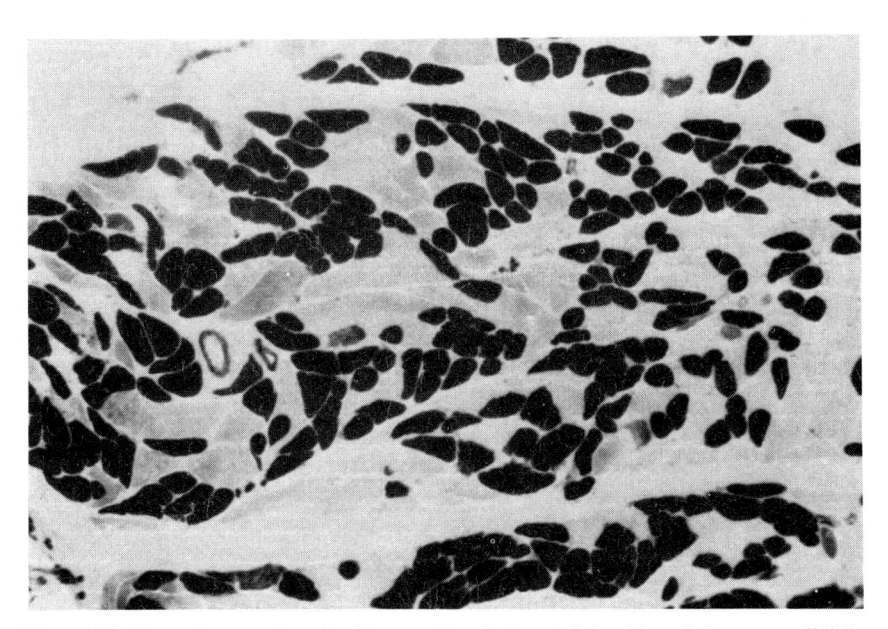

Figure 11. Normal external anal sphincter. The darker-staining Type 1 fibres are slightly smaller than the paler Type 2 fibres, and there is Type 1 fibre predominance. ATPase, pH 4.3, × 140.

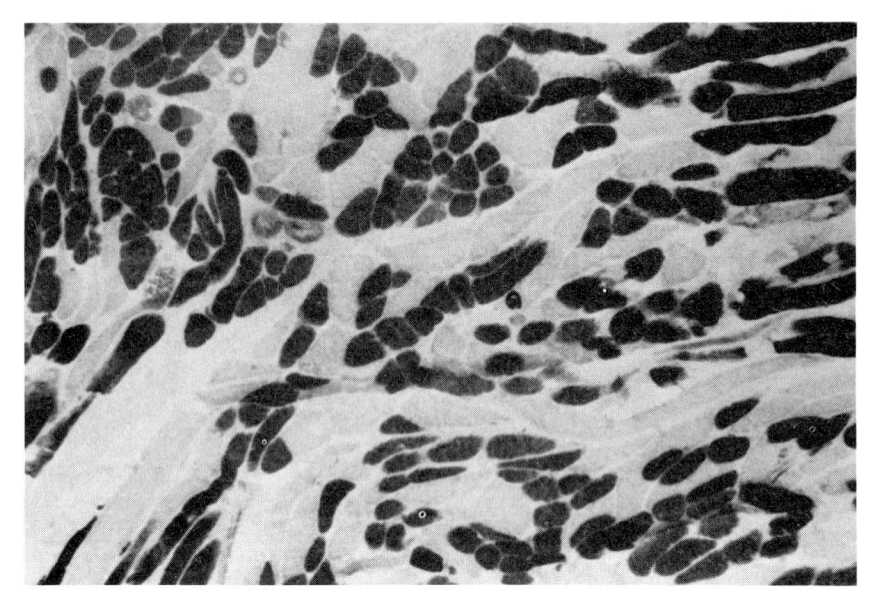

Figure 12. Normal puborectalis. The features are similar to those found in the external anal sphincter. ATPase, pH 4.3, × 130.

neuromuscular disorders, can be excluded on both clinical and histological criteria.

In the incontinent patients the mean diameters of both Type 1 and Type 2 fibres were increased in all the muscles studied. This fibre hypertrophy was most prominent in the puborectalis and it affected Type 2 fibres more than Type 1 fibres, both in this muscle and in the external anal sphincter. In the levator ani both fibre types were slightly hypertrophied, but in women with anorectal incontinence, hypertrophy of Type 1 fibres was less marked in this muscle. Since there was marked Type 1 fibre predominance, slightly greater in patients with incontinence than in control subjects, the functional significance of Type 1 fibre hypertrophy must outweigh that of Type 2 fibre hypertrophy. Fibre hypertrophy in the external anal sphincter and puborectalis muscles was accompanied by increased variability in fibre diameter, shown by increased interquartile range of mean diameter in the incontinent patients.

Histograms of fibre size, plotted separately for Type 1 and Type 2 fibres, showed that there was an abnormal range of fibre diameter, including both very small and very large fibres in the external anal sphincter and puborectalis muscles. Furthermore, the fibre-size histograms in these muscles revealed multiple peaks of fibre diameter, an observation providing additional support for the concept that the primary cause of damage to these muscles was damage to their nerve supply (see Beersiek, Parks and Swash, 1979).

In both external anal sphincter and puborectalis muscles, there was a marked loss of fibres, but this was usually more severe in the former muscle

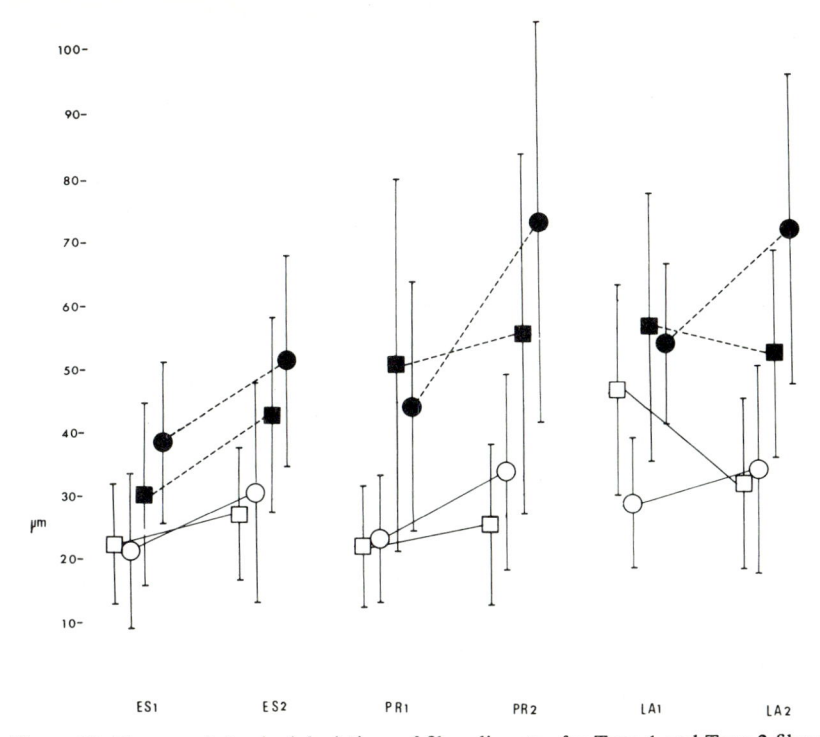

Figure 13. Means and standard deviations of fibre diameter for Type 1 and Type 2 fibres in external anal sphincter, puborectalis and levator ani muscles of normal subjects and incontinent patients of either sex. See text for discussion. Filled symbols = incontinent patients; open symbols = normal subjects; square symbols = male; round symbols = female; ES1 = external sphincter Type 1 fibres; ES2 = external sphincter Type 2 fibres; PR = puborectalis, etc.; LA = levator ani, etc.

(see Parks, Swash and Urich, 1977). In some of our patients with incontinence the external anal sphincter was largely destroyed.

COMMENT

Although the puborectalis and external anal sphincter muscles bear the brunt of the histological changes observed in anorectal incontinence, fibre hypertrophy was far more prominent in the puborectalis than in the external anal sphincter muscles. Type 1 fibre predominance was increased to a similar degree in both muscles. There were no histological differences between patients in whom no cause was evident for incontinence, those in whom there was a prominent history of defaecation straining, and those in whom there was perianal sensory impairment, but those patients who had experienced a difficult or precipitate childbirth accounted for most of the cases in which no evidence of fibre-type grouping was found. Fibre-type grouping is indicative of reinnervation of a muscle and is thus suggestive of damage to the nerve supply to the muscle.

Type 1 fibre predominance is a characteristic feature of muscles with a tonic, postural function, for example, soleus and tibialis anterior (Johnson et al, 1973). It may also occur in certain neuromuscular disorders (Dubowitz and Brooke, 1973) but there were no features of such disorders in our incontinent subjects. Type 1 muscle fibres, dependent on oxidative metabolic pathways, have relatively slow twitch characteristics, and are capable of sustained contraction (Burke et al, 1971). The external anal sphincter has been shown to be in a state of continuous partial activity, even during sleep (Floyd and Walls, 1953; Porter 1962), a characteristic consistent with Type 1 fibre predominance.

In patients in whom the external anal sphincter has been virtually destroyed, as in most of the patients with faecal incontinence in this series, continence must depend almost entirely on the puborectalis, and on the caudal fibres of the levator ani muscle. When damage occurs to the external anal sphincter and puborectalis muscles, whatever its cause, continence can be maintained only if the remaining innervated fibres of these muscles can contract sufficiently strongly, both to maintain the anorectal angulation and to close the anal canal. There is thus an increased functional load on the remaining fibres in these muscles. This leads to fibre hypertrophy (Edgerton, 1970; Schwartz, Sargeant and Swash, 1976). However, this may itself lead to secondary degenerative changes in muscles (Swash and Schwartz, 1977) and thus to failure of compensation.

In those patients in whom histological abnormalities in the external anal sphincter and puborectalis muscles were gross it was not possible to be certain of the cause of the abnormality. Anorectal incontinence is clearly a syndrome with more than one cause and denervation is not a factor in all cases. Direct trauma to the puborectalis and external sphincter muscles during childbirth, associated with various surgical procedures, with inflammatory bowel disease or as a result of fistula formation, is also an important causative factor. However, there was histological evidence of a neurogenic disorder in 75 per cent of incontinent patients. Parks, Swash and Urich (1977) have suggested that damage to the nerve supply to these muscles may result from obstetric trauma, and from repeated stretch injury to the pudendal nerves during perineal descent, itself induced by excessive defaecation straining (see also Porter, 1962; Parks, Porter and Hardcastle, 1966), and have put forward the hypothesis that entrapment of these nerves in the pelvis, beneath the sacrospinous ligaments, may be important in some cases. The changes found in small nerve branches innervating the external anal sphincter and puborectalis muscles are consistent with this hypothesis, and in dissection of the pudendal nerves in cadavers we have found that this nerve is often tightly bound in connective tissue as it leaves the pelvis and enters the pudendal canal, passing beneath the sacrospinous ligament (Figure 14). Normal nerves are vulnerable to stretching forces greater than about 12 per cent of their length (Sunderland, 1978), and the combination of nerve entrapment in the pelvis with perineal descent induced during defaecation straining might be sufficient to lead to recurrent injury to the pudendal nerves, and so to progressive denervation atrophy of the external anal sphincter and puborectalis muscles.

In recent physiological studies, we have found that the latency of the anal reflex measured by an electrophysiological technique (Henry and Swash, 1978) is markedly increased in patients with anorectal incontinence (Henry, Parks and Swash, 1980). Furthermore, single-fibre electromyogram (EMG)

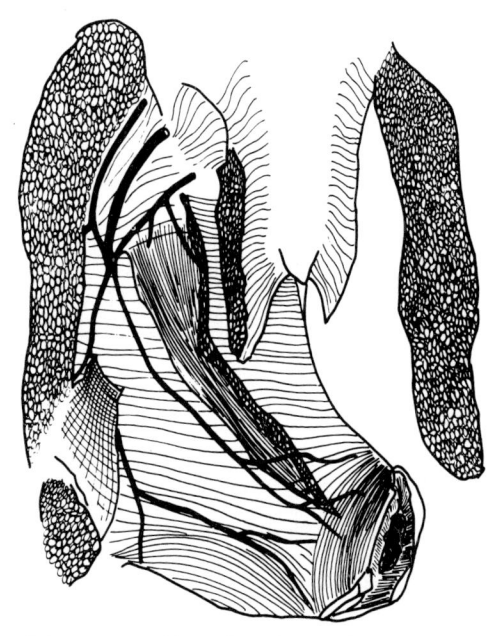

Figure 14. Drawing of the course and branches of the pudendal nerve; from a dissection. The posterior part of the external anal sphincter is innervated by branches of the inferior rectal nerve, and the anterior part from the perineal nerve. Both these nerves are branches of the pudendal nerve. The inferior rectal nerve also contains cutaneous afferent fibres which are distributed to the lower part of the anal canal and to the skin between the anus and coccyx. The perineal nerve also supplies motor innervation to the puborectalis part of the levator ani muscles and to other perineal muscles. A direct branch of the motor root of S4 supplies the external sphincter in some patients.

studies of the external anal sphincter muscle in these patients (Neill and Swash, 1980; Neill, Parks and Swash, 1980) show abnormalities consistent with reinnervation, and these can be correlated quantitatively with the severity of the incontinence. In normal elderly subjects these single-fibre EMG studies reveal abnormalities which approach those found in younger subjects incontinent only to liquid stool, suggesting that similar abnormalities may occur in the voluntary anal sphincter musculature of normal aged people, which may predispose to the development of faecal incontinence (Neill and Swash, 1979). There is thus an increasing body of evidence to support the concept that 'idiopathic' anorectal (faecal) incontinence is commonly due to damage to the innervation of the voluntary anal sphincter musculature, but further work is needed to test the hypothesis that this is usually the result of stretch-induced damage to the pudendal nerves, associated with entrapment of these nerves in the pelvis.

ACKNOWLEDGEMENTS

This work has been carried out in collaboration with Mr R.J. Lane, Mr F. Beersiek, Mr M.M. Henry, Mr M.E. Neill and Mr T. Teramoto during their tenure as Research Fellows at St Mark's Hospital, London, and with Sir Alan Parks. Financial support has been provided by the St Mark's Hospital Research Fund, The London Hospital Research Fund and the Wellcome Trust.

Figures 3, 5 and 10 are reproduced from Beersiek, Parks and Swash (1979), with kind permission of the editor of *Journal of the Neurological Sciences*; Figures 4, 6, 7, 8 and 9 are reproduced from Parks, Swash and Urich (1977), with kind permission of the editor of *Gut*.

REFERENCES

Beersiek, F., Parks, A.G. & Swash, M. (1979) Pathogenesis of ano-rectal incontinence: a histometric study of the anal sphincter musculature. *Journal of the Neurological Sciences*, **42**, 111-127.

Bennett, R.C. & Duthie, H.L. (1964) The functional importance of the internal anal sphincter. *British Journal of Surgery*, **51**, 355-357.

Burke, R.E., Levine, O.N., Zajac, F.E., Tsairis, P. & Engel, W.K. (1971) Mammalian motor units; physiological histochemical correlation in three fibre types in cat gastrocnemius muscle. *Science*, **174**, 709-712.

Butler, E.C.B. (1954) Complete rectal prolapse following removal of tumours of the cauda equina. *Proceedings of the Royal Society of Medicine*, **47**, 521-522.

Cihak, R., Guttmann, E. & Hanzlikova, V. (1970) Involution and hormone-induced persistence of the M. sphincter (levator) ani in female rats. *Journal of Anatomy*, **106**, 93-101.

Dubowitz, V. & Brooke, M.H. (1973) *Muscle Biopsy — a Modern Approach*. London: W.B. Saunders.

Duthie, H.L. (1971) Progress report: anal continence. *Gut*, **12**, 844-852.

Edgerton, V.R. (1970) Morphology and histochemistry of the soleus muscle from normal and exercised rats. *American Journal of Anatomy*, **127**, 81-87.

Engel, W.K. (1971) 'Ragged-red fibres' in ophthalmoplegia syndromes and their differential diagnosis (abstract) In *Second International Congress on Muscle Diseases, Perth*. I.C.S. p. 237. Amsterdam: Excerpta Medica.

Floyd, W.F. & Walls, E.W. (1953) Electromyography of the sphincter ani externus in man. *Journal of Physiology* (London), **122**, 599-609.

Goligher, J.C., Leacock, A.G. & Brossy, J.J. (1953) The surgical anatomy of the anal canal. *British Journal of Surgery*, **43**, 51-61.

Hakelius, L. (1975) Free autogenous muscle transplantation in two cases of total anal incontinence. *Acta Chirurgica Scandinavica*, **141**, 69-76.

Henry, M.M. & Swash, M. (1978) Assessment of pelvic floor disorders and incontinence by electrophysiological recording of the anal reflex. *Lancet*, **i**, 1290-1291.

Henry, M.M., Parks, A.G. & Swash, M. (1980) The anal reflex in idiopathic faecal incontinence: an electrophysiological study. Submitted for publication.

Johnson, M.A., Polgar, J., Weightman, D. & Appleton, D. (1973) Data on the distribution of the fibre types in thirty-six human muscles: an autopsy study. *Journal of the Neurological Sciences*, **18**, 111-129.

Kerremans, R. (1969) *Morphological and Physiological Aspects of Anal Continence and Defaecation*. Brussels: Editions Arscia.

Neill, M.E. & Swash, M. (1979) Is faecal incontinence in the elderly neurogenic? *Lancet*, **ii**, 364.

Neill, M.E. & Swash, M. (1980) Increased motor unit fibre-density in the external anal sphincter muscle in ano-rectal incontinence: a single fibre E.M.G. study. *Journal of Neurology, Neurosurgery and Psychiatry*, in press.

Neill, M.E., Parks, A.G. & Swash, M. (1980) Assessment of the pelvic floor in faecal incontinence and rectal prolapse: clinical features, anal pressure studies and electrophysiological tests. Submitted for publication.

Parks, A.G. (1975) Anorectal incontinence. *Proceedings of the Royal Society of Medicine*, **68**, 681-690.

Parks, A.G. & Swash, M. (1979) Denervation of the anal sphincter causing idiopathic anorectal incontinence. *Journal of the Royal College of Surgeons of Edinburgh*, **24**, 94-96.

Parks, A.G., Porter, N.H. & Hardcastle, J.D. (1966) The syndrome of the descending perineum. *Proceedings of the Royal Society of Medicine*, **59**, 477-482.

Parks, A.G., Porter, N.H. & Melzack, J. (1962) Experimental study of the reflex mechanism controlling the muscles of the pelvic floor. *Diseases of the Colon and Rectum*, **5**, 407-414.

Parks, A.G., Swash, M. & Urich, H. (1977) Sphincter denervation in ano-rectal incontinence and rectal prolapse. *Gut*, **18**, 656-665.

Phillips, S.G. & Edwards, D.A.W. (1965) Some aspects of anal continence and defaecation. *Gut*, **6**, 396-406.

Porter, N.H. (1962) A physiological study of the pelvic floor in rectal prolapse. *Annals of the Royal College of Surgeons of London*, **31**, 379-401.

Schuster, M.M. (1975) The riddle of the sphincters. *Gastroenterology*, **69**, 249-262.

Schwartz, M.S., Sargeant, M.K. & Swash, M. (1976) Longitudinal fibre splitting in neurogenic muscular disorders; its relation to the pathogenesis of 'myopathic' change. *Brain*, **99**, 617-636.

Sunderland, S. (1978) *Nerve and Nerve Injuries*. 2nd edn, pp. 62-66. Edinburgh: Churchill-Livingstone.

Swash, M. & Fox, K.P. (1974) The pathology of the human muscle spindle; effect of denervation. *Journal of the Neurological Sciences*, **22**, 1-24.

Swash, M. & Schwartz, M.S. (1977) Implications of longitudinal fibre splitting in neurogenic and myopathic disorders. *Journal of Neurology, Neurosurgery and Psychiatry*, **40**, 1152-1159.

Thompson, P. (1899) *The Myology of the Pelvic Floor*. Newton: McCorquodale.

PART TWO

Inflammatory Disease

6

Immunological Mechanisms in the Small Intestine

ANNE FERGUSON
ALLAN MOWAT

The immune apparatus of the gastrointestinal tract has several features which differentiate it from the systemic immune system. Not only are there many areas of organized lymphoid tissues — the Peyer's patches, appendix, and mesenteric lymph nodes draining the gut — but there are many cells with immunological functions dispersed under and within the epithelium. Examination of the properties of the cells concerned, and in particular studies of lymphocyte traffic, have shown that the gut-associated lymphoid tissues (GALT) are populated by gut derived and gut-seeking cells, separate categories from the T and B cells associated with the systemic immunological organs. The immunoglobulins secreted by plasma cells at mucosal surfaces, including those of the gut, are predominantly IgA with some IgM, in contrast to the immunoglobulins secreted by plasma cells in other parts of the body. Specific immune reactions in the mucosae, including those of the gut, are complemented and supplemented by various non-specific immune factors such as lysozyme and mononuclear phagocytes. Additionally, physical factors such as the gastric acid, mucus, and the state of continuous exfoliation of the epithelium into the lumen, enhance non-specific immunity.

The nature of antigen exposure in the gastrointestinal tract is unique, when compared with other lymphoid organs. Whereas most cells and the extracellular fluid are in general sterile, the epithelium of the gastrointestinal tract is continuously exposed to many antigens, living and nonliving, the majority of which are entirely harmless. Nevertheless, several times a year at least, pathogens ranging in size and complexity from viruses to tape worms will induce a variety of immune reactions in the gut and elsewhere. It is therefore hardly surprising that an enormous spectrum of immunological reactions can be induced in the gut, and that in any intestinal infection a variety of host-parasite relationships may be found within an individual patient at different stages of the illness and between one patient and another, even though they have been infected with the same organism.

The immunological properties of the small intestine, the subject of this paper, cannot be considered in isolation from the digestive and other

© 1980 W.B. Saunders Company Ltd.

physiological and pathological aspects of this large and complex organ. For example, it has been clearly demonstrated in experimental animals that a small fraction of protein, given orally, will cross the epithelium of the gut as intact molecules to reach the bloodstream or lymphatics. One of the results of a mucosal immune response of the IgA class is that the amount of 'macromolecular' uptake is reduced although not completely eliminated (Walker, Isselbacher and Bloch, 1977; Swarbrick, Stokes and Soothill, 1979). When, as a result of disease of the stomach or pancreas, protein digestion is impaired the small bowel mucosa will be exposed to very much greater quantities of protein antigen than normal. This is likely to influence both the amount and the molecular structure of antigen presented to the intestinal immune system and may therefore influence not only whether or not an immune reaction is induced, but also the magnitude, time-course and length of gut involved, when immune reactions occur on subsequent antigen challenge. Thus such factors as pancreatic function may influence the extent of bowel affected by the enteropathy of food hypersensitivities, coeliac disease and cows' milk protein intolerance.

Since the immune apparatus of the small intestinal mucosa includes humoral antibody (locally synthesized and from the bloodstream), T and B lymphocytes (derived from the gut-seeking T and B immunoblasts) and small numbers of mononuclear phagocytes, mast cells and eosinophils, the elements are present to allow the occurrence in the mucosa of a variety of types of immune reactions. From our work on cell-mediated immune reactions in the intestine, it is clear that local immune reactions may influence non-lymphoid tissues of the gut such as the epithelium. Since the pathologist is frequently presented with small biopsies of intestinal mucosa from patients thought to have allergic or inflammatory gastrointestinal diseases, we have collected together in this paper the published information on the effects, on the small bowel mucosa, when immune reactions of the reaginic, immune complex or T cell-mediated type evolve in this tissue. Virtually all of the work described below has been carried out in small animals. Nevertheless, we hope that the facts outlined below, cautiously applied to the interpretation of human disease states, will have relevance to the pathogenesis and pathology of a number of gastrointestinal diseases.

EFFECTS OF LOCAL HYPERSENSITIVITY REACTIONS ON THE SMALL INTESTINAL MUCOSA IN EXPERIMENTAL ANIMALS

Unsuccessful attempts to induce local immune reactions in the intestinal mucosa are unlikely to be published. For example, at various times in the last eight years, members of our research group have successfully rendered animals immune to bovine serum albumin (some animals having reaginic antibody, others precipitating antibody), other milk proteins, gluten, α-gliadin, tuberculin, oxazolone and dinitrochlorobenzene. However, in the majority of these experiments, oral or intralumenal antigen challenge produced no clinical histopathological or other reaction in the mucosa of the immune animal. Our only limited success was the production of an anaphylactic reaction in the mucosa in some immunized mice, and an immune complex reaction when antigen was placed in isolated loops of gut in animals with high titres of circulating antibody (Ferguson, 1976). It is also unfortunate that the methods used to examine the histopathology, function, permeability, etc., of the intestine have not been applied in any consistent way to the spectrum of hypersensitivity reactions used. Thus there are very considerable gaps in the information available. Furthermore, facts such as the nature of gut flora, presence or absence of the chronic parasite infections often found in experimental animals and the diet of the animals concerned are often not provided. Finally, new research work may require a thorough re-examination of some of the earlier papers. For example, in helminth parasite infections of the gut, an IgE class immune response is induced and there is considerable expansion of the number of mast cells in the tissue at the time of worm expulsion. These factors, together with the presence of oedema in parasitized gut, have led to the widely-held belief that many of the features of the parasitized small intestine are caused by reaginic hypersensitivity mechanisms—for example, gastrointestinal protein loss. However, the recent careful study by Nawa (1979) has indicated that the leak of plasma proteins into the gut lumen in *Nippostrongylus brasiliensis* infection is due to factors secreted by the worms and does not correlate with the presence of the immune response. Thus some of the facets of reaginic hypersensitivity, which have been deduced from experiments involving parasite infections, will certainly require reappraisal.

REAGINIC HYPERSENSITIVITY

Several clearly documented and carefully controlled models have been used to examine the effects of an antigen/IgE response on the intestine.

The small intestine in systemic anaphylaxis. An IgE class immune response is induced in an animal (usually a rat) by appropriate immunization, the titre of antibody being measured by passive cutaneous anaphylaxis. The primed animal is then challenged with an intravenous dose of antigen, and a dye such as Evans blue is also given intravenously to detect leak of plasma proteins into the tissues and into the lumen. The resulting anaphylaxis varies in severity from mild to fatal, and the effect on the gut can be seen macroscopically by the extravasation of Evans blue (Barth, Jarrett and Urquhart, 1966) or by measuring changes in vascular and mucosal permeability by using radio-iodine-labelled protein markers (Bloch et al, 1979).

Oral challenge of primed animals. Rats primed for IgE antibody production were challenged by feeding antigen, in the work of Byars and Ferraresi (1976). They used radio-iodine-labelled protein to measure intestinal permeability, and were able to demonstrate a reduction in 'intestinal anaphylaxis' in animals treated with agents which stabilize the mast cell membrane.

Passive intestinal anaphylaxis. By using a method similar to that for inducing passive cutaneous anaphylaxis a local reaginic hypersensitivity reaction can be produced in the wall of the small bowel or colon. This technique was used for some human work in the 1940s, in which the site of passive immunization was the ileum or colon in patients with ileocolostomies, and the rectal mucosa was also studied, by using direct injection of the rectum at proctoscopy (reviewed in *Lancet*, 1975).

Macroscopically, the studies in passive intestinal anaphylaxis correlate quite well with observations in animals. Within five or ten minutes of antigen challenge there is oedema and reddening of the mucosa, and mucus is secreted but the tissue appears entirely normal by one to two hours. In histopathological examination of tissues from rats and mice, the findings may be completely normal, or the appearances may be very similar to the early post-mortem changes which develop rapidly in these small animals. There is some oedema in the core of the villus, the base of epithelial cells may separate from the basement membrane and a small bleb may form at the villus tip. Furthermore, it should be emphasized that these changes are inconsistent even in areas of the gut which, macroscopically, have definite lesions demonstrated, for example by blue discoloration in animals given Evans blue (Barth, Jarrett and Urquhart, 1966; Ferguson, 1976; Kleinman, 1979).

In view of the recent interest in macromolecular transport across the gut epithelium, the findings of Bloch et al (1979) are of interest in that they were able to demonstrate a greatly increased uptake of immunoreactive bovine serum albumin from the gut lumen into venous blood when rats were subjected to mild systemic anaphylaxis.

Although it seems likely that a morphological feature of these reactions will be degranulation of mast cells, with eosinophil infiltrate in the tissue, studies of reaginic hypersensitivity reactions have in the main not included carefully controlled histopathological observations. In addition, it must be emphasized that many of the gut mast cells are in the submucosa in the vicinity of the muscularis mucosa rather than in the villi, and immune reactions at this rather deeper level of the gut have been largely neglected to date.

CYTOTOXIC HYPERSENSITIVITY

We are not aware of any reported work on the effects of cytotoxic immune reactions on the small bowel of experimental animals. Circumstantial evidence that anti-intestinal antibody is unlikely to cause substantial damage to the villi and epithelium has been provided by the work of Rabin and Rogers (1976). They immunized rabbits with various intestinal extracts, and were able to show, by immunofluorescence, the presence of anti-intestinal antibodies. However, although various pathological lesions were produced, including stunting of the villi and infiltration with plasma cells and lymphocytes, this enteropathy did not correlate with the presence of anti-intestinal antibody and the authors concluded that cellular immune mechanisms were more likely to be the pathological mechanism. There is a clinical report, of a patient with IgA deficiency and a malabsorption syndrome, in whom the jejunal biopsy showed villous atrophy with crypt hyperplasia. However, the patient did not respond to treatment for coeliac disease and immunological investigation showed the presence of an autoantibody to intestinal epithelial cells (McCarthy et al, 1978).

IMMUNE COMPLEX HYPERSENSITIVITY

Several animal models have been used to examine this aspect of intestinal mucosal immunology. The effects sought by the different research groups, and therefore those demonstrated, have varied considerably in the different systems.

Antigen within ligated loops. In pigs, actively immunized by injections of bovine serum albumin (BSA) in complete Freund's adjuvant, or passively immunized, the effect of interaction between antigen in the lumen and antibody in the circulation were examined in ligated loops of small intestine. Antigen, and various control substances, were injected into the lumen of the loops and the tissues examined four hours later. Intradermal injection of antigen in the same animals was used and classical Arthus reactions were produced in the skin with oedema, haemorrhage, thrombosis and perivascular accumulation of neutrophils. However, in the ligated loops the only pathological features observed were accumulation of neutrophils focally in the epithelium of the villi, and in the capillaries lying immediately under the epithelium. In a small group of animals studied for 24 hours, the tissue had returned to complete normality by 24 hours. Bellamy and Nielsen suggest that in this model, some antigen penetrates the epithelium, interacts with antibody in the vicinity of the basement membrane, polymorphs then phagocytose small amounts of antigen-antibody complexes, release their lysosomal contents and there is desquamation of a few epithelial cells nearby so that a stream of neutrophils may enter the intestinal lumen through this small breach. There were extremely large numbers of polymorphs in the lumena of these ligated loops and the authors suggest that this may in fact be a mechanism to recruit polymorphs into a site of intestinal infection (Bellamy and Nielsen, 1974a, 1974b). Functional studies on water, sodium and chloride absorption were carried out in these animals and were normal, indicating that immune complex-mediated reactions, in these pigs, did not impair at least one function of the intestinal mucosa (Bellamy and Hamilton, 1977).

Systemic immune complex disease. Accinni and his colleagues have produced immune complex disease in rabbits by frequent injections of antigen. Immune complexes were found by immunofluorescence and electron microscopy in many organs, including the gut. Examination of the small intestinal mucosa showed granular deposits in the walls of blood vessels, mucosal and submucosal, and also, in the villi, in capillary walls and in lacteals. Deposits were also seen near the epithelial cells. However, the only histopathological features observed on light microscopy were slight to moderate oedema of the mucosa and submucosa, and 'mild infiltration with inflammatory cells'. The electron microscope revealed degranulated basophils, mast cells and neutrophils in mucosal and submucosal intestinal areas. However, even with electron microscopy, surface epithelial cells appeared normal (Accinni et al, 1978).

Although Hodgson and his colleagues (1978) have not examined the small intestine, their work on immune complex mediated colitis in rabbits should be mentioned here. They have produced a more extensive colonic injury in the rabbit than is found in standard immune complex disease, by using the Auer technique. Immune complexes, formed in antigen excess, are given intravenously to rabbits and the complexes are localized in the rectum by the mild trauma produced by instillation of dilute formalin. Clearly this is another example of the interaction between the immune system and non-immunological intestinal injury, both of which are likely to be involved in the induction of many inflammatory gastrointestinal diseases.

Immune complexes and goblet cells. As a chance finding during their experiments on absorption of antigen across the mucosa of intestine, Walker, Wu and Bloch (1977) found that immune complexes formed in antibody excess, and injected into the duodenum of normal rats, caused a marked increase in the number of disrupted goblet cells, and an increase in ^{35}S-labelled mucus recovery. They suggested that enhanced mucus release could have a role in clearing the surface of the intestine of complexes, or in reducing macromolecular access to the epithelial cells. Further studies, involving infusion of antigen into the intestine of previously immunized rats, have shown that after systemic immunization mucus was not released on intraduodenal infusion of antigen, whereas there was release of goblet cell mucus when orally immunized animals were stimulated by intraduodenal antigen infusion (Lake et al, 1979).

It seems unlikely that conditions favourable for the development of immune complexes will be present in the intestines of man and animals who are eating food in normal quantities and who have normal digestive enzymes. Nevertheless, in the rather artificial situation of antigen perfusion of the small intestine in a diseased individual (with coeliac disease or cows' milk protein intolerance) immune complexes have indeed been demonstrated. However, immune complexes are not normally found in the jejunal mucosa of a patient with untreated coeliac disease, and polymorphs are not a feature of the pathology. It is not known whether immune complexes are deposited in the small intestinal mucosa in patients with systemic immune complex diseases, nor, if these complexes are present, whether there is any effect on intestinal absorption.

T CELL-MEDIATED HYPERSENSITIVITY

The small intestinal mucosa is a dynamic organ, for in addition to the very considerable amounts of fluid which cross the epithelium in both directions, there is also continuous renewal of the epithelial and connective tissue cells. Since cell-mediated immune (CMI) reactions take one or more days to evolve, it might be argued that conditions will rarely be appropriate for the evolution of a T cell-mediated reaction in this organ. However, there are a number of antigens which will persist in or adjacent to the small bowel mucosa for days, for example micro-organisms and parasites, invasive or adherent to the surface epithelium; particulate material firmly attached to the connective tissue, stroma or the surfaces of cells; and histocompatibility antigens, autoantigens and organ-specific antigens. It is also conceivable that certain foods which are ingested regularly may be involved in CMI reactions and there is clinical evidence of this in coeliac disease (wheat and other glutens) and in the malabsorption syndrome of infants with cows' milk protein intolerance. We have used a number of models to examine the effects of a local CMI reaction on the intestinal mucosa, and these include graft-versus-host disease, rejection of transplanted allografts of intestine, parasite infections in T cell-depleted hosts, and oral challenge with antigen after animals have been orally immunized.

Rejection of small intestinal allografts. Small fragments of intestine from fetal mice or rats can be transplanted heterotopically into adult recipients of the same or different strains. For most of our work, we have used the technique of heterotopic transplantation of grafts of fetal small intestine under the kidney capsules of mice (Ferguson and Parrott, 1972). Isografts grow normally for months, but allografts are infiltrated with lymphocytes and the tissue is destroyed one to three weeks after transplantation, the timecourse depending on immunological status of the host and histocompatibility differences between donor and host strains (Ferguson and Parrott, 1973). The effects on the small bowel mucosa of the T cell-mediated reaction in allograft rejection have been examined by conventional light microscopy, electron microscopy, morphometry, counts of lymphoid cells, and by epithelial cell kinetic studies using a stathmokinetic technique (MacDonald and Ferguson, 1976, 1977; Ferguson et al, 1978). The earliest pathological feature is infiltration of lymphocytes in the lamina propria, with lymphocytes also present between the epithelial cells of the villi. Crypts become hyperplastic, and crypt cell production rate increases to five times that of isografts. Later there is villus shortening and finally ulceration and necrosis of the tissue. Throughout, until they are exfoliated into the lumen, surface enterocytes appear essentially normal.

Transplantation of long segments of the small intestine as allografts attached to the mesentery has been carried out in larger experimental animals such as dogs (Holmes et al, 1971) and also in seven human patients (Stanffer, 1977). The histopathological changes in these segments of intestine have in general been examined only subjectively, but are similar to those described above in mice.

Graft-versus-host disease. When graft-versus-host disease is induced in small rodents by the injection of allogeneic lymphocytes into neonatal recipients, or of parenteral lymphocytes into F_1 hybrid recipients, adults or neonates, an enteropathy with diarrhoea and malabsorption is produced, varying in severity according to immunological and other factors (Reilly and Kirsner, 1965; Hedberg, Reiser and Reilly, 1968).

We examined the histopathology and epithelial cell kinetics of neonatal mice suffering graft-versus-host disease, and found the pathology and crypt cell kinetics to be similar to those of allograft rejection (MacDonald and Ferguson, 1977). However, in recent experiments in which graft-versus-host disease has been induced in adult mice, and in which the recipient mice do not suffer from diarrhoea, at least for the first two weeks after spleen cell injection, examination of the jejunum has shown no abnormality apart from an increase in crypt cell production rate and a rise in the number of intra-epithelial lymphocytes. In particular, villi are of normal size. A similar situation, with crypt hyperplasia preceding the development of villus damage, was seen in young mice at about five days after induction of graft-versus-host disease.

We postulated that the changes in intestinal architecture in allograft rejection and in graft-versus-host disease were due to lymphokines secreted by T cells, and not due to cytotoxic cells (Ferguson and MacDonald, 1977). Support for the existence of these proposed 'enteropathic' lymphokines has been provided by the work of Elson, Reilly and Rosenberg (1977). They induced graft-versus-host in F_1 hybrid recipient mice by injection of parental-strain spleen cells. Graft-versus-host disease could also be induced in grafts of F_1 small intestine implanted under the kidney capsule of the hosts, but similar damage to the villi was found in grafts of parental-strain intestine implanted under the other kidney capsule of the same animal. The proposed explanation of this phenomenon was that in the traffic of lymphocytes through the mucosa, parental-strain lymphocytes mixed with host lymphocytes and the lymphokines secreted by the injected parental lymphocytes produced villus shortening, etc., although the lymphocytes and epithelium of the graft were entirely histocompatible.

On the basis of the results of these and other experiments, we have proposed that the architecture of the small intestine may be affected in two ways by a local CMI reaction.

Phase 1 is hyperplasia of the crypts of Lieberkühn, with rapid transit of enterocytes up the sides of the villi but with no atrophy or shortening of villi. This lesion can only be detected by cytokinetic techniques, and subjective examination of the histological preparation is usually normal. (Counts of intra-epithelial lymphocytes may, however, be high.) In Phase 1 the only possible adverse effect on the host will be relative immaturity of enterocytes, with a risk of deficiency of enzymes involved in nutrient and electrolyte transport across the mucosa. Benefit to the host, in infection, will be conferred if the pathogen is present within epithelial cells, or is adherent to the epithelium. Phase 1 is likely also to produce more rapid healing of abrasions or small ulcers in the mucosa.

Phase 2 is a more severe, and clinically relevant, lesion in which hyperplasia of the crypts is accompanied by collapse of the stroma of villi, loss of adhesion of epithelial cells to the basement membrane and therefore 'villous atrophy'. The reduction in surface area is likely to cause diarrhoea and malabsorption. Nevertheless, we have not produced the cuboidal epithelial cells, with grossly abnormal brush border, which are so typical of untreated coeliac disease, and therefore the question as to whether a CMI reaction can under certain circumstances damage individual enterocytes is at present unanswered.

HYPERSENSITIVITY IN PARASITE INFECTIONS

The immune response to parasites is complex and involves humoral, cellular and many non-specific factors in addition to direct cytotoxic effects of parasites and their secretions. Nevertheless, there is evidence that at least some of the enteropathy in intestinal parasite infections is the result of the thymus-dependent component of the immune response (probably the cell-mediated component). In *Nippostrongylus brasiliensis* infection of rats, *Trichinella spiralis* infection of mice, and *Giardia muris* infection of mice, the enteropathy has been shown to be much less severe or even absent in animals depleted of T lymphocytes (Ferguson and Jarrett, 1975; Roberts-Thomson and Mitchell, 1978; Manson-Smith, Bruce and Parrott, 1979). However, the methods used to examine enteropathy in these models have been confined to morphometry of tissue sections. Epithelial cell kinetic studies have not been carried out, and these will be required in order to elucidate precisely the relative contributions by parasites and by the immune response at different times after infection and in the recovery phase after parasite elimination.

CONCLUSIONS

The effect of reaginic, immune complex and T cell-mediated immune reactions on the small intestine of experimental animals has not been fully documented. Changes in intestinal structure have been carefully examined in CMI reactions, but not in the antibody-mediated hypersensitivities. There is a relative dearth of information on fluid and electrolyte transport, absorption and malabsorption, and studies on mucosal permeability have been confined to models of reaginic hypersensitivity. The various lymphoid cell types have in the main been merely described, and subjective observations reported. Nevertheless, a number of features of intestinal pathology as may be seen in jejunal biopsies can, on the basis of the above, be attributed to local hypersensitivity reaction. These are summarized in Figure 1. Reaginic and immune complex hypersensitivity reactions will be more readily demonstrated by using a variety of tests in peripheral blood, and by the clinical effects of antigen challenge on organs other than the gastrointestinal tract— for example, the skin and the respiratory tract. When a patient is suspected of having an intestinal hypersensitivity reaction, and the jejunal biopsy is abnormal with crypt hyperplasia and villus shortening, we would propose that the immunological mechanism involved is likely to be T cell mediated. There is as yet no evidence that intestinal mucosal T cells are cytotoxic, and the effects are probably mediated by lymphokines which stimulate crypt mitosis, damage the stroma of the villi and recruit other cells of the immune series into the mucosa.

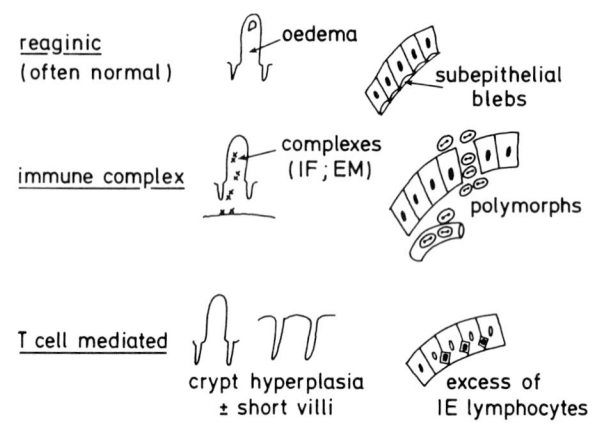

Figure 1. Features of small intestinal mucosal pathology which (on the basis of animal experiments) may provide evidence of local hypersensitivity reactions. IF = Immunofluorescence; EM = electron microscopy; IE = intra-epithelial.

REFERENCES

Accinni, L., Brentjens, J.R., Albini, B., Ossi, E., O'Connell, D.W., Pawlowski, I.B. & Andres, G.A. (1978) Deposition of circulating antigen-antibody complexes in the gastrointestinal tract of rabbits with chronic serum sickness. *Digestive Diseases*, 23, 1098-1106.

Barth, E.E.E., Jarrett, W.F.H. & Urquhart, G.M. (1966) Studies on the mechanism of the self cure reaction in rats infected with *Nippostrongylus brasiliensis*. *Immunology*, 10, 459-464.

Bellamy, J.E.C. & Hamilton, D.L. (1977) Effects of immune mediated enteroluminal neutrophil emigration on intestinal function in pigs. *Canadian Journal of Comparative Medicine*, 41, 36-40.

Bellamy, J.E.C. & Nielsen, N.O. (1974a) Immune mediated emigration of neutrophils into the lumen of the small intestine. *Infection and Immunity*, 9, 615-619.

Bellamy, J.E.C. & Nielsen, N.O. (1974b) A comparison between the active cutaneous Arthus reaction and immune mediated enteroluminal neutrophil emigration in pigs. *Canadian Journal of Comparative Medicine*, 38, 193-202.

Block, K.J., Bloch, D.B., Stearns, M. & Walker, W.A. (1979) Intestinal uptake of macromolecules. VI. Uptake of protein antigen *in vivo* in normal rats and in rats injected with *Nippostrongylus brasiliensis* or subjected to mild systemic anaphylaxis. *Gastroenterology*, 77, 1039-1044.

Byars, N.E. & Ferraresi, R.W. (1976) Intestinal anaphylaxis in the rat as a model of food allergy. *Clinical and Experimental Immunology*, 24, 352-356.

Elson, C.O., Reilly, R.W. & Rosenberg, I.H. (1977) Small intestinal injury in the graft-versus-host reaction: an innocent bystander phenomenon. *Gastroenterology*, 72, 886-889.

Ferguson, A. (1976) Models of intestinal hypersensitivity. *Clinics in Gastroenterology*, 5, 271-288.

Ferguson, A. & Jarrett, E.E.E. (1975) Hypersensitivity reactions in the small intestine. 1. Thymus dependence of experimental 'partial villous atrophy'. *Gut*, 16, 114-117.

Ferguson, A. & MacDonald, T.T. (1977) Effects of local delayed hypersensitivity on the small intestine. *Ciba Foundation Symposium*, No. 46. pp. 305-327. Amsterdam: Elsevier North-Holland.

Ferguson, A. & Parrott, D.M.V. (1972) Growth and development of 'antigen-free' grafts of foetal mouse intestine. *Journal of Pathology*, **106**, 95-101.

Ferguson, A. & Parrott, D.M.V. (1973) Histopathology and time-course of rejection of allografts of mouse small intestine. *Transplantation*, **15**, 546-554.

Ferguson, A., Carr, K.E., MacDonald, T.T. & Watt, C. (1978) Hypersensitivity reactions in the small intestine. 4. Influence of allograft rejection on small intestinal mucosal architecture: a scanning and transmission electron microscope study. *Digestion*, **18**, 56-63.

Hedberg, C.A., Reiser, S. & Reilly, R.W. (1968) Intestinal phase of the runting syndrome in mice. 2. Observations on nutrient absorption and certain disaccharidase abnormalities. *Transplantation*, **6**, 104-110.

Hodgson, H.J.F., Potter, B.J., Skinner, J. & Jewell, D.P. (1978) Immune complex mediated colitis in rabbits. An experimental model. *Gut*, **19**, 225-232.

Holmes, J.T., Klein, M.S., Winawer, S.J. & Fortner, J.C. (1971) Morphological studies of rejection in canine jejunal allografts. *Gastroenterology*, **61**, 693-706.

Kleinman, R.E. (1979) Relationship of uptake and transport of protein by the immature intestine to antigenicity of infant formulas. In *The Mast Cell* (Ed.) Pepys, J. & Edwards, A.M. pp. 371-374. Tunbridge Wells: Pitman Medical.

Lake, A.M., Bloch, K.J., Neutra, M.R. & Walker, W.A. (1979) Intestinal goblet cell mucus release. II. *In vivo* stimulation by antigen in the immunised rat. *Journal of Immunology*, **122**, 834-837.

Lancet (anonymous) (1975) Allergy in the gastrointestinal tract. *Lancet*, **ii**, 1021-1023.

MacDonald, T.T. & Ferguson, A. (1976) Hypersensitivity reactions in the small intestine. 2. Effects of allograft rejection on mucosal architecture and lymphoid cell infiltrate. *Gut*, **17**, 81-91.

MacDonald, T.T. & Ferguson, A. (1977) Hypersensitivity reactions in the small intestine. 3. The effects of allograft rejection and of graft-versus-host disease on epithelial cell kinetics. *Cell Tissue Kinetics*, **10**, 301-312.

McCarthy, D.M., Katz, S.I., Gazze, L., Waldmann, T.A., Nelson, D.L. & Strober, W. (1978) Selective IgA deficiency associated with total villous atrophy of the small intestine and an organ-specific anti-epithelial cell antibody. *Journal of Immunology*, **120**, 932-938.

Manson-Smith, D.F., Bruce, R.G. & Parrott, D.M.V. (1979) Villous atrophy and expulsion of intestinal *Trichinella spiralis* are mediated by T-cells. *Cellular Immunology*, **47**, 285-292.

Nawa, Y. (1979) Increased permeability of gut mucosa in rats infected with *Nippostrongylus brasiliensis*. *International Journal of Parasitology*, **9**, 251-255.

Rabin, B.S. & Rogers, S.J. (1976) Non pathogenicity of anti-intestinal antibody in the rabbit. *American Journal of Pathology*, **83**, 269-282.

Reilly, R.W. & Kirsner, J.B. (1965) Runt intestinal disease. *Laboratory Investigation*, **14**, 102-107.

Roberts-Thomson, I.C. & Mitchell, G.F. (1978) Giardiasis in mice. 1. Prolonged infection in certain mouse strains and in hypothymic (nude) mice. *Gastroenterology*, **75**, 42-46.

Stanffer, U.G. (1977) The present state of small bowel transplantation in animal research and in man. *Zeitschrift für Kinderchirurgie und Grenzgebiete*, **22**, 241-248.

Swarbrick, G.T., Stokes, C.R. & Soothill, J.F. (1979) Absorption of antigens after oral immunisation and the simultaneous induction of specific systemic tolerance. *Gut*, **20**, 121-125.

Walker, W.A., Isselbacher, K.J. & Bloch, K.J. (1977) Intestinal uptake of macromolecules: effect of oral immunisation. *Science*, **177**, 608-610.

Walker, W.A., Wu, M. & Bloch, K.J. (1977) Stimulation by immune complexes of mucus release from goblet cells of the rat small intestine. *Science*, **197**, 370-372.

7
Viral Infections

C.R. MADELEY

The mammalian gut has been described as a perfect culture vessel for a variety of organisms (Flewett, 1976). It is a tube kept at a constant temperature, supplied with a frequent supply of nutrients, and kept well mixed by peristalsis. It is lined by cells in different stages of maturity having a considerable variety of functions and making a diversity of products. Few animals (including man) live in a sterile environment and attempts will be made to colonize this attractive milieu. Since the gut is far from sterile clearly the commensal organisms succeed in doing so and survival of the body as a whole depends considerably on their activities both in providing necessary by-products of their own metabolism and by helping to keep unwanted additional invaders out.

It is apparent from this that the presence of a micro-organism in the faeces discharged from the gut does not, of itself, indicate that something is amiss. It is necessary to establish the significance of such a finding, particularly with bacteria. With viruses the question appears to be easier since no one has been able to ascribe a positive benefit to their presence other than the rather vague one that a virus not causing disease may, by taking up the available cells for its own replication, prevent superinfection by another more virulent one.

Nevertheless, the question is still valid and it is necessary to make a distinction between *infection* (i.e., a virus is present, and comparatively easy to prove) and *affection* (i.e., that a virus is not only present but is also causing significant disease; this is much more difficult to prove). The distinction may be one of degree because the presence of a virus replicating inside a cell is unlikely to leave it totally unaffected functionally but the sum total of this dysfunction may not be significant to the patient or animal as a whole. *De minimis non curat lex*; medicine, too, should not be too quick to ascribe significance.

THE VIRUSES

Viruses, bacteria and protozoa all infect the gut and all may be associated with gut dysfunction. Bacteria and protozoa inhabit the lumen and do not have to invade the cells of the gut wall but viruses must penetrate into living

© 1980 W.B. Saunders Company Ltd.

cells in order to replicate and therefore will have some effect on the metabolism of these cells. The cells affected may be the host cells or bacterial ones in the lumen. There is, however, no direct evidence so far that bacterial viruses (bacteriophages) can precipitate gut disease either through killing off large numbers of bacteria or by enhancing the pathogenic capacity of otherwise harmless bacteria, commensal or invading, by a transduction process similar to that found in diphtheria. However, such a process cannot yet be ruled out and the possible roles of bacteriophages will be discussed later.

Apart from the bacteriophages, the other viruses to be found in the human gut fall into two groups. Group I viruses are those that are found most regularly in the gut but cause disease, if at all, only elsewhere in the body. These include the polioviruses, Coxsackie A and B viruses, echoviruses, reoviruses and some adenoviruses (Table 1). They share one other attribute, that they were all discovered by growth in some form of culture system (day-old mice or cell cultures). Because they can be grown they have mostly now been well characterized both physicochemically and antigenically.

The viruses in Group II (Table 1), on the other hand, were all discovered by direct electron microscopy of stool extracts and do not grow in the routine culture systems used to isolate the Group I viruses. They have not been found elsewhere in the body and appear to be confined to the gut. Failure to

Table 1. *Viruses found in stools*

Group	No. of serotypes
I Viruses that can be grown and passaged	
(a) Enterovirus	
Polio types 1-3	3
Coxsackie A types 1-22, 24	23
Coxsackie B types 1-6	6
Echo types 1-9, 11-17, 19-34	32
Enterovirus types 68-71	4
(b) Adenovirus types 1-35[a]	35
(c) Reovirus types 1-3	3
Total	106
II Viruses detected by electron microscopy	
(a) Norwalk types 1-3[b]	3
(b) Rotavirus types 1-4?	4?
(c) Adenovirus	?
(d) Astrovirus	?
(e) Coronavirus	?
(f) Calicivirus	?
(g) Small round viruses[c]	?
III Bacteriophages	
(a) Isometric (e.g., ΦX 174)	Multiple
(b) Tailed	Multiple

[a] Not all adenovirus types have been reported as faecal isolates.
[b] Assuming Norwalk, Montgomery County and Hawaii to be different.
[c] A heterogeneous group including the following: W agent, Appleton and Higgins' agent, Ditchling agent, cockle virus.

find them in other parts, particularly the respiratory tract, may be due to the insensitive methods available to detect them. However, as with the Group I viruses, they have also been observed in the stools of normal babies and the conditions necessary for them to initiate disease are still unknown.

In the context of enteroviruses (polio, Coxsackie A and B and echo) it is well accepted that 'infection' and 'disease' are not synonymous terms. Surveys of day nurseries (Patterson and Bell, 1963) and babies in the tropics (Parks, Queiroga and Melnick, 1967) have shown that excretion of these viruses by apparently normal infants is common. The excretion of Group I viruses is rarely accompanied by diarrhoea, though occasional outbreaks have been reported, for example by echo 18 virus (Eichenwald et al, 1958). Nevertheless, the same virus has been isolated from babies without diarrhoea much more frequently. However, a considerable amount of non-bacterial diarrhoeal disease in children and adults has been observed and the existence of another group of viruses was postulated long before any of the Group II viruses were recognized. The first to be described was Norwalk agent which was recognized as an agent of disease (Dolin et al, 1971) some time before the virus itself was observed in the electron microscope (Kapikian et al, 1972). As the virus was present in the faeces of patients and volunteers in small numbers and was difficult to identify even by immune electron microscopy (IEM), these findings attracted comparatively little attention. Shortly afterwards the more readily visible rotavirus was recognized and a serious search of faecal extracts for virus particles began.

Rotavirus was first recognized in gut biopsies from babies with diarrhoea (Bishop et al, 1973) but was then found readily in preparations of stool extracts. It has since been observed throughout the world wherever it has been sought, with stool extracts frequently containing very large numbers of virus particles. Consequently it is often easy to find and can be identified with certainty when particles with the complete outer rim (Figure 1a; Flewett et al, 1974) are present. Without this outer rim the particles are smaller and can be confused with the very similar but slightly larger reovirus (Figure 1b), particularly if the calibration and stability of the microscope are unknown. Differentiation requires careful scrutiny of individual particles but is rarely a serious problem as reoviruses are seen very infrequently in crude stool extracts and usually only in small numbers. Very large numbers will almost certainly be rotaviruses.

Adenoviruses were also seen with comparative ease and were even easier to identify. However, they were only very rarely seen in stools from which an adenovirus could be grown in cell culture. Morphologically they are absolutely typical adenoviruses (Figure 1 c and d) and no visible coating of antibody or other material can be seen to account for their failure to grow. Typing of adenoviruses by IEM is not very satisfactory and Flewett et al (1975) obtained only suggestive evidence that the viruses they found in faeces from an outbreak in a long-stay children's ward were of type 7. Since this is a common serotype which normally grows readily in cell culture this finding was strange. There was also a paradox in that the more adenovirus there was in the stool the less likely was it to grow. These and other points about stool adenoviruses are discussed further below.

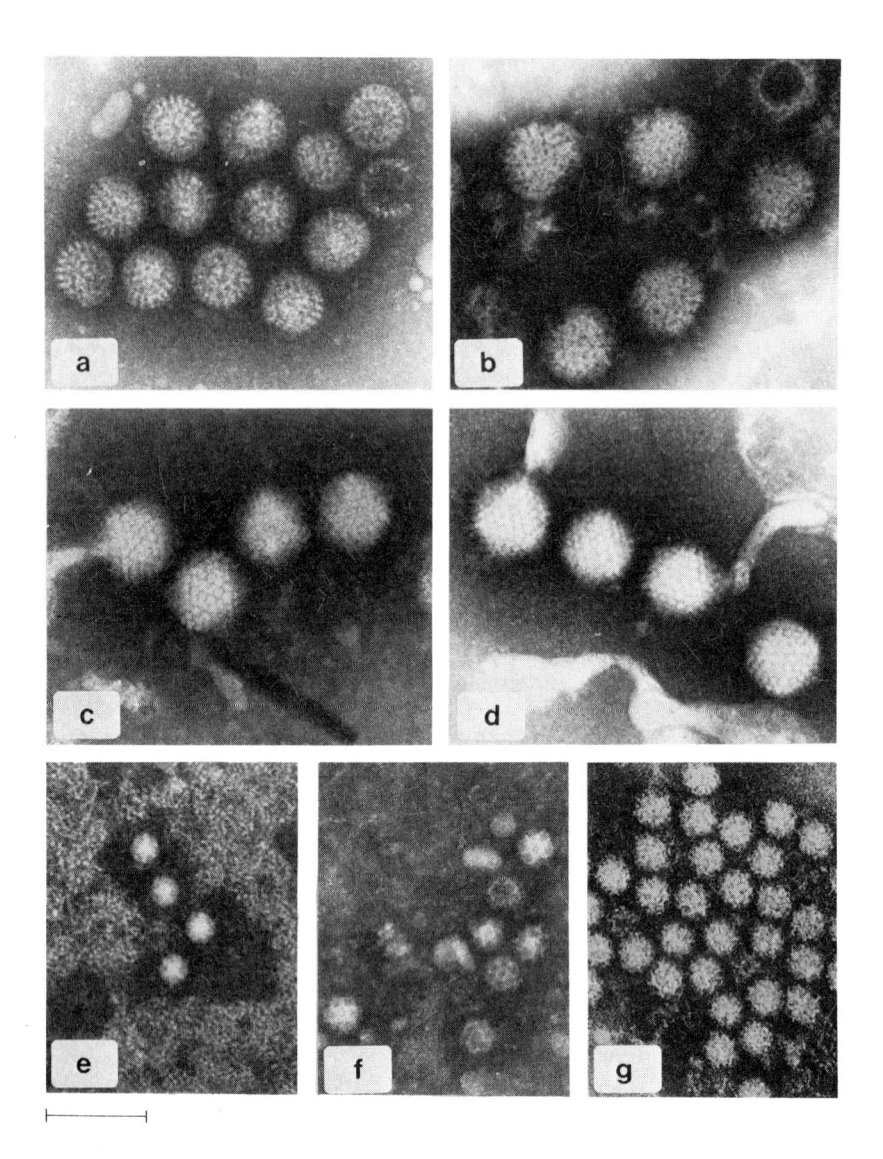

Figure 1. The viruses found in stools. (a) Rotaviruses from stool. Note complete outer membrane in the majority of particles. (b) Reovirus type 3 from cell culture. Note absence of outer membrane on any particle. (c) Adenoviruses from stool, untyped and failed to grow in cell culture. (d) Adenovirus type 3 from stool, cultured in cells and indistinguishable from (c). (e) Astroviruses from stool. Note smooth outline and absence of central hollow on the particles. (f) Caliciviruses from stool. Note slightly larger size compared with astroviruses, central hollow on five of the particles, and Star-of-David on the uppermost particle. (g) Norwalk agent mixed with acute-phase serum from Kapikian et al (1972), with kind permission of the authors and the editor of *Journal of Virology*. All viruses stained with 3 per cent potassium phosphotungstate, pH 7.0, and printed at a final magnification of 140 000 ×. Scale bar = 100 nm.

From Madeley (1979a), by kind permission of the editor of *Journal of Clinical Pathology*.

Microscopists with good high-resolution machines were then able to see a variety of small round virus-like objects. In size, they were between 22 and 33 nm in diameter but careful inspection of the pictures taken of these particles has shown that they may be divided into groups on a basis of size and details of surface morphology. Because of the problems inherent in calibrating microscopes (at the magnification used to find virus) and in measuring particles accurately and reproducibly, differences of sizes reported by different operators are probably not significant unless they exceed about 20 per cent of the measured value. Differentiation on morphological grounds is more objective and at least four types have been described (Table 2). They fall into two groups: (a) those with entire smooth

Table 2. *Morphological types of small round viruses*

Group	Outline	Size (nm)	Appearance
1	Smooth	20-22	Adeno-associated virus
2	Smooth	25-27	Enterovirus
3	Smooth	28	Astrovirus
4	Feathery	30-33	Calicivirus
5	Feathery	30-33	Norwalk Minireovirus Minirotavirus

edges and (b) those with irregular ones. The smaller entire-edged particles often have an outline suggesting a hexagon, may be found in the same stool as an adenovirus and may be adenovirus-associated virus (AAV). An adenovirus is not always observed, however, and these may not be AAVs. Slightly larger particles with circular outline may show no surface features. These are indistinguishable from enteroviruses (Figure 2a) but only rarely is an enterovirus grown from such a stool. This suggests that the majority are not known enteroviruses.

Astroviruses (Madeley and Cosgrove, 1975) are distinguishable from this second type by the presence of a star-shaped surface structure with the star showing either five or six points (Figure 2e; Madeley, 1979b). Like rotaviruses, astroviruses are often found in stools in very large numbers but by no means all the particles show surface stars. Usually enough will be present to make the identification, though frequently the operator is most sure at the first glance; certainty ebbs away with more prolonged scrutiny.

The feathery-edged particles divide into two groups: (a) definite caliciviruses and (b) others, some of whom may be caliciviruses but which do not show typical calicivirus morphology. The caliciviruses have an identifiable structure (Figure 1f; Madeley and Cosgrove, 1976; Madeley, 1979b) which is characteristic and indistinguishable from already established animal viruses (swine, pinniped and feline strains have been described). The human strains differ, however, in failing to grow in cell culture. With feline strains the majority of particles show typical morphology but recent evidence (Caul, Ashley and Pether, 1979) suggests that not all feline strains show

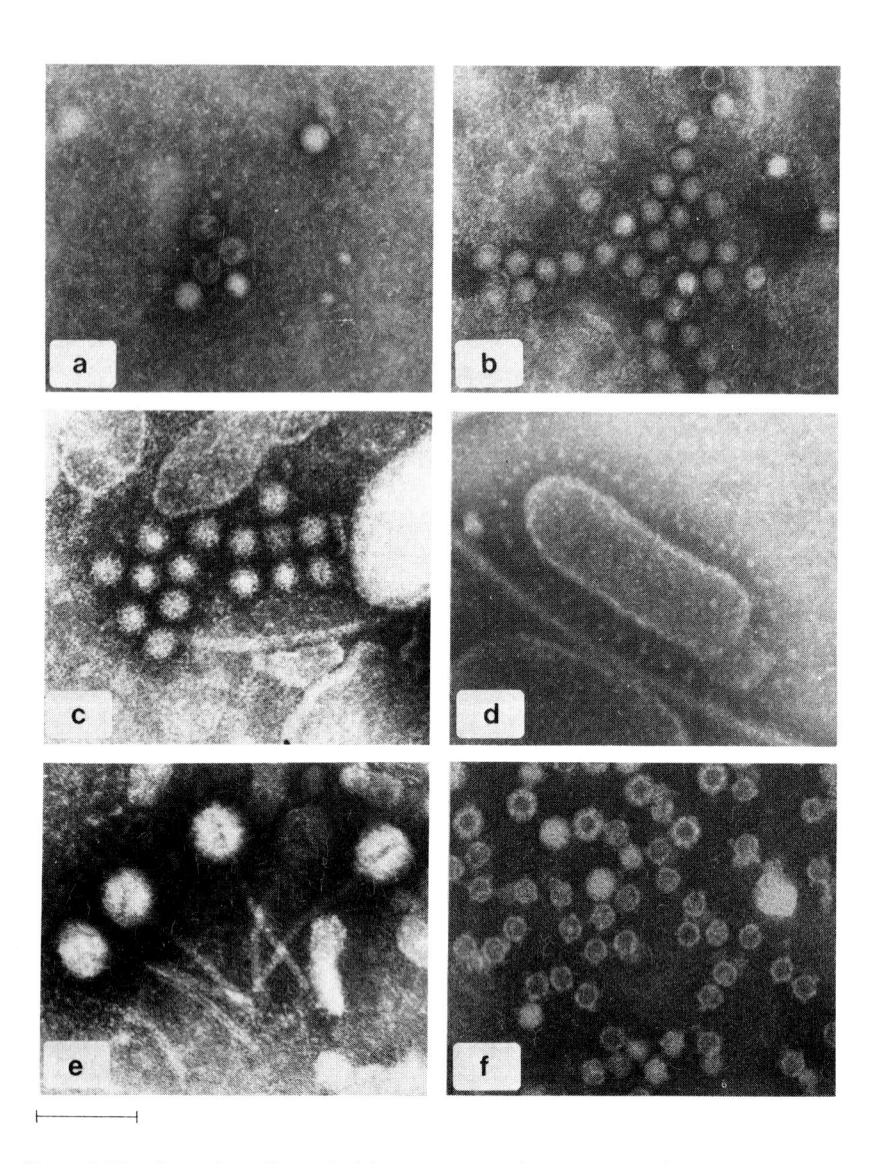

Figure 2. The viruses found in stools. (a) Enteroviruses (echovirus type 5) from cell culture. All enteroviruses have identical morphology and cannot be distinguished from each other in the electron microscope. (b) Small round viruses (SRVs) from stool, approximately 25 nm in diameter with a smooth outline. (c) SRVs from stool, approximately 30 nm in diameter with a 'feathery' outline. (d) Coronavirus from stool. Note long surface projections with spherical knob at end. (e) Tailed bacteriophages from stool. (f) Bacteriophage ΦX 174 from lysed culture of *Escherichia coli*. (e) and (f) represent two types of bacteriophages likely to be present in stools, and the ΦX 174 would be classed as an SRV. All viruses stained with 3 per cent potassium phosphotungstate, pH 7.0, and printed at a final magnification of 140 000 ×. Scale bar = 100 nm.

From Madeley (1979a), with kind permission of the editor of *Journal of Clinical Pathology*.

typical calicivirus structure and a proportion of the particles are very similar to the other group. This includes Norwalk and related viruses (Hawaii and Montgomery County), minireoviruses (Middleton, Szymanski and Petric, 1977), mini rotaviruses (Spratt et al, 1978) and other unnamed articles. At Ruchill, Glasgow, we have referred collectively to these as 'fuzzy-wuzzies' for want of a better name. Whether these are atypical caliciviruses, as some believe (Curry and Roberts, 1980), or all different cannot be decided at present. None of the published pictures shows a clear-cut calicivirus morphology and, despite the careful examination of many good quality pictures, it has not proved possible to link them unequivocally with the caliciviruses. Worse still, since it is far from being uncommon to find more than one virus in a stool, the finding of definite caliciviruses in an extract together with equally definite fuzzy-wuzzies can be interpreted with equal logic as two viruses or one virus showing two morphologies. In the absence of any definite evidence one way or the other I prefer the former interpretation as not prejudging the issue.

Another possible interpretation is that the feathery viruses are smooth-edged ones with antibody on their surfaces. This seems unlikely as it does not explain why one virus found in the acute stage of diarrhoea is coated with 'antibody' and another is not. While conceding that this begs the question of causation, the point seems as valid as others asserted as fact in this uncertain area. Proof one way or the other will have to await discovery of how to grow these and other stool viruses in cell culture.

Coronaviruses are well established as causes of diarrhoea in piglets (transmissible gastroenteritis) (Woode, 1969) and the morphology of the virions of this disease is indistinguishable from the original coronaviruses found in respiratory infections of man (Almeida and Tyrrell, 1967) and chickens (Berry et al, 1964). Coronavirus-like particles have been found in human faeces in India, England, South Africa and Australia. They have surface projections which are longer and more knob-like and whose connecting stalk may often be too narrow to be visible in the microscope (Figure 2d). Though resembling pieces of membranous debris they are sufficiently different to present little problem in indentification (Caul, Ashley and Egglestone, 1977).

Finally there are bacteriophages. Only two morphological forms that might be bacteriophages are seen in any quantity in faecal extracts (Figure 2 e and f). Some of the 'small round viruses' may be isometric bacteriophages but only rarely do they resemble ΦX 174. If they are bacteriophages their host species is unknown and finding out is a task of daunting magnitude requiring considerable luck to succeed.

The lollipop-shape of the tailed bacteriophages has not been found among the animal viruses, and since their structure reflects their method of infecting cells by injection of their nucleic acid there is no reason to doubt their identity as bacteriophages. The numbers that may be present in a faecal extract vary considerably and most, but not all, extracts contain small numbers. An occasional extract, however, contains very large numbers which may reach levels similar to those found with rotaviruses and adenoviruses.

INFECTION AND DISEASE

There are two traditional bases for the diagnosis of viral disease. These are demonstration of the virus and/or demonstration of an antibody response at the relevant time. These are so well established that to call them in question risks the charge of heresy. However, this question is very relevant in deciding causation and has to be examined.

The finding of a virus in an ill patient has been accepted in most instances as indicating that it is the causative organism of the disease, particularly if it has been isolated from the affected organ. This acceptance has been due to the rarity of commensal carriage and no such carriage has been found in some of the major virus diseases such as rabies, smallpox, measles and influenza. Investigation of others, however, including polio, has shown that children in particular may excrete enteroviruses without overt disease.

Seroconversion means that the immune mechanisms have received a stimulus big enough to trigger a response but does not necessarily mean that the body's function has been disturbed. This is clearly shown, for instance, in the use of killed vaccines where seroconversion can be demonstrated without any multiplication of the virus and rarely any systemic upset. In this context we should also remember that in babies under six months of age the mechanisms of immunity are developing and may not react fully to a stimulus.

If, therefore, a virus is observed in the faeces in large numbers we should not be surprised to find that an antibody response has taken place but we should be wary of over-interpreting the significance of this finding. Stimulus does not equate with damage.

It is against this background that we have to try to establish which viruses cause diarrhoea (or some other bodily dysfunction) and under what circumstances. It is a difficult task because non-bacterial diarrhoea (i.e., where no known pathogenic strain of bacterium has been isolated and which is severe enough to threaten life) occurs in babies young enough to have residual maternal immunity, to have variably competent immune responses of their own, to be still establishing their own patterns of gut function, and often to be in the process of weaning. Finally, they will be too young to be ethically usable for experiment.

This last point means that the evidence will come directly from observations of natural challenge and indirectly from animal experiments. Let us examine it:

Evidence of excretion. This may come from electron microscopic visualization of virus, detection of viral antigens by various methods and, in some cases, partial virus growth in cell cultures. (For recent reviews of these methods see Madeley (1979a) and Holmes (1979).) Each of these methods may detect different components of the viruses and they are not therefore quantitatively comparable one with another. Due to the practical difficulties of obtaining a standard stool extract, the amount of virus detected in the test used will not bear a constant relationship to the amount of virus in the faeces in the rectum. Conclusions about the quantity of virus observed have therefore to be drawn with caution. A large number of particles or a large amount of viral antigen observed in a test on a faecal extract is therefore not necessarily of greater significance than a small number.

Rotavirus has been by far the most commonly recorded virus in faeces. It has been found in all countries, tropical and temperate, rich and poor, where it has been sought. It has been found more in children than in adults but has none the less been observed in all ages. It has also been found more often in the stools of patients with diarrhoea than in those without and has been referred to as the commonest cause of infantile diarrhoea. Seroconversion following excretion has also been demonstrated.

Not all rotavirus excretions have been observed in patients with diarrhoea. Several groups (Totterdell, Chrystie and Banatvala, 1976; Murphy, Albrey and Crewe, 1977; Madeley, Cosgrove and Bell, 1978) have observed excretion by normal neonates. Excretion of morphologically normal virus takes place over several days and no obvious antibody is seen to be attached to it (Madeley, Cosgrove and Bell, 1978). Similar excretion by older babies has also been reported in a small number of babies followed up at home (see below).

In comparison, the other viruses have been observed less frequently, but different patterns emerge if epidemics are compared with endemic diarrhoea. Norwalk and other small round viruses (SRV) have been implicated more in outbreaks in both schools and adults than rotavirus, which in comparison has only rarely been found in association with common-source outbreaks (Hara et al, 1978; Lycke et al, 1978). This distinction may not be as great as it seems and may reflect only the difficulty of recognizing with certainty small numbers of more or less featureless SRVs in cases of endemic diarrhoea. Recent studies by Greenberg et al (1979) have suggested that Norwalk and related viruses may be more common than had been thought.

Astroviruses have been found in association with endemic diarrhoea (Madeley et al, 1977), in localized outbreaks (Kurtz, Lee and Pickering, 1977) and in normal babies (Madeley, Cosgrove and Bell, 1978). The proportion of recognizates associated with disease was very similar to that for rotavirus in a similar population (Madeley, 1979a), and neither was found to be an inevitable pathogen. They have so far been observed only by some workers throughout the world and it is not clear whether this reflects differences in distribution or the difficulties of making a positive identification without a high-resolution microscope in good working order.

Caliciviruses have a less strong association with endemic diarrhoea (Madeley, 1979a) but have been implicated in two common-source school outbreaks in England (McSwiggan, Cubitt and Moore, 1978) and Japan (Chiba et al, 1980). The close morphological similarity of other viruses (Norwalk, minireoviruses, minirotaviruses, etc.) means that there is considerable uncertainty here.

Coronaviruses have also been observed only by a few workers. Again it is uncertain whether this reflects differences in distribution or differences in preparation since it is easy to strip the projections by rough handling or prolonged storage. They have been found in the faeces of adults more than in those of children and excretion over several months has been observed (Clarke, Caul and Egglestone, 1979). Consequently their role in causation is even less clear than that of the other viruses.

The adenoviruses pose an even more complex problem of interpretation. It has long been possible to isolate strains of this virus from stools by culture and most of the known 35 serotypes have been isolated from this source. However, electron microscopy (EM) has revealed that a considerable number of stools contain typical adenoviruses which do not grow in the routine cell cultures used to isolate the established serotypes. It has been estimated that 5 to 8 per cent of children's stools contain adenoviruses detectable by EM (Davidson et al, 1975; C.R. Madeley, 1978, unpublished observations). Repeated excretions detected either by isolation (Bell et al, 1961) or by EM (Scott et al, 1979) are common but there have been several reports (Flewett et al, 1975; Tufvesson and Johnsson, 1976; Whitelaw, Davies and Parry, 1977; Richmond et al, 1979) of outbreaks where the only virus that could be implicated was an EM-detectable adenovirus. There is now evidence that some of these adenoviruses form at least one new serotype (Johansson et al, 1980) so that conclusions over their role in diarrhoea are premature at the moment.

The Group I viruses (Table 1), despite their preference for gut cells, have not been found to be commonly associated with diarrhoea. Very occasionally a virus has been found in a common-source outbreak but it is not clear whether it was a cause or taking the opportunity to spread in a closed community.

There has been a great deal of published work on the role of rotaviruses in animal diarrhoea. Strains have been recovered from almost every species in which they have been sought, and the rotavirus appears to be almost the most ubiquitous virus of all. Experiments on gnotobiotic animals have shown that they can precipitate diarrhoea in a wide variety of species. Reports include detailed histopathology from which it is apparent that the virus infects the distal two-thirds of the intestinal villus, causing considerable sloughing of the mucosa followed by regeneration and return to normality. However, as soon as a normal gut flora is introduced into the equation the results become much less clear-cut and it may be difficult to demonstrate any ability to cause diarrhoea at all in the field (Logan, Pearson and McNulty, 1979). Far from helping to potentiate rotavirus in causing diarrhoea, a normal flora may even, it seems, prevent either colonization or disease.

None the less, the potential for causing diarrhoea under artificial conditions is undeniable and this has been extrapolated to man somewhat uncritically. In at least one respect the parallel is not exact, in that overt diease may be induced in newborn animal neonates but they become refractory a week to ten days after birth. Newborn humans are susceptible to infection but do not develop disease. They are apparently most liable to suffer diarrhoea after several weeks or months of life and to become refractory months or years later. Whether this is equally true with all serotypes of the human virus remains to be shown but the pattern does seem to differ from that in animals.

An astrovirus similar in appearance to the human one has been described in lambs. In gnotobiotic animals it causes a mild diarrhoea but does not cause a major problem in normal farm animals (Snodgrass and Gray, 1977). Another virus whose identity as an astrovirus is less certain has been associated with diarrhoea in calves (Woode and Bridger, 1978) but it, too, does not appear to cause severe problems in the field.

Transmissible gastroenteritis due to a swine coronavirus is, on the other hand, well established as a pathogen in contrast to the human counterpart where prolonged excretion makes a pathogenic role more difficult to define.

Possible mechanisms for bacteriophages in causing diarrhoea in man have been mentioned already. Although there is no direct evidence to link them with disease it seems reasonable to think that the variation in the amount present (from occasional to approximately 500 virions per 400-mesh grid square) may sometimes reflect some significant process in the gut, even if it is only a predominance of one type of bacterium not necessarily recognized as pathogenic.

The possibility of transduction by bacteriophages is intriguing, and might help to resolve the uncertainty about the role of toxin production in diarrhoea associated with some strains of *Escherichia coli*. Proving such a role will not be easy, and it also raises the possibility of synergism between an altered commensal and a virus. Studies in which virology is combined with bacteriology and parasitology do not identify a microbiological cause for up to one-third of infantile diarrhoea cases admitted to hospital (Madeley et al, 1977). While some of these cases are probably not truly infective in origin, some could be due to a commensal bacterium not normally recognized as a pathogen but with a pathogenic potential transduced into it by infection by a bacteriophage. This potential could then be enhanced by the presence of another human virus, and it is not uncommon to find both kinds of viruses in the same stool.

Serological surveys. It is easier to look for antibodies in the sera of a population than for virus in its stools. Most of the published surveys have been for antibody to rotavirus and have been conducted in the United States of America (Kapikian et al, 1975), the United Kingdom (Elias, 1977) and Australia (Ghose, Schnagl and Holmes, 1978). The results are all very similar whether from complement fixation, immunofluorescence or ELISA (enzyme-linked-immunosorbent assay). Antibody is acquired from about six months of age and by five years over 90 per cent of the population has detectable antibody and, though the level shows some decline in middle and old age, it does not drop much below 60 per cent, as shown in Figure 3. These findings by complement fixation are not readily paralleled with other viruses. Complement-fixing antibodies usually decline after about one year, remaining undetectable thereafter. Consequently these data suggest, firstly, that rotavirus infection is extremely common and, secondly, that reinfection probably occurs. Kim et al (1977) reported that circulating antibody is probably not protective and therefore immunity may be either short-lived or outflanked by other serotypes, allowing re-stimulation of the immune mechanisms. However, only a minority of those infected suffer diarrhoea severe enough to warrant hospitalization so that the majority of rotavirus infections are probably trivial or asymptomatic. Only a small survey of astrovirus antibody has been reported so far and it shows a pattern similar to that found with rotaviruses (Kurtz and Lee, 1978). It would be interesting to see whether these results were confirmed with larger numbers and, if so, they would indicate that astroviruses are commoner and more widespread than their relative infrequency of sighting would imply.

In contrast, antibody to Norwalk is acquired more slowly (Figure 3), with the 50 per cent positive level not being reached until the 40 to 49 year age group. This indicates that the virus is not so widespread and therefore that a higher proportion of infections result in disease. These results therefore highlight the distinction between infection and affection.

No serological surveys on adenoviruses, caliciviruses, coronaviruses or other small round viruses have been reported. It would be technically difficult at present and, in the case of coronaviruses, would be difficult to interpret.

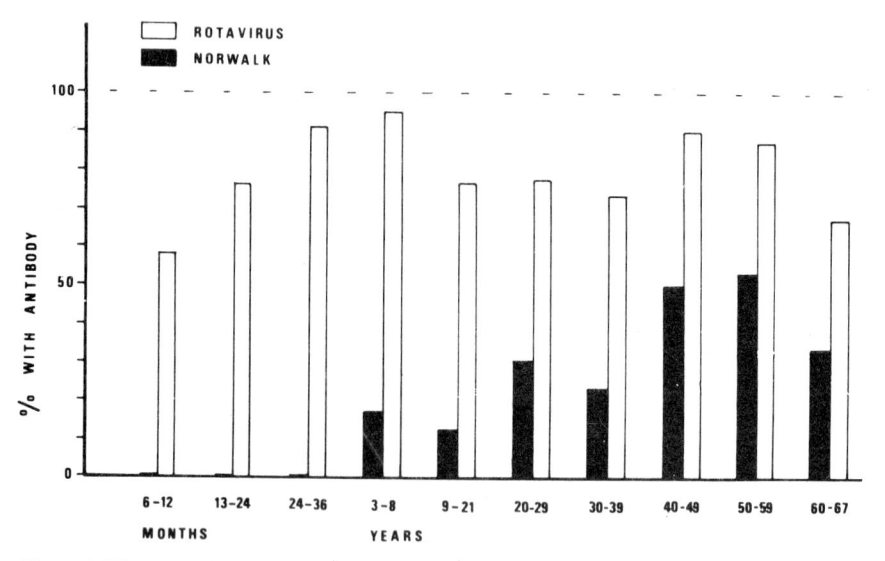

Figure 3. Histogram showing the acquisition of antibody to rotavirus and Norwalk agent by age groups in a population in the USA. The test used was immune adherence haemagglutination. Adapted from Greenberg and Kapikian (1978).

COMMUNITY STUDIES

The illnesses that cause children to be admitted to hospital are acquired at home. It is therefore logical to look at the ecology of the viruses in that environment. Excellent studies have been carried out by Bell and his colleagues at Junior Village (Bell et al, 1961), Fox and his colleagues in New York and Seattle (The Virus Watch Program, Fox et al, 1966) and several others. These authors used culture methods to look for viruses and found that virus infections are common, particularly where there is overcrowding.

These results were born out by Mata et al (1977), who found excretion of enteroviruses and adenoviruses to be commonplace among Guatemalan children, but the authors make no mention of disease being associated with this excretion. The viruses recorded included echo-, polio- and Coxsackie viruses as well as adenoviruses. No electron microscopy (EM) was attempted due to lack of facilities.

These investigations are difficult, laborious and time consuming by culture methods. They are even more so by EM, and this may account for few such studies being reported so far. Full details of our study have already been published (Scott et al, 1979) and only the general conclusions will be presented here.

Twenty-seven babies from a single poor-housing area in Glasgow were followed up at home between March 1976 and March 1977. A weekly stool specimen regardless of the baby's health was collected by the mother from the nappy and a history of the baby's health was also obtained from the mother. As can be seen from Figure 4 over 300 stools were collected and examined. A considerable number of viruses were detected by EM of which the most common morphological type was an adenovirus. It was not possible to grow or type these and it is not known whether the recognizates from any one patient were the same or different serotypes. Admissions to hospital are represented by the black and white boxes in the figure. The illnesses that led to admission were varied and were by no means all diarrhoea. More details of these admissions are given later (see Figure 6).

The viruses observed by EM were related to illness in the home, as shown in Figure 5. Viruses, where observed, were not always associated even with trivial illness in the home. All the morphological types of viruses were observed in the stools of babies that were apparently normal, as well as in those with illness which could be diarrhoeal, repiratory or a combination of the two.

A weekly stool is clearly too infrequent to be certain of detecting viruses excreted in association with an illness during the intervening six days and it is more than likely that many viruses were missed. However, the absence of illness associated with recorded virus excretion is interesting and does not confirm that even rotaviruses are inevitable pathogens. The rotavirus recognizates were not typed and it is possible that the ones excreted by babies 18 and 22 were type 1 and not type 2. Yolken et al (1978) have published evidence that, in Guatemala at least, type 2 is more virulent than type 1.

The extent to which weekly stools may miss virus excretion is shown by the amount of virus excretion detected in these follow-up babies, and others from the same housing area which were not being followed up, when they were admitted to hospital (Figure 6). This part of the study showed two things: firstly, that the babies frequently excreted EM-detectable viruses and that the morphological type changed frequently and, secondly, that a significant diarrhoea is hard to define. Most of the babies listed in Figure 6 had at least one episode of diarrhoea, or loose or frequent stools. Most of these episodes did not require treatment and one (baby 7 in November 1976) had 'diarrhoea' lasting three weeks, excreted a succession of viruses and did not require specific treatment.

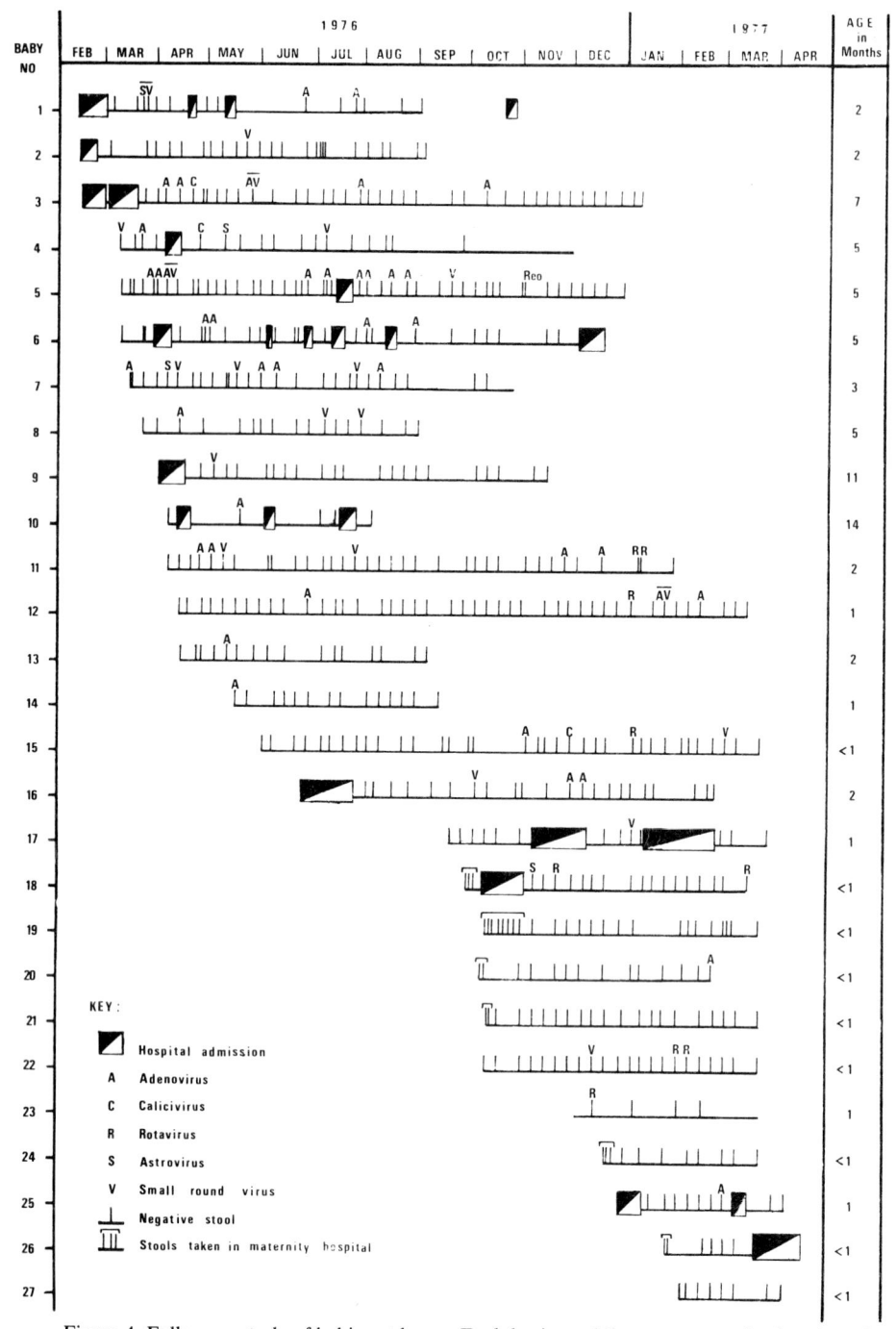

Figure 4. Follow-up study of babies at home. Each horizontal line represents the duration of follow-up; each vertical represents a stool specimen examined by electron microscopy (EM); each letter over the vertical is a virus (or viruses) detected by EM, with their identity indicated by the key. From Scott et al (1979), with kind permission of the editor of *Journal of Hygiene*.

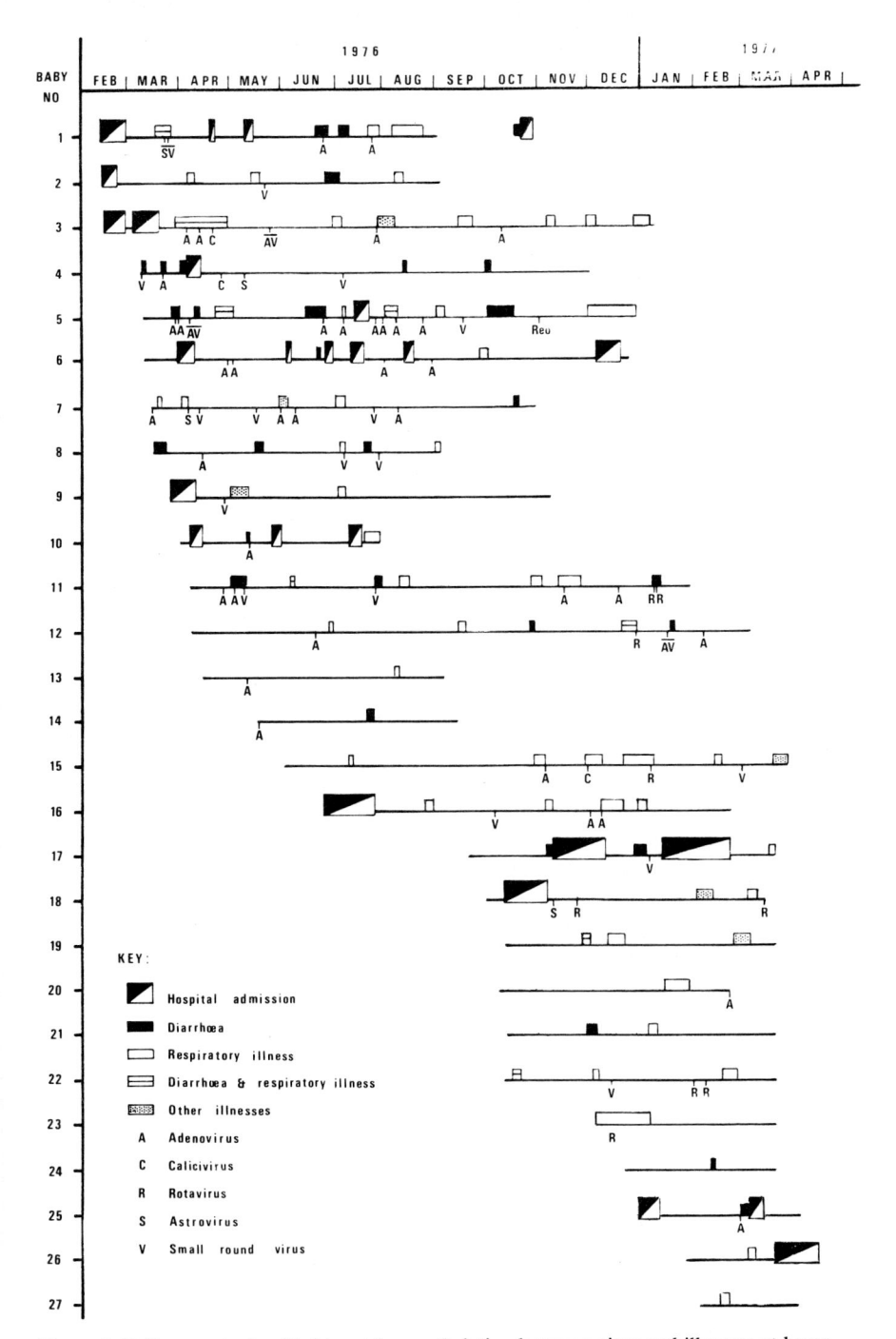

Figure 5. Follow-up study of babies at home. Relation between virus and illnesses at home. Only the virus-positive stools from Figure 4 are shown below the lines. The illnesses reported by the mother are shown above the line. From Scott et al (1979), with kind permission of the editor of *Journal of Hygiene*.

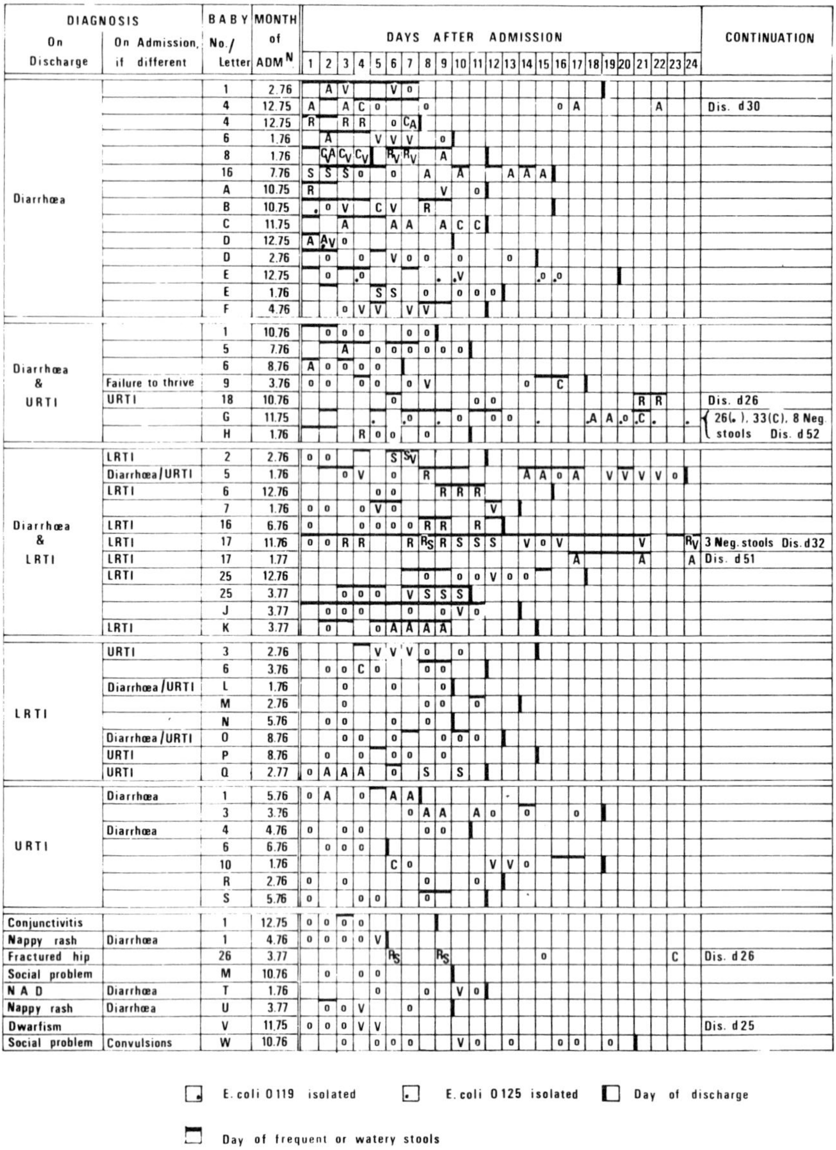

Figure 6. Hospital admissions of follow-up babies. Letters represent days on which stool specimens were obtained. Those where no virus was found by EM are indicated by '0'. Virus-positive stools are indicated by the appropriate letter (for a key see Figure 4). From Scott et al (1979), with kind permission of the editor of *Journal of Hygiene*.

How much of this copious virus excretion was the result of hospital-acquired infection is unknown. The babies were admitted to three different hospitals but we were not aware at any time of any one virus spreading through any of the wards. From other (unpublished) results, it is likely that these faecal viruses can spread through cubicalized infectious-disease wards where the staff are experienced enough to prevent cross-infection with bacterial pathogens. A comparison of Figures 5 and 6 suggests that considerable viral acquisition also occurs at home, is probably greater than our weekly sampling could show and, by analogy with previous work, the turnover is likely to be increased in overcrowded conditions. It would, however, have been very interesting to have had a record of the viruses excreted by these babies during the week immediately prior to their admission to hospital.

All these babies came from one small area of the city, consisting of four or five streets of council flats. It was a close-knit community with a great deal of close contact between households. This situation would facilitate spread of all micro-organisms as well as viruses and it does not follow that the pattern would be repeated in other areas where the families keep more apart. Much of the world lives in poor overcrowded housing so the findings in this study may have relevance to other areas where diarrhoea and other diseases are major problems.

The frequency of excretion of adenoviruses is particularly interesting. Most babies excreted them at one time or another and it is not clear whether different recognizates represent reinfections or recrudescences. It will become possible to say with certainty when one episode ends and another begins only when it is possible to grow and type them in cell culture. This seems as far away as ever since no one has discovered the trick of growing most of the EM-detectable recognizates.

MECHANISMS OF CAUSATION

From the results that we and others have obtained it is becoming clear that the presence of virus alone may not be sufficient to initiate diarrhoea. The observation of virus has to be seen in context, and the context is that of individual babies. Even in a newborn baby there is constant shedding of very large numbers, in absolute terms, of cells from the tips of the intestinal villi. Consequently a virus must damage a large number of cells if it is going to add significantly to this loss and upset the equilibrium of the baby's gut. Though it is not possible to assess accurately the total number of virus particles excreted in one bowel motion, the numbers seen in some stool extracts can be very high. The numbers of Group I viruses, which do not cause diarrhoea, rarely reach EM-detectable levels and this may mean that fewer cells are infected.

The simple explanation that diarrhoea is a quantitative phenomenon (the more cells infected the more the diarrhoea) is not good enough. Very large numbers may be found in stool extracts from normal babies and may be rotaviruses, adenoviruses, astroviruses or even tailed bacteriophages. The question is qualitative as well as quantitative. How many of what kind of cell are not only *in*fected but *aff*ected?

Animal experiments have shown that, with rotaviruses at least, it is the cells of the distal two-thirds of the intestinal villus that are infected and it is these cells that have differentiated the most. This part has cells with the most diverse functions and is the part that is sloughed in response to infection.

The functions of the cells of the villi will vary from time to time in an individual and probably with his or her diet. Individual viruses may infect selectively cells with different characteristics in terms of surface antigens, secretory products, metabolic activity and senescence. Whether such infection has a detectable effect on the patient will depend on the number of cells infected, the importance to the patient at that time of the types of cell affected or their products and, probably, the duration of that infection.

It follows from this argument that the potential of different viruses to cause diarrhoea will probably be different and will vary between different subjects and in one subject from time to time. It further follows, therefore, that formal 'proof' of causation will be difficult to obtain except in general terms and the general significance of each kind of virus and maybe each serotype of that virus will have to be established by patient epidemiology.

QUESTIONS TO BE ANSWERED

There are several questions that we should try to answer if we are going to understand diarrhoea and the role of viruses in causing it.

1. Are particular cells affected by each virus?
2. If so, what are their characteristics?
3. Are all strains of each virus equally capable of inducing diarrhoea?
4. How much structure and/or function can be damaged before diarrhoea develops?
5. Are there 'diarrhoeal' babies (i.e. those with a genetic, or induced, tendency to get diarrhoea)?
6. Are there dietary (quantitative as well as qualitative) factors?
7. Can we/should we try to prevent diarrhoea in infants and, if so, how?
8. What is the secret of persuading these stool viruses to grow in cell cultures?

The answer to question 8 will facilitate finding answers to the other seven. It seems just as elusive now as it did prior to 1973.

The list is by no means exhaustive; other workers with different interests will have no difficulty in adding to it.

REFERENCES

Almeida, J.D. & Tyrrell, D.A.J. (1967) The morphology of three previously uncharacterized human respiratory viruses that grow in organ culture. *Journal of General Virology*, **1**, 175-178.

Bell, J.A., Huebner, R.J., Rosen, L., Rowe, W.P., Cole, R.M., Mastrota, F.M., Floyd, T.M., Chanock, R.M. & Shvedoff, R.A. (1961) Illness and microbial experiences of nursery children at Junior Village. *American Journal of Hygiene*, **74**, 267-292.

Berry, D.M., Cruickshank, J., Chu, H.P. & Wells, R.J.H. (1964) The structure of infectious bronchitis virus. *Virology*, **23**, 403.

Bishop, R.F., Davidson, G.P., Holmes, I.H. & Ruck, B.J. (1973) Virus particles in epithelial cells of duodenal mucosa from children with acute non-bacterial gastroenteritis. *Lancet*, **ii**, 1281-1283.

Bruce-White, G.B. & Stancliffe, D. (1975) Viruses and gastroenteritis. *Lancet*, **ii**, 703.

Caul, E.O., Ashley, C.R. & Egglestone, S.I. (1977) Recognition of human enteric coronaviruses by electron microscopy. *Medical Laboratory Science*, **34**, 259-263.

Caul, E.O., Ashley, C. & Pether, J.V.S. (1979) Norwalk-like particles in epidemic gastroenteritis in the U.K. *Lancet*, **ii**, 1292.

Chiba, S., Sakuma, Y., Akihara, M., Kogasaka, R., Horino, K., Nakao, T. & Fukui, S. (1979) An outbreak of gastroenteritis associated with calicivirus in an infant home. *Journal of Medical Virology*, **4**, 249-254.

Clarke, S.K.R., Caul, E.O. & Egglestone, S.I. (1979) The human enteric coronaviruses. *Postgraduate Medical Journal*, **55**, 135-142.

Curry, A. & Roberts, J.L. (1980) Realistic look at small round faecal viruses found by electron microscopy. *Lancet*, **i**, 99.

Davidson, G.P., Bishop, R.F., Townley, R.R.W., Holmes, I.H. & Ruck, B.J. (1975) Importance of a new virus in acute sporadic enteritis in children. *Lancet*, **i**, 242-246.

Dolin, R., Blacklow, N.R., DuPont, H.L., Formal, S., Buscho, R.F., Kasel, J.A., Chames, R.P., Hornick, R. & Chanock, R.M. (1971) Transmission of acute infectious nonbacterial gastroenteritis to volunteers by oral administration of stool filtrates. *Journal of Infectious Diseases*, **123**, 307-312.

Eichenwald, H.F., Ababio, A., Arky, A.M. & Hartman, A.P. (1958) Epidemic diarrhea in premature and older infants caused by echo virus type 18. *Journal of the American Medical Association*, **166**, 1563-1566.

Elias, M.M. (1977) Distribution and titres of rotavirus antibodies in different age groups. *Journal of Hygiene*, **79**, 365-372.

Flewett, T.H. (1976) In *Acute Diarrhoea in Childhood*, Ciba Foundation Symposium No. 42 (new series), pp. 237-250. Amsterdam: Elsevier, Excerpta Medica, North Holland.

Flewett, T.H., Bryden A.S., Davies, H.A., Woode, G.N., Bridger, J.C. & Derrick, J.M. (1974) Relation between viruses from acute gastroenteritis of children and new born calves. *Lancet*, **ii**, 61-63.

Flewett, T.H., Bryden, A.S., Davies, H.A. & Morris, C.A. (1975) Epidemic viral enteritis in a long stay children's ward. *Lancet*, **i**, 4-5.

Fox, J.P., Elveback, L.R., Spigland, I., Frothingham, T.E., Stevens, D.A. & Huger, M. (1966) The Virus Watch Program: a continuing surveillance of viral infections in metropolitan New York families. I. Overall plan, methods of collecting and handling information and a summary report of specimens collected and illnesses observed. *American Journal of Epidemiology*, **83**, 389-412.

Ghose, L.H., Schnagl, R.D. & Holmes, I.H. (1978) Comparison of an enzyme-linked immunosorbent assay for quantitation of rotavirus antibodies with complement fixation in an epidemiological survey. *Journal of Clinical Microbiology*, **8**, 268-276.

Greenberg, H.B. & Kapikian, A.Z. (1978) Detection of Norwalk agent antibody and antigen by solid-phase radioimmunoassay and immune adherence hemagglutination assay. *Journal of the American Veterinary Medical Association*, **173**, 620-623.

Greenberg, H.B., Valdesuso, J., Yolken, R.H., Gangarosa, E., Gary, W., Wyatt, R.G., Konno, T., Suzuki, H., Chanock, R.M. & Kapikian, A.Z. (1979) Role of Norwalk virus in outbreaks of non-bacterial gastroenteritis. *Journal of Infectious Diseases*, **139**, 564-568.

Hara, M., Mukoyama, J., Tsuruhara, T., Ashiwara, Y., Saito, Y. & Tagaya, I. (1978) Acute gastroenteritis among schoolchildren associated with reovirus-like agent. *American Journal of Epidemiology*, **107**, 161-169.

Holmes, I.H. (1979) Viral gastroenteritis. *Progress in Medical Virology*, **25**, 1-36.

Johansson, M.E., Uhnoo, I., Kidd, A.H., Madeley, C.R. & Wadell, G. (1980) Direct identification of enteric adenovirus, a candidate new serotype, associated with infantile gastroenteritis by enzyme-linked immunosorbent assay. *Journal of Clinical Microbiology*, in press.

Kapikian, A.Z., Wyatt, R.G., Dolin, R., Thornhill, T.S., Kalica, A.R. & Chanock, R.M. (1972) Visualization by immune electron microscopy of a 27-nm particle associated with acute infectious nonbacterial gastroenteritis. *Journal of Virology*, **10**, 1075-1081.

Kapikian, A.Z., Cline, W.L., Mebus, C.A., Wyatt, R.G., Kalica, A.R., James, H.D., VanKirk, D.A., Chanock, R.M. & Kim, H.W. (1975) New complement fixation test for the human reovirus-like agent of infantile gastroenteritis. *Lancet*, **i**, 1056-1061.

Kim, H.W., Brandt, C.D., Kapikian, A.Z., Wyatt, R.G., Arrobio, J.O., Rodriguez, W.J., Chanock, R.M. & Parrott, R.H. (1977) Human reovirus-like agent infection. *Journal of the American Medical Association*, **238**, 404-407.

Kurtz, J.B. & Lee, T.W. (1978) Astrovirus gastroenteritis. Age distribution of antibody. *Medical Microbiology and Immunology*, **166**, 227-230.

Kurtz, J.B., Lee, T.W. & Pickering, D. (1977) Astrovirus associated gastroenteritis in a children's ward. *Journal of Clinical Pathology*, **30**, 948-952.

Logan, E.F., Pearson, G.R. & McNulty, M.S. (1979) Quantitative observations on experimental reo-like virus (rotavirus) infection in colostrum-deprived calves. *Veterinary Record*, **104**, 206-209.

Lycke, E., Blomberg, J., Berg, G., Eriksson, A. & Madsen, L. (1978) Epidemic acute diarrhoea in adults associated with infantile gastroenteritis virus. *Lancet*, **ii**, 1056-1057.

Madeley, C.R. (1979a) Viruses in the stools. *Journal of Clinical Pathology*, **32**, 1-10.

Madeley, C.R. (1979b) A comparison of the features of astroviruses and caliciviruses seen in samples of faeces by electron microscopy. *Journal of Infectious Diseases*, **139**, 519-524.

Madeley, C.R. & Cosgrove, B.P. (1975) 28 nm particles in faeces in infantile enteritis. *Lancet*, **ii**, 451-452.

Madeley, C.R. & Cosgrove, B.P. (1976) Caliciviruses in man. *Lancet* **i**, 199-200.

Madeley, C.R., Cosgrove, B.P. & Bell, E.J. (1978) Stool viruses in babies in Glasgow. 2. Investigations into normal babies in hospital. *Journal of Hygiene* (Cambridge), **81**, 285-294.

Madeley, C.R., Cosgrove, B.P., Bell, E.J. & Fallon, R.J. (1977) Stool viruses in babies in Glasgow. 1. Hospital admissions with diarrhoea. *Journal of Hygiene* (Cambridge), **78**, 261-273.

Mata, L., Urrutia, J.J., Serrato, G., Mohs, E. & Chin, T.D.Y. (1977) Viral infections during pregnancy and in early life. *American Journal of Clinical Nutrition*, **30**, 1834-1842.

McSwiggan, D.A., Cubitt, D. & Moore, W. (1978) Calicivirus associated with winter vomiting disease. *Lancet*, **i**, 1215.

Middleton, P.J., Szymanski, M.T. & Petric, M. (1977) Viruses associated with acute gastroenteritis in young children. *American Journal of Diseases of Children*, **131**, 733-737.

Murphy, A.M., Albrey, M.B. & Crewe, E.B. (1977) Rotavirus infections of neonates. *Lancet*, **ii**, 1149-1150.

Parks, W.P., Queiroga, L.T. & Melnick, J.L. (1967) Studies of infantile diarrhoea in Karachi, Pakistan. *American Journal of Epidemiology*, **85**, 469-478.

Patterson, W.J. & Bell, E.J. (1963) Poliomyelitis in a nursery school in Glasgow. *British Medical Journal*, **i**, 1574-1576.

Richmond, Shirley J., Caul, E.O., Dunn, S.M., Ashley, C.R., Clarke, S.K.R. & Seymour, N.R. (1979) An outbreak of gastroenteritis in young children caused by adenovirus. *Lancet*, **i**, 1178-1180.

Scott, T.M., Madeley, C.R., Cosgrove, B.P. & Stanfield, J.P. (1979) Stool viruses in babies in Glasgow. 3. Community studies. *Journal of Hygiene* (Cambridge), **83**, 469-485.

Snodgrass, D.R. & Gray, E.W. (1977) Detection and transmission of 30 nm virus particles (astroviruses) in faeces of lambs with diarrhoea. *Archives of Virology*, **55**, 287-291.

Spratt, H.C., Marks, M.I., Gomersall, M., Gill, P. & Pai, C.H. (1978) Nosocomial infantile gastroenteritis associated with minirotavirus and calicivirus. *Journal of Pediatrics*, **93**, 922-926.

Totterdell, B.M., Chrystie, I.L. & Banatvala, J.E. (1976) Rotavirus infections in a maternity unit. *Archives of Disease in Childhood*, **51**, 924-928.

Tufvesson, B. & Johnsson, T. (1976) Occurrence of reo-like viruses in young children with acute gastroenteritis. *Acta Pathologica et Microbiologica Scandinavica*, *B*, **84**, 22-28.

Whitelaw, A., Davies, H. & Parry, J. (1977) Electron microscopy of fatal adenovirus gastroenteritis. *Lancet*, **i**, 361.

Woode, G.N. (1969) Transmissible gastroenteritis of swine. *Veterinary Bulletin*, **39**, 239-248.

Woode, G.N. & Bridger, J.C. (1978) Isolation of small viruses resembling astroviruses and caliciviruses from acute enteritis of calves. *Journal of Medical Microbiology*, **11**, 441-452.

Yolken, R.H., Wyatt, R.G., Zissis, G., Brandt, C.D., Rodriguez, W.J., Kim, H.W., Parrot, R.H., Urrutia, J.J., Mata, L., Greenberg, H.B., Kapikian, A.Z. & Chanock, R.M. (1978) Epidemiology of human rotavirus types 1 and 2 as studied by enzyme-linked immunosorbent assay. *New England Journal of Medicine*, **299**, 1156-1161.

8
Bacterial Infections of the Gastrointestinal Tract

H.P. LAMBERT

It is now possible to distinguish several forms of pathogenesis in infective gastroenteritis, and those relevant to the bacterial diarrhoeas are the subject of this presentation. Some of the discoveries of the last decade, notably the advances in oral repletion in cholera and other forms of gastroenteritis, have made a huge impact on clinical management; others do not so far have much application. Nor can it be claimed that the newer knowledge of diarrhoeal disease is yet matched by increased precision of clinical diagnosis. Certainly polar groups can be distinguished, notably cholera as the type of small bowel disturbance caused by acute imbalances of water and salt transport without bacterial invasion or systemic illness, and acute bacillary dysentery, at any rate in its severe form, as the type of acute bacterial colitis. But between these extremes lies a great mass of diarrhoeal disease, the pathogenesis of which cannot be defined at the bedside; indeed, the clinician is often at a loss even to know at what site or sites in the bowel the main disturbance arises. Again, although a number of newly identified causes of bacterial diarrhoea, such as *Campylobacter* and *Yersinia*, have been added to the traditional list, no bacterial or viral aetiology can yet be assigned in a substantial proportion of acute bowel disturbances thought to be infective in orgin.

Cholera

Modern work on the pathogenesis of cholera is well known, and an excellent monograph by Barua and Burrows (1974) can be consulted for all aspects of the disease. The account here will be limited to a brief summary to serve as an introduction to the newer work on diarrhoea caused by *Escherichia coli*. After decades of controversy cholera can now be regarded as an example of a 'toxin' disease just as much as can diphtheria and tetanus. The vibrio extensively colonizes, but does not invade, the bowel and produces a toxin which is present in culture filtrates. The effects are those of isotonic loss of small bowel fluid with consequent shrinkage of the extracellular fluid and metabolic acidosis, but only trivial histological changes, with none of the signs of acute inflammation, can be found in the mucosa to which the organisms attach. All manifestations of the illness can be ascribed to this disturbance of small bowel transport mechanisms. Choleragen bound to the enterocyte acts by stimulating adenylcyclase, leading to increased intracellular concentration of adenosine 3′,5′-cyclic monophosphate (cyclic AMP) which in turn leads to the defects of ionic transport, namely, increased secretion of Cl^- and possibly HCO_3^- and decreased coupled influx of Na^+ and Cl^-.

Escherichia coli

This organism constitutes one of the main components of the normal aerobic flora of the lower bowel. The evidence that some strains of *E. coli*, which came to be known as enteropathogenic serotypes, are important in the aetiology of infant diarrhoea, was derived mainly from epidemiological studies. The role of *E. coli* in diarrhoeal disease has now been much extended. Diarrhoea caused by *E. coli* is evidently not confined to the 'enteropathic' strains. *E. coli* can cause diarrhoea in adults and older children as well as in infants, and at least three pathogenic mechanisms are involved; but the pathogenesis of the form of *E. coli* diarrhoea first described, that caused by enteropathic *E. coli* in infancy, has proved a most elusive problem. These lines of progress in human diarrhoeas have been initiated chiefly by the work on cholera and by parallel advances in the study of *E. coli* diarrhoeas of farm animals.

Enterotoxic *E. coli*

The methods used in the assay of cholera toxin were gradually refined, extended and applied to the measurement of other bacterial toxins. These developments showed that certain strains of *E. coli* of human bowel origin did produce toxins with characteristics similar to those found in *E. coli* from animal diarrhoeas (Smith and Halls, 1967). One is heat labile (LT), a protein with some antigenic relationship to cholera toxin and acting in a similar way by activation of cyclic AMP. The other is heat stable (ST), a polypeptide, poorly antigenic and inactive in the tissue culture systems used to detect the action of LT on adenylcyclase activity. ST is thought to act by stimulating cyclic guanosine monophosphate (GMP) in the bowel mucosa (Hughes et al, 1978). Strains producing these toxins are known as enterotoxigenic *E. coli* (ETEC) and may produce ST or LT alone, or both types of toxin. Toxin production is mediated by a heterogeneous group of plasmids (Gyles, So and Falkow, 1974); by contrast, production of cholera toxin is chromosomally determined.

Identification of toxigenic *E. coli* on any scale is technically demanding and, until recently, had been used by relatively few researchers, so that epidemiological evidence of the role of these organisms in human disease was slow to develop. It has now become evident that ETEC are an important cause of travellers' diarrhoea. Two of the largest studies are that of Gorbach et al (1975), with evidence of acquisition of a toxigenic *E. coli* in 26 of 38 subjects developing diarrhoea and in six of 41 controls, and that of Merson et al (1976), with toxigenic strains in 23 of 59 patients and six of 62 controls. Another important group of diarrhoeas in which ETEC have been implicated are the non-cholera diarrhoeas of tropical countries; they have been identified in all age groups and in a number of countries (Nalin et al, 1975; Sack et al, 1977). By contrast, the role of ETEC in infantile diarrhoea in wealthy countries is still uncertain since they have been found with variable frequency, and some studies have revealed no strains of this sort (Echeverria, Blacklow and Smith, 1975; Gurwith and Williams, 1977). Moreover, ETEC were rarely found in two studies in which jejunal fluid was examined, although in one of them LT-producing strains were found in 10 of 64 stool specimens (Sack et al, 1975; Ellis-Pegler et al, 1979).

Mucosal attachment. Studies in animal diarrhoeas revealed that enterotoxigenic strains also require the capacity to adhere to the mucosal surface of the small bowel in order to exhibit full pathogenicity (Smith and Linggood, 1971; Jones and Rutter, 1972). This property, which like toxigenicity is determined by transmissible plasmids, is mediated by specialized pili visible on electron microscopy. A number of plasmid-controlled adhesion factors has also been identified in *E. coli* strains of human origin. One was revealed by its capacity to colonize the rabbit bowel, and a similar but antigenically distinct colonization factor antigen (CFA I and CFA II) was later defined; most toxigenic strains of *E. coli* produce one or other, but not both, of these antigens (Evans and Evans, 1978). Another antigenically distinct adherence factor has been studied in *E. coli* 026 and found to be transferred coordinately with resistance to a number of antibiotics (Williams et al, 1978).

Mucosal attachment has been studied especially in *E. coli* but such factors are certainly important in other pathogenic bowel bacteria. The attachment of *Vibrio cholerae* has been studied in great detail (Freter and Jones, 1976) and attachment factors are now also being examined in other species, notably in *Shigellae* and *Salmonellae*.

Enteroinvasive *E. coli*

In the late 1960s Japanese workers identified strains of *E. coli*, generally sharing cross-reacting O antigens with *Shigella* serotypes as the cause of outbreaks of diarrhoea with dysenteric features. Their pathogenic role, and evidence for colonic inflammation rather than small bowel colonization as a feature of their pathogenesis, were established in the volunteer studies of Dupont et al (1971). The epidemiological importance of these strains is apparently substantially smaller than that of the enterotoxigenic serotypes, but is none the less well established for at least two of them. *E. coli* 0124 has been associated with a number of outbreaks of diarrhoea including a notable episode in which at least 400 people in the USA were infected by imported French cheese heavily contaminated by this organism (Marier et al, 1973). Another 'dysenteric' serotype, *E. coli* 0164, has also been identified in several outbreaks in several countries.

Enteropathogenic *E. coli* (EPEC)

Although the classical enteropathogenic serotypes of *E. coli* do not appear to impose as great a threat to infant health as when they were first identified in the 1940s, recent work has confirmed older epidemiological evidence of their relationship to infantile gastroenteritis. Paradoxically, the mechanisms of their pathogenicity are still obscure, since they do not produce enterotoxins, nor do they appear to act like the 'dysenteric' strains. Two possible mechanisms have been postulated. Klipstein et al (1978) showed EPEC strains to induce disturbance of water and electrolyte transport in the perfused rat jejunum although giving negative results in the standard tests of LT or ST enterotoxin; so perhaps EPEC are indeed also enterotoxigenic if tested by suitable methods. Another possible mechanism is suggested by the cytotoxic action which some of these strains display on Vero cells in tissue culture. The significance of the effect remains uncertain since only 25 of 253 strains of EPEC isolated from infants with diarrhoea showed this property, and strains giving positive results in the perfused rat jejunum were negative in the Vero test system (Scotland et al, 1980). Cytotoxicity has been established in an *E. coli* infection in rabbits by Cantey and Blake (1977), who showed, by electron microscopy, the action of their strain in destroying the microvillous border and adhering to the enterocyte.

Shigella

The *Shigella* species are confined in their pathogenicity to man and some primates, and are spread by the faecal-oral route, with secondary environmental contamination. Volunteer studies have, however, shown an important difference between shigellosis and other bacterial infections of the human gut, such as typhoid, cholera or enterotoxic *E. coli*. Whereas the infecting dose of the latter organisms (at least under the conditions of the experiment but perhaps not in natural circumstances) is high, of the order of 10^5 to 10^{10} organisms, *Shigella dysenteriae* type 1 is able to induce infection and disease in volunteers in the minute inoculum of 10 to 100 organisms (Levine et al, 1973).

Shigella infections are classically associated with an acute colitis and this clinical evidence of invasive capacity is matched by experimental analogues in which the organisms are shown to penetrate epithelial cells in tissue culture and in the guinea pig cornea. But just as *Salmonella* infections are now recognized to affect the colon as well as the small bowel, so too has evidence been accumulated of small bowel as well as colonic involvement in shigellosis. Several strains of *Shigella* induce intestinal fluid secretion in model systems for the detection of enterotoxin, apparently by activation of jejunal adenylcyclase (Charney et al, 1976). These two sites of action are sometimes detectable in the clinical syndrome in which watery diarrhoea in the early stages is followed later by the dysenteric component of cramps and bloody mucoid stools.

The nature of *Shigella* toxin and its relevance in pathogenesis have been extensively studied by Keusch and his colleagues. It appears that invasiveness rather than toxigenicity is the chief determinant of virulence but, since patients do develop antitoxic antibody and the toxin has been shown to bind to a cell membrane receptor, small amounts of toxin may yet be important in pathogenesis at the cellular level (Keusch, 1979). Certainly small bowel secretion is an important component of experimental shigellosis in the rhesus monkey (Rout et al, 1975).

Salmonella

The traditional account of the pathology of non-typhoid salmonellosis describes a disease confined to the small intestine, and characterized by inflammation, accumulation of both polymorphonuclear leucocytes and macrophages, and oedema affecting mainly the lamina propria. Clinicians have long noted that patients with acute salmonella gastroenteritis, and from whom no other pathogen has been recovered, often have bloody stools and other features suggestive of colonic involvement. Boyd's early work on the colon in salmonellosis has been confirmed and extended by Mandal and Mani (1976) who found colonic inflammation in 21 of 23 patients in hospital with salmonella diarrhoea. Rout et al (1974) showed similar changes in the salmonella-infected rhesus monkey. Additional work by Day, Mandal and Morson (1978) detailed the colonic changes in human salmonellosis. Acute inflammatory changes were present in the mucosa and submucosa, with polymorphonuclear leucocytes and sometimes more chronic inflammatory cells in the lamina propria, while crypt abscesses and mucus depletion were seen in a few biopsies.

Current interest in enterotoxins has been extended to the salmonellas. Koupal and Deibel (1975) characterized an enterotoxin produced by *Salmonella enteritidis* and showing properties common to the LT and ST toxins of *E. coli*, and evidence of enterotoxin production has been obtained in a number of test systems, but experiments designed to decide if enterotoxin production is important in the pathogenesis of salmonella gastroenteritis have given conflicting results. Adherence factors are also being studied, as with cholera and *E. coli*, and Tannock, Blumershine and Savage (1975) have published fascinating data on the mechanism of attachment and penetration of the ileal mucosa of mice by *Salmonella typhimurium*. A comprehensive review of all aspects of salmonellosis has recently been provided by Turnbull (1979).

Campylobacter

This has been known for years in veterinary practice and occasionally isolated from human blood cultures. Successful techniques were finally developed by Butzler (1973) in Belgium and by Skirrow (1977) in England for selecting these fastidious bacteria from the bowel flora. A flood of interesting information has followed showing this organism as a common cause of acute gastrointestinal illness in all countries able to detect its presence. More than 6000 isolates were reported to the Communicable Diseases Surveillance Centre in 1978. Although, as with other pathogens, subclinical carriage occurs as do mild illnesses with no special features, fully developed *Campylobacter* enteritis has a number of features which allow at least a tentative clinical diagnosis. A febrile prodromal illness is found in about half the patients, abdominal colic is common, and initial watery diarrhoea is often followed by a colitic phase with blood and leucocytes in the stool. One important feature is accounted for by the predilection shown by this organism for the terminal small bowel. The clinical features may lead to exploration of the abdomen for 'acute appendicitis', when the jejunum and ileum are found to be acutely inflamed and the mesenteric nodes enlarged. The disease may also simulate typhoid and ulcerative colitis. The pathogenesis has not yet been examined in great detail but seems to involve chiefly direct invasion of the target organs, heat-stable but not heat-labile enterotoxin being produced by only a few strains.

Campylobacter is usually found in the stool for a few weeks after the first identification, but human-to-human infection seems to be uncommon in adults. Small children may act as a source and nursery outbreaks have been observed. Most human *Campylobacter* infections seem to arise from animal sources, especially from dogs and chickens; waterborne and milkborne outbreaks, the latter of course from unpasteurized milk, are described but the organism does not often appear to be foodborne.

Yersinia enterocolitica

A wide range of syndromes has now been associated with infection by this organism. As far as the bowel is concerned, the association with acute diarrhoeal disease is still uncertain; more definite is its relationship with terminal ileitis which may closely simulate acute appendicitis in its clinical presentation. In contrast to the more familiar bacterial bowel pathogens, symptoms may continue for some weeks or months. The more prolonged forms of disease as seen in specialist gastroenterological practice are exemplified by the description of Vantrappen et al (1977) who saw 37 adults with abdominal pain and diarrhoea lasting between one week and several months; 40 per cent of them had appendicitis-like syndromes. The terminal ileum showed a coarse nodular pattern and colonoscopy revealed colitis-like changes, with inflammatory changes and ulceration. A 'follicular ileitis' often persisted for several months.

Yersinia enterocolitis appears to be an invasive rather than a toxin disease; in an experimental model in mice, infection is initiated in the Peyer's patches, followed by caseous necrosis of the mesenteric glands, and septicaemic spread to other sites.

Clostridial Bowel Disease

The common form of food poisoning caused by certain strains of *Clostridium perfringens* type A has been well recognized for many years. So has a very different disease, 'pig-bel', a necrotizing enteritis common in Papua New Guinea and associated with infections by *Cl. perfringens* type C, and against which an effective vaccine has now been produced (Lawrence et al, 1979) in the form of an absorbed toxoid.

Evidence of clostridial involvement has now also been obtained in two other human bowel diseases. *Clostridium butyricum* is one of the contenders for a bacterial aetiology in necrotizing enterocolitis of the newborn (Howard et al, 1977), although many other organisms have been involved and the pathogenesis of the syndrome is still uncertain. Stronger evidence comes from another syndrome, pseudomembranous colitis, first described before the antibiotic era, but now most commonly associated with antimicrobial drugs. Colitis was most frequently associated with lincomycin and clindamycin but the syndrome has followed administration of ampicillin, other penicillins, cephalosporins, co-trimoxazole and metronidazole. Earlier reports of antibiotic-associated colitis especially implicated tetracyclines and chloramphenicol. Stools of patients with this type of colitis contain a heat-labile toxin active against many cell lines, and this cytotoxin can be neutralized by antibody against *Clostridium sordellii*. Search for a candidate *Clostridium* sp, however, revealed that *Clostridium difficile*, but not *Clostridium sordellii*, could often be found in the stools of patients with antibiotic colitis. This paradox was resolved when it was found that antitoxin raised against *Cl. sordellii* cross-reacts with the cytotoxin of *Cl. difficile*. There appears to have emerged a strong association between the development of antibiotic colitis and the presence of *Cl. difficile* and its toxin in the stools (Bartlett et al, 1978; Larson, Price and Honour, 1978). The concept of *Cl. difficile* and its toxin as the cause of antibiotic colitis has led to successful trials of treatment with vancomycin, to which the organism is susceptible, but many problems remain. The organism is only occasionally isolated from the stools of healthy adults, but neonates can apparently maintain high populations of the organism without ill effect; and although selection of the bowel flora is thought important in its emergence as a pathogen, *Cl. difficile* is sometimes found in the stools of patients with colitis who have received antibiotics inhibitory to the strain.

CONCLUSION

In parallel with advances on viral involvement in bowel infection, knowledge of bacterial bowel infection has progressed enormously in the last decade. New important pathogens have been identified and several strands of pathogenesis disentangled. There is thus a real hope, as more becomes known of relevant bacterial components and of pathogenic mechanisms, that oral or injected vaccines against bacterial gut infections may be developed to follow the example of the recent pig-bel vaccine. As always, application of existing knowledge is slow and difficult; general use of the oral rehydration regimens developed by the World Health Organization and others would yield a huge gain to child health in developing countries.

This presentation has been confined to acute bacterial infections of the gut. Just as fascinating are the developments in chronic bowel disease. Some are familiar themes, such as bowel involvement in tuberculosis and actinomycosis. The probable microbial aetiology of Whipple's disease and its response to antimicrobial drug treatment is well recorded. The current debate about the possible role of atypical mycobacteria in Crohn's disease has still to be resolved. Above all, the role of bacteria in sprue, and in the development of malnutritional syndromes of childhood in developing countries, provide an important challenge in future work.

REFERENCES

Bartlett, J.G., Chang, T.W., Gurwith, M., Gorbach, S.L. & Onderdonk, A.B. (1978) Antibiotic-associated pseudomembranous colitis due to toxin producing clostridia. *New England Journal of Medicine*, **298**, 531-534.

Barua, D. & Burrows, W. (1974) *Cholera*. Philadelphia: W.B. Saunders.

Butzler, J.P., Dekeyser, P., DeTrain, M. & DeHaen, F. (1973) Related vibrios in stools. *Journal of Pediatrics*, **82**, 493-495.

Cantey, J.R. & Blake, R.K. (1977) Diarrhoea due to *Escherichia coli* in the rabbit: a novel mechanism. *Journal of Infectious Diseases*, **135**, 454-462.

Charney, A.N., Gots, R.E., Formal, S.B. & Gianella, R.A. (1976) Activation of intestinal mucosal adenylate cyclase by *Shigella dysenteriae* I enterotoxin. *Gastroenterology*, **70**, 1085-1090.

Day, D.W., Mandal, B.K. & Morson, B.C. (1978) The rectal biopsy appearances in salmonella colitis. *Histopathology*, **2**, 117-131.

DuPont, H., Formal, S.B., Hornick, R.B., Snyder, M.J., Libonati, J.P., Sheahan, D.G., Labrec, E.H. & Kalas, J.P. (1971) Pathogenesis of *Escherichia coli* diarrhea. *New England Journal of Medicine*, **285**, 1-9.

Echeverria, P., Blacklow, N.R. & Smith, D.H. (1975) Role of heat-labile toxigenic *Escherichia coli* and Reovirus-like agent in diarrhoea in Boston children. *Lancet*, **ii**, 1113-1116.

Ellis-Pegler, R.B., Lambert, H.P., Rowe, B. & Gross, R.J. (1979) *Escherichia coli* in gastroenteritis of children in London and Jamaica. *Journal of Hygiene* (Cambridge), **82**, 115-121.

Evans, D.G. & Evans, D.J. (1978) New surface-associated heat-labile colonization factor antigen (CFA/11) produced by enterotoxigenic *Escherichia coli* of serogroups 06 and 08. *Infection and Immunity*, **21**, 638-647.

Freter, R. & Jones, G.W. (1976) Adhesive properties of *Vibrio cholerae*: nature of the interaction with intact mucosal surfaces. *Infection and Immunity*, **14**, 246-256.

Gorbach, S.L., Kean, B.H., Evans, D.G., Evans, D.J. & Bessudo, D. (1975) Travellers' diarrhoea and toxigenic *Escherichia coli*. *New England Journal of Medicine*, **296**, 1210-1213.

Gurwith, M.J. & Williams, T.B. (1977) Gastroenteritis in children — a two-year review in Manitoba. I. Aetiology. *Journal of Infectious Diseases*, **136**, 239-247.

Gyles, C.L. So, M. & Falkow, S. (1974) The enterotoxin plasmids of *Escherichia coli*. *Journal of Infectious Diseases*, **130**, 40-49.

Howard, F.M., Flynn, D.M., Bradley, J.M., Noone, P. & Szawatkowski, M. (1977) Outbreak of necrotising enterocolitis caused by *Clostridium butyricum*. *Lancet*, **ii**, 1099-1102.

Hughes, J.M., Murad, F., Chang, B. & Guerrant, R.L. (1978) Role of cyclic GMP in the action of heat-stable enterotoxin of *Escherichia coli*. *Nature*, **271**, 755-756.

Jones, G.W. & Rutter, J.M. (1972) Role of K88 antigen in the pathogenesis of neonatal diarrhoea caused by *Escherichia coli* in piglets. *Infection and Immunity*, **6**, 918-927.

Keusch, G.T. (1979) Specific membrane receptors: pathogenetic and therapeutic implications in infectious diseases. *Review of Infectious Diseases*, **1**, 517-529.

Klipstein, F.A., Rowe, B., Engert, R.F., Short, H.B. & Gross, R.J. (1978) Enterotoxigenicity of enteropathogenic serotypes of *Escherichia coli* isolated from infants with epidemic diarrhoea. *Infection and Immunity*, **21**, 171-178.

Koupal, L.R. & Deibel, R.H. (1975) Assay, characterization, and localization of an enterotoxin produced by salmonella. *Infection and Immunity*, **11**, 14-22.

Larson, H.E., Price, A.B. & Honour, P. (1978) *Clostridium difficile* and the aetiology of pseudomembranous colitis. *Lancet*, **i**, 1063-1066.

Lawrence, G., Shann, F., Freestone, D.S. & Walker, P.D. (1979) Prevention of necrotising enteritis in Papua New Guinea by active immunisation. *Lancet*, **1**, 227-230.

Levine, M.M., DuPont, H.L., Formal, S.B., Hornick, R.B., Takeuchi, A., Gangarosa, E.J., Snyder, M.J. & Libonati, J.P. (1973) Pathogenesis of *Shigella dysenteriae* 1 (Shiga) dysentery. *Journal of Infectious Diseases*, **127**, 261-270.

Mandal, B.K. & Mani, V. (1976) Colonic involvement in salmonellosis. *Lancet*, **i**, 887-888.

Marier, R., Wells, T.G., Swanson, R.C., Callahan, W. & Mehlman, I.J. (1973) An outbreak of enteropathogenic *Escherichia coli* food-borne disease traced to imported French cheese. *Lancet*, **ii**, 1376-1378.

Merson, M.H., Morris, G.K., Sack, D.A., Wells, J.G., Feeley, J.C., Sack, R.B., Creech, W.B., Kapikian, A.Z. & Gangarosa, E.J. (1976) Travellers' diarrhea in Mexico. A prospective study of physicians and family members attending a Congress. *New England Journal of Medicine*, **294**, 1299-1305.

Nalin, D.R., Rahaman, M., McLaughlin, J.C., Yunus, M. & Curlin, G. (1975) Enterotoxigenic *Escherichia coli* and idiopathic diarrhoea in Bangladesh. *Lancet*, **ii**, 1116-1119.

Rout, W.R., Formal, S.B., Dammin, G.J. & Giannella, R.A. (1974) Pathophysiology of salmonella diarrhoea in the rhesus monkey: intestinal transport, morphological and bacteriological studies. *Gastroenterology*, **67**, 59-70.

Rout, W.R., Formal, S.B., Fiannella, R.A. & Dammin, G.J. (1975) Pathophysiology of shigella diarrhoea in the rhesus monkey: intestinal transport, morphological and bacteriological studies. *Gastroenterology*, **68**, 270-278.

Sack, R.B., Hirschhorn, N., Brownlee, I., Cash, R.A., Woodward, W.E. & Sack, D.A. (1975) Enterotoxigenic *Escherichia coli*-associated diarrhoeal disease in Apache children. *New England Journal of Medicine*, **292**, 1041-1045.

Sack, D.A., McLaughlin, J.C., Sack, R.B., Orskov, F. & Orskov, I. (1977) Enterotoxigenic *Escherichia coli* isolated from patients at a hospital in Dacca. *Journal of Infectious Diseases*, **135**, 275-280.

Scotland, S.M., Day, N.P., Willshaw, G.A. & Rowe, B. (1980) Cytotoxic enteropathogenic *Escherichia coli* (correspondence). *Lancet*, **i**, 90.

Skirrow, M.B. (1977) Campylobacter enteritis — a 'new' disease. *British Medical Journal*, **ii**, 9-11.

Smith, H.W. & Halls, S. (1967) Studies on *Escherichia coli* enterotoxin. *Journal of Pathology and Bacteriology*, **93**, 531-542.

Smith, H.W. & Linggood, M.A. (1971) The transmissible nature of enterotoxin production in a human enteropathogenic strain of *Escherichia coli*. *Journal of Medical Microbiology*, **4**, 301-305.

Tannock, G.W., Blumershine, R.V. & Savage, D.C. (1975) Association of *Salmonella typhimurium* with, and its invasion of, the ileal mucosa in mice. *Infection and Immunity*, **11**, 365-370.

Turnbull, P.C.B. (1979) Food poisoning with special reference to salmonella — its epidemiology, pathogenesis and control. *Clinics in Gastroenterology*, **8** (3), 663-714.

Vantrappen, G., Agg, H.O., Ponette, E., Geboes, K. & Bertrand, L. (1977) Yersinia enteritis and enterocolitis: gastroenterological aspects. *Gastroenterology*, **72**, 220-227.

Williams, P.H., Sedgwick, M.I., Evans, N., Turner, P.J., George, R.H. & McNeish, A.S. (1978) Adherence of enteropathogenic *Escherichia coli* to human intestinal mucosa is mediated by colicinogenic conjugative plasmid. *Infection and Immunity*, **22**, 393-402.

9
Plasmid-Mediated and Other Characteristics of *Escherichia coli* Enteropathogenic for Domestic Mammals: Their Influence on Small Intestinal Colonization

H. WILLIAMS SMITH

Escherichia coli is an important cause of diarrhoea in calves, lambs, piglets and recently-weaned pigs, the clinical disease in these domestic mammals closely resembling that in human beings. Because many experiments likely to yield important information on *E. coli* diarrhoea, by their very nature, cannot be performed on human beings, the hope has been that conclusions drawn from such experiments in domestic mammals would be applicable to human beings and this indeed has turned out to be the case. The acquisition of the information has been greatly aided, or only made possible, by the discovery that several characteristics of enteropathogenic *E. coli* are borne on transferable plasmids. Exploiting the fact that plasmids can be transferred from one bacterium to another and can also be removed from them, lines of bacteria have been constructed that, as far as could be determined, were isogenic apart from possessing different combinations of the plasmids found in enteropathogenic strains. The administration of these bacteria (Smith and Linggood, 1971, 1972; Jones and Rutter, 1972; Smith and Huggins, 1978) or of extracts of them (Smith and Gyles, 1970) to domestic mammals revealed that not only were some of these plasmid-borne characters importantly involved in the pathogenesis of *E. coli* diarrhoea but that were it not for them the disease would be of little significance. The more important findings of these experiments are summarized in Table 1 and they provide a basic explanation of the pathogenesis of *E. coli* diarrhoea. This is that for a bacterium to be enteropathogenic it must possess at least two properties: it must be able to proliferate in the small intestine, which it does by adhering to the epithelium, and, when proliferating there, it must produce enterotoxin which provokes the movement of fluid from the body into the alimentary tract, giving rise to the acute severe diarrhoea which is the main characteristic of the disease.

Many incompletely-explored aspects of the pathogenesis of *E. coli* diarrhoea

Table 1. *Summary of effects of plasmids in enteropathogenic* E. coli

Plasmids present		Effect	
'Adhesive'[a]	Enterotoxin	Small intestinal proliferation	Diarrhoea
−	−	−	−
−	+	−	−
+	−	++	+ or −
+	+	++	++

[a] 88 for piglets; 99 for calves, lambs and piglets

in domestic mammals, of course, remain: for example, the part played by bacterial components other than the plasmid-determined 88 and 99 antigens in small intestine proliferation. The 987P antigen, which has not been shown to be plasmid-mediated, has now been found important in this respect in some enteropathogenic piglet strains (Isaacson, Nagy and Moon, 1977; Nagy, Moon and Isaacson, 1977) but many enteropathogenic strains exist, especially those that infect recently-weaned pigs, that possess neither the 88, 99 or 987P antigens. The K antigens, too, appear essential for some piglet strains to express their full enteropathogenicity (Nagy, Moon and Isaacson, 1976; Isaacson, Nagy and Moon, 1977; Nagy, Moon and Isaacson, 1977). The available evidence, too, indicates that organisms possessing the 99 or the 987P antigen may only be able to proliferate in the more posterior parts of the small intestine of piglets whereas 88^+ organisms can proliferate throughout it. This is undoubtedly important in determining the severity of the diarrhoea produced by enteropathogenic *E. coli* because, as Table 2 shows, the anterior part of the small intestine is much more susceptible to enterotoxin than the posterior part. Nearly all 88^+ strains possess transmissible Raf genes (Smith and Parsell, 1975), identifiable by ability to ferment raffinose, and molecular studies (Shipley, Gyles and Falkow, 1978) confirm that they are located on the same plasmid as the 88 genes; whether they are

Table 2. *Susceptibility of different parts of pig small intestine to* E. coli *enterotoxin*

Part	Volume of exudate (ml) in ligated segment in that part	Part	Volume of exudate (ml) in ligated segment in that part
1	60	8	5
2	60	9	5
3	40	10	5
4	50	11	0
5	20	12	0
6	10	13	0
7	10		

Part 1 was next to the stomach and part 13 was next to the caecum; a ligated segment in each part was inoculated with 1 ml of a broth culture of a porcine enteropathogenic strain, that produced heat-labile and heat-stable enterotoxin, 24 hours before the pig was killed.

implicated in the aetiology of diarrhoea is not known. The picture is further complicated by the fact that some pigs have an hereditary resistance to infection with strains possessing the 88 antigen. At least two phenotypes exist, one that permits adhesion of 88⁺ organisms to the small intestinal epithelium and one that does not. The phenotypes are the product of two alleles at a single locus inherited in a simple Mendelian manner, the product of the 'adhesive' allele being dominant over the product of the non-adhesive allele (Sellwood et al, 1974, 1975; Rutter et al, 1975). Whether 88-resistant piglets could be infected with 88⁻ enteropathogens was not known.

More information on the subjects referred to above, and especially on the relative importance of different bacterial components in promoting colonization of the small intestine of different species of domestic mammals, was clearly necessary and it was obtained by inoculating animals orally with laboratory-constructed forms of strains that differed from each other, as far as could be ascertained, only by the presence or absence of one or more of these components; the results of these experiments are discussed below. Because of the many genetic and other variations that exist among young animals of the same species, the sets of laboratory-constructed forms of the same strain were studied in the *same* experimental animal. Spontaneous mutants of the forms, each resistant to a different antibiotic, were used so that the concentration of each in the different parts of the alimentary tract could be estimated by performing bacterial counts on appropriate antibiotic-containing culture media; preliminary studies had revealed that such mutants survived or multiplied in the alimentary tract to an extent similar to that of the strains from which they were derived. Colostrum-deprived experimental animals were used to negate the unequal influence that antibody might exert on the multiplication of the different forms in the alimentary tract; furthermore, the animals were all fed on the same diet, heat-sterilized cows' milk, three times daily by stomach tube, those of the same species receiving the same amount. The availability of 88-susceptible (S) piglets, kindly supplied by Dr R. Sellwood of the Agricultural Research Council Institute for Research on Animal Disease, and of 88-resistant (R) piglets provided information on their differing susceptibility to the colonizing factors that were studied. All experimental animals were inoculated within eight hours of birth. Because *E. coli* multiplies profusely in the stomach of piglets in the first 16 hours or so of life and floods into the small intestine (Smith and Jones, 1963) they, and the other animals, were given an inoculum in their first feed in which the *E. coli* strains under study were always greatly outnumbered by organisms of a non-pathogenic *E. coli* strain called P403 and by lactobacilli. This ensured that the numbers of enteropathogenic *E. coli* in the stomach were never high enough to produce sufficient enterotoxin to cause diarrhoea when it entered the small intestine and that the number of organisms entering that organ was too low to give a false impression of colonization. After inoculation, the animals were inspected at frequent intervals for evidence of diarrhoea and its severity assessed. If death appeared imminent they were killed. Otherwise, they were killed 28 to 32 hours after inoculation, previous experience having revealed that diarrhoea seldom commences after this time. Immediately after they were killed, the concentrations of viable organisms of each of the inoculated *E. coli* strains in the contents of the stomach, seven equal-sized portions of small intestine, the caecum, colon and rectum and in scrapings of the walls of the seven small intestinal portions were estimated by performing counts on sets of plates of MacConkey's agar containing such antibiotics as were necessary to distinguish all the inoculated strains from each other. The spleen was also examined to confirm that bacterial invasion of the body had not occurred.

All the animals that had diarrhoea when they were killed were found to have at least 10^8 enterotoxigenic (Ent$^+$) *E. coli* organisms per gram of their posterior small intestinal contents. In general, the further forward in the small intestine these organisms proliferated the more severe was the diarrhoea and the more pronounced were the clinical signs of dehydration, an observation that was in agreement with the data presented in Table 2. Most of the animals that had to be killed before the end of the customary 28 to 32 hours observation period because they were near to death had high concentrations of the infecting organisms in their anterior small intestine; they included many piglets that had been given 88$^+$ organisms. Concentrations of *E. coli* greater than 10^7 per gram of contents were seldom found in the stomachs of the experimental animals. They consisted mainly of organisms of the non-pathogenic strain P403 which had formed the major *E. coli* component of the inoculum. These organisms were present in the small intestines in low concentrations only, those in the wall scrapings of a particular part being about 10 times lower than those in its contents. By contrast, organisms of strains that proliferated in the small intestine were often 10 times more numerous in the wall scrapings of a particular part than in its contents.

The Effect of the Ent, 88 and 99 Plasmids on Small Intestinal Colonization by an O9:K36:H19 Non-Pathogenic Strain of *E. coli*

Different combinations of the 88, 99 and Ent plasmids were implanted in a non-pathogenic O9:K36:H19 *E. coli* strain isolated originally from the faeces of a healthy pig; the Ent plasmid coded for heat-labile (LT) and heat-stable (ST) enterotoxins as defined by Smith and Gyles (1970). The results of giving these forms of the O9:K36:H19 strain orally to an 88S and an 88R piglet and to a calf and lamb are summarized in Table 3. The 88S piglet, the calf and the lamb developed diarrhoea which was associated with proliferation of 88$^+$99$^-$Ent$^+$ organisms throughout the small intestine of the piglet and with proliferation of 88$^-$99$^+$Ent$^+$ organisms in the middle and posterior parts of the small intestines of the calf and lamb. The 88R piglet remained healthy and the concentrations of 88$^+$99$^-$Ent$^+$ organisms in its small intestine, as in the case of the calf and lamb, were no higher than those of 88$^-$99$^-$Ent$^+$ organisms. 88$^-$99$^+$Ent$^+$ organisms were present only in low concentrations in the small intestines of the 88S and 88R piglets. When the experiment was repeated in two 88S piglets employing a dose of 10^9 viable organisms of each of the four forms of the O9:K36:H19 strain instead of the customary 10^7, the 88$^-$99$^+$Ent$^+$ form proliferated to a moderate degree in

Table 3. *The concentration of organisms in different parts of the alimentary tract of an 88S[a] and an 88R[a] piglet, a calf and a lamb given orally a mixture of forms of a non-pathogenic O9:K36:H19 strain in which had been implanted 88, 99 and Ent plasmids[b]*

Animal	Forms of strain in mixture	stomach contents	\multicolumn{4}{c}{wall scrapings of small intestine, part[c]}	colon contents
			1	3	5	7	
88S piglet[a]	88⁻99⁻Ent⁻	6.6	5.9	5.6	6.2	6.3	6.8
	88⁻99⁻Ent⁺	5.2	4.0	4.2	4.6	5.0	5.5
	88⁺99⁻Ent⁺	6.4	9.0	9.2	9.4	9.4	8.5
	88⁻99⁺Ent⁺	4.7	4.3	4.0	4.7	5.0	5.0
88R piglet[a]	88⁻99⁻Ent⁻	5.8	3.0	5.0	7.6	6.6	8.3
	88⁻99⁻Ent⁺	4.5	3.0	5.2	6.4	5.6	6.8
	88⁺99⁻Ent⁺	3.0	<2.0	2.3	3.2	3.0	4.7
	88⁻99⁺Ent⁺	3.5	2.0	4.0	5.2	5.0	6.0
Calf	88⁻99⁻Ent⁻	5.3	4.4	4.6	5.2	5.9	7.9
	88⁻99⁻Ent⁺	4.6	4.2	4.4	4.5	5.3	6.4
	88⁺99⁻Ent⁺	2.7	2.6	2.7	3.5	4.2	5.9
	88⁻99⁺Ent⁺	3.5	4.6	7.7	8.6	8.5	9.2
Lamb	88⁻99⁻Ent⁺	4.2	3.0	2.5	3.0	3.6	4.2
	88⁺99⁻Ent⁺	<2.0	2.5	3.0	3.0	3.2	3.2
	88⁻99⁺Ent⁺	3.7	3.6	8.5	8.3	8.0	8.7

Number of organisms of stated form ($\log_{10}$ per g)

Data from Smith and Huggins (1978), with kind permission of the editor of *Journal of Medical Microbiology*.
[a]88S = 88 susceptible; 88R = 88 resistant.
[b]The piglets had been given 10^7 viable organisms of each of the four forms; the dose of each for the calf was 10^9 and for the lamb 10^8 viable organisms. All animals were also given a non-pathogenic *E. coli* strain, P403, and a lactobacillus strain, 10^9 of each for the piglets and the lamb and 10^{10} of each for the calf; the animals were killed 28 to 32 hours after inoculation.
[c]The small intestine was divided into seven equal parts for counting; part 1 was nearest to the stomach and part 7 to the colon.

the posterior small intestine of one of them. The concentrations present in parts 1, 3, 5 and 7 of this piglet were, $\log_{10}$ per gram, 5.2, 6.2, 7.6 and 8.6, respectively, compared with 5.6, 5.4, 5.8 and 5.9 in the case of the 88⁻99⁻Ent⁺ form. The corresponding figures, though, for the 88⁺99⁻Ent⁺ form were 9.2, 8.5, 9.0 and 9.2.

88⁻99⁻Ent⁺ organisms, if anything, were present in lower concentrations in the small intestines of all the animals that had been inoculated with the O9:K36:H19 forms than were 88⁻99⁻Ent⁻ organisms, confirming that Ent was playing no part in the proliferative process.

The Effect of the Ent, 88 and 99 Plasmids on the Colonization of the Small Intestine by an *E. coli* K12 Strain

When the experiments with the O9:K36:H19 strain were repeated with an *E. coli* K12 strain, an 88S and three 88R piglets and three calves showed no signs of ill health after inoculation, thus revealing that there is more to enteropathogenicity than the mere possession of an appropriate small intestinal colonizing factor and the ability to produce enterotoxin; the K12 strain employed was lac^-, required proline, histidine, tryptophane and phenylalanine for growth and, like all K12 strains, was O^- and K^-. Only low concentrations of the $88^+99^-Ent^+$, $88^-99^+Ent^+$, $88^-99^-Ent^+$ and $88^-99^-Ent^-$ forms of the K12 strain were present in their alimentary tracts, none of the plasmid-containing forms surviving better than the $88^-99^-Ent^-$ form or the non-pathogenic P403 strain; the results of some of these examinations are summarized in Table 4. A fourth calf included in these experiments developed mild diarrhoea. Although the concentrations of the

Table 4. *The concentration of organisms in different parts of the alimentary tract of an 88S and an 88R piglet and a calf given orally a mixture of forms of an* E. coli *K12 strain in which had been implanted 88, 99 and Ent plasmids*

Animal	Forms of strain in mixture	stomach contents	1	3	5	7	colon contents
88S piglet	$88^-99^-Ent^-$	<2.0	3.3	4.0	4.8	5.8	7.9
	$88^-99^-Ent^+$	<2.0	<2.0	<2.0	3.9	<2.0	<2.0
	$88^+99^-Ent^+$	<2.0	<2.0	<2.0	5.3	3.7	6.6
	$88^-99^+Ent^+$	<2.0	<2.0	<2.0	5.5	4.4	7.0
88R piglet	$88^-99^-Ent^-$	5.4	<2.0	<2.0	<2.0	<2.0	6.3
	$88^-99^-Ent^+$	4.5	<2.0	<2.0	<2.0	<2.0	4.2
	$88^+99^-Ent^+$	5.3	<2.0	<2.0	<2.0	3.3	6.0
	$88^-99^+Ent^+$	5.5	<2.0	<2.0	<2.0	4.0	5.9
Calf	$88^-99^-Ent^-$	4.8	4.5	5.3	5.0	6.4	5.3
	$88^-99^-Ent^+$	3.0	3.9	4.3	4.0	5.7	4.0
	$88^+99^-Ent^+$	4.3	4.5	4.6	4.5	4.6	5.5
	$88^-99^+Ent^+$	4.3	4.3	5.3	5.5	6.9	5.0

Number of organisms of stated form ($\log_{10}$ per g) in wall scrapings of small intestine, part

Data from Smith and Huggins (1978), with kind permission of the editor of *Journal of Medical Microbiology*.
For other details see Table 3.

$88^-99^+Ent^+$ form in its small intestine were not high, they were higher than those of the other three forms which, in all parts of the small intestine, were less than, $\log_{10}$ per gram, 2.0; the figures for the $88^-99^+Ent^+$ form in the wall scrapings of parts 1 to 7 were 2.9, 3.2, 3.4, 4.0, 6.2, 6.8 and 6.8, respectively, five to 100 times lower than those for the non-pathogenic P403 strain.

The failure of *E. coli* K12 to permit full expression of the colonizing plasmids, and thereby of Ent, in the alimentary tract were further demonstrated by giving a calf the four forms of this strain and, at the same dose level, a O8:K85,99 calf enteropathogenic strain. The calf developed severe diarrhoea and the concentrations of the O8:K85,99 strain in parts 1 to 7 of its small intestine were, $\log_{10}$ per gram, 4.4, 5.0, 5.5, 5.8, 9.0, 9.5 and 9.5, respectively. The corresponding figures for the four K12 forms were all less than 2.0. In a similar experiment in an 88S piglet the corresponding figures for an O141:K85,88 pig pathogenic strain that was substituted for the

O8:K85,99 strain were 9.3, 9.0, 9.3, 9.5, 9.3, 9.6 and 9.6, respectively. Those for the 88⁺99⁻Ent⁺ form of the K12 strain were 4.0, 3.7, 5.0, 5.3, 5.6, 5.3 and 5.0, respectively. They were 10 to 100 times higher than those for the 88⁻99⁺Ent⁺ form and about 100 to 1000 times higher than those for the 88⁻99⁻Ent⁻ form.

The Effect of the 88 and 99 Plasmids on the Colonization of the Alimentary Tract by an O141:K85,88 Piglet Enteropathogenic Strain

Mixtures of an O141:K85,88 piglet enteropathogenic strain that produced LT and ST, an 88⁻ form of it and this form in which had been implanted a 99 plasmid were given to four 88S and four 88R piglets and two calves (Table 5). As expected, the 88⁺99⁻ form did not proliferate in any part of the small

Table 5. *The concentration of organisms in different parts of the alimentary tract of an 88S and an 88R piglet and a calf given orally a mixture of forms of an O141:K85,88 piglet enteropathogenic strain possessing different combinations of the 88 and 99 plasmids*

Animal	Forms[a] of strain in mixture	stomach contents	wall scrapings of small intestine, part 1	3	5	7	colon contents
88S piglet	88⁻99⁻	6.0	5.5	4.0	5.6	5.4	6.6
	88⁺99⁻	6.8	9.3	9.4	9.6	9.8	9.5
	88⁻99⁺	6.0	5.0	6.7	8.0	8.0	8.5
88R piglet	88⁻99⁻	3.3	3.0	3.8	3.0	3.0	4.4
	88⁺99⁻	3.3	2.6	3.4	2.5	2.4	3.7
	88⁻99⁺	3.7	4.5	4.4	8.5	8.8	8.6
Calf	88⁻99⁻	5.3	3.0	3.8	3.6	4.5	6.4
	88⁺99⁻	6.2	4.3	4.8	4.4	5.5	6.8
	88⁻99⁺	6.9	5.9	6.5	8.9	9.2	9.3

Number of organisms of stated form ($\log_{10}$ per g) in

[a] All forms were Ent⁺. For other details see Table 3.
Data from Smith and Huggins (1978), with kind permission of the editor of *Journal of Medical Microbiology*.

intestine of the 88R piglets but it proliferated throughout the small intestine of the 88S piglets. By contrast, there was no difference, as a group, between the 88S and 88R piglets in the susceptibility of their small intestines to proliferation by the 88⁻99⁺ form, confirming that the intestinal receptors of the 99 antigen were quite different from those of the 88 antigen. The parts of the small intestine of both the 88S and 88R piglets in which 88⁻99⁺ proliferation occurred, however, did vary from piglet to piglet; high concentrations of this form were found in parts 2 to 7 of one, in parts 3 to 7 of two and in parts 5 to 7 of four. In the lower parts of the small intestine of two 88S piglets organisms of this form were as numerous as those of the 88⁺99⁻ form. In the calves, only the 88⁻99⁺ form proliferated, in parts 3 to 7 in one and in parts 5 to 7 in the other.

The Effect of the 88 and 99 Plasmids on the Colonization of the Alimentary Tract by an O8:K85,99 lamb Enteropathogenic Strain

Forms of an O8:K85,99 lamb enteropathogenic strain that produced only ST and an 88^-99^- and an 88^+99^- form of it were given to two 88S and six 88R piglets and to eight calves (Table 6). High concentrations of the 88^+99^- form were found throughout the small intestine of the two 88S piglets but only low concentrations were present in the 88R piglets and the calves. Apart from part 7 of the small intestine of the 88S piglet illustrated in Table 6, only low

Table 6. *The concentration of organisms in different parts of the alimentary tract of an 88S and an 88R piglet and a calf given orally a mixture of forms of an O8:K85,99 lamb enteropathogenic strain possessing different combinations of the 88 and 99 plasmids*

Animal	Forms of strain in mixture	stomach contents	1	3	5	7	colon contents
88S piglet	88^-99^-	4.8	3.3	3.9	5.6	5.8	5.4
	88^+99^-	5.7	7.7	7.6	8.3	8.9	7.7
	88^-99^+	3.9	2.9	3.2	6.0	8.4	7.5
88R piglet	88^-99^-	<2.0	3.2	3.3	4.3	7.8	9.2
	88^+99^-	<2.0	2.5	2.5	4.0	6.9	8.2
	88^-99^+	<2.0	2.0	2.7	4.3	5.6	8.7
Calf	88^-99^-	6.7	5.7	6.2	8.2	8.3	8.2
	88^+99^-	6.6	5.3	5.5	6.3	6.6	7.2
	88^-99^+	6.7	5.6	8.3	9.5	9.6	9.3

Columns 1–7 show the number of organisms of stated form ($\log_{10}$ per g) in wall scrapings of small intestine, part.

Data from Smith and Huggins (1978), with kind permission of the editor of *Journal of Medical Microbiology*.
For other details see Tables 3 and 5.

concentrations of the 88^-99^+ form were found in the small intestines of all the 88S and 88R piglets. This is in general agreement with the results obtained with the similar form of the O9:K36:H19 strain but not with the similar forms of the O141:K85,88 and the O9:K30,99 strains (see Table 9) because these two forms proliferated in the small intestine of all the 88S and 88R piglets indicating that, 'crippled' strains like *E. coli* K12 apart, the 99 antigen was able to express itself in some *E. coli* strains only as a small intestinal colonizing agent in piglets. This was not the case in calves because the antigen always expressed itself in the O9:K36:H19 strain, the O141:K85,88 strain, the O9:K30,99 strain (see Table 9) and other strains as well as in the O8:K88,99 strain. The latter strain proliferated only in the middle and lower parts of the small intestine of six of the seven calves to which it had been given but in the seventh it proliferated throughout this organ. Proliferation on 99^+ strains throughout the small intestine of calves was also observed in subsequent experiments and this, together with the results reported here on calves and piglets, suggests that receptors of the 99 antigen are present throughout the small intestine but that adhesion may be more difficult to obtain in the anterior small intestine because the speed of chyme flow there is greatest. The fact that proliferation of the 88⁺ forms of all the strains tested, except *E. coli* K12, usually occurred throughout the small intestine of the 88S piglets not only implies that 88 receptors are present throughout the small intestine of these piglets but that 88 adhesion is more efficient than 99 adhesion.

In the experiments with the O8:K85,99 strain, the 88⁻99⁻ form was found in unexpectedly high concentrations in the small intestine of several of the calves, these concentrations only being five to ten times lower than those of the 88⁻99⁺ form. Because of this finding, the 88⁻99⁻ form of this strain and of the O141:K85,88, O9:K36:H19 and K12 strains and of an O149:K91,88:H19 piglet enteropathogenic strain were given to a calf. The calf developed diarrhoea, and high concentrations of the 88⁻99⁻ form of the O8:K85,99 strain, but not of the other strains, were found in its small intestine (Table 7),

Table 7. *The concentration of organisms in different parts of the alimentary tract of a calf given orally a mixture of laboratory-prepared and wild 99⁻ or 88⁻ strains of* E. coli

Material examined	Number of organisms ($\log_{10}$ per g) present of strain					
	O8:K85,99	O141:K85,88	O149:K91,88:H19	O9:K36:H19	K12	P403
Stomach contents	6.6	5.2	<2.0	6.3	<2.0	5.3
Wall scrapings of small intestine, part						
1	7.5	3.6	<2.0	4.2	<2.0	4.6
2	7.0	3.7	2.0	4.2	<2.0	5.0
3	6.8	3.7	2.3	4.2	<2.0	4.5
4	7.8	3.7	3.5	4.0	<2.0	4.6
5	9.0	3.7	<2.0	4.4	<2.0	4.5
6	9.3	3.7	2.3	4.4	<2.0	4.3
7	9.5	4.8	2.6	5.0	<2.0	5.4
Colon contents	8.5	6.0	4.5	7.0	<2.0	6.2

Data from Smith and Huggins (1978), with kind permission of the editor of *Journal of Medical Microbiology*.
For other details see Tables 3 and 5.

indicating quite clearly that under certain conditions special colonizing factors, like 88 and 99, although still able to increase the degree of colonization, are not essential for sufficient colonization to occur to give rise to diarrhoea. It is noteworthy that when this experiment was repeated in an 88R piglet, the piglet remained healthy and only low concentrations of the infecting organism were found in its small intestines; one further example of the differences between the small intestine of the calf and piglet in regard to *E. coli* colonizing ability.

The Effect of the 987P and 88 Antigens on the Colonization of the Alimentary Tract by O9:K103,987P Piglet Enteropathogenic Strains

The results of inoculating two 88S and two 88R piglets and two calves with forms of an O9:K103,987P strain possessing either the 987P or 88 antigen or neither (Table 8) confirmed the observations of Moon and his co-workers

Table 8. *The concentration of organisms in different parts of the alimentary tract of an 88S and an 88R piglet and a calf given orally a mixture of forms of an O9:K103,987P piglet-enteropathogenic strain possessing different combinations of the 987P and 88 antigen*

Animal	Forms of strain in mixture	stomach contents	\multicolumn{4}{c}{wall scrapings of small intestine, part}	colon contents
			1	3	5	7	
88S piglet	987P⁻88⁻	3.7	5.0	5.3	5.3	4.6	5.8
	987P⁺88⁻	3.6	4.9	5.9	9.3	9.4	9.7
	987P⁻88⁺	2.8	4.3	6.8	8.4	8.7	8.8
88R piglet	987P⁻88⁻	2.0	2.9	4.0	2.9	3.3	4.2
	987P⁺88⁻	2.7	4.2	4.5	9.5	9.8	9.0
	987P⁻88⁺	3.3	3.5	4.2	3.0	4.4	5.5
Calf	987P⁻88⁻	<2.0	3.4	3.7	4.0	5.2	8.5
	987P⁺88⁻	<2.0	<2.0	3.6	4.0	5.4	8.7
	987P⁻88⁺	<2.0	<2.0	3.6	4.0	5.2	7.8

Number of organisms of stated form ($\log_{10}$ per g).

Data from Smith and Huggins (1978), with kind permission of the editor of *Journal of Medical Microbiology*.
For other details see Tables 3 and 5.

(Isaacson, Nagy and Moon, 1977; Nagy, Moon and Isaacson, 1977) that 987P is a potent small intestinal colonizing factor in the piglet. The O9:K103,987P strain and its 987P⁻ mutant had been received from Dr Harley Moon; the 88 plasmid had been implanted in it in this laboratory but we had failed to implant a 99 plasmid in it. Colonization of the 987P⁺88⁻ form was confined to the posterior small intestine. Interestingly, this was also the case with the 987P⁻88⁺ form, revealing that, at least in one strain, 88 antigen adhesion, like 99 and 987P antigen adhesion, is more difficult to achieve in the anterior than in the posterior small intestine. Neither form of the O9:K103,987P strain proliferated in the calves, results that were confirmed with another strain of the same antigenic formula, both strains being used in increased dosage. Thus it appears that the 987P antigen, like the 88 plasmid, is not a small intestinal colonizing factor for these animals. In an additional experiment in which three 88R piglets were given a 987P⁺88⁺ and 987P⁺88⁻ form, the concentrations of the former form in the small intestines were 10 to 100 times less than that of the latter form, indicating that the combined effect of the two factors in 88R piglets was to depress intestinal colonization. In an 88S piglet the 987P⁺88⁺ form proliferated to a greater extent than the 987P⁺88⁻ form.

The Effect of the O and K Antigens on the Colonization of the Alimentary Tract by Calf, Piglet and Lamb Enteropathogenic Strains

The results of estimating the concentrations of the inoculated organisms in the alimentary tracts of an 88S and an 88R piglet and a calf given different forms of an O9:K30,99 calf-enteropathogenic strain that produced ST only (Table 9) demonstrated the important part played by the K30 antigen in

Table 9. *The concentration of organisms in different parts of the alimentary tract of an 88S and an 88R piglet and a calf given orally a mixture of forms of an O9:K30,99 calf-enteropathogenic strain possessing different combinations of O, K, 88 and 99 antigens*

	Forms of strain in mixture	stomach contents	1	3	5	7	colon contents
88S piglet	O⁻K⁻99⁻	<2.0	<2.0	2.0	5.7	3.3	3.6
	O⁻K⁻99⁺	4.0	5.2	5.7	7.4	7.3	7.7
	O⁺K⁻99⁻	<2.0	2.8	3.0	6.4	4.2	4.6
	O⁺K⁻99⁺	7.2	5.5	5.9	7.3	7.9	6.6
	O⁺K⁺99⁻	6.3	5.2	4.6	8.9	8.3	7.9
	O⁺K⁺99⁺	6.6	6.2	6.2	9.9	9.9	9.9
	O⁺K⁺99⁻88⁺	7.5	9.4	9.6	9.8	9.9	9.9
88R piglet	O⁻K⁻99⁻	<2.0	<2.0	<2.0	4.4	2.0	4.8
	O⁻K⁻99⁺	2.7	2.5	3.3	6.8	8.3	6.9
	O⁺K⁻99⁻	2.0	2.0	2.3	5.7	4.0	5.9
	O⁺K⁻99⁺	4.5	3.6	4.3	6.9	8.5	7.3
	O⁺K⁺99⁻	2.0	2.5	3.3	8.4	7.6	7.5
	O⁺K⁺99⁺	4.5	4.5	4.6	9.5	9.2	8.4
Calf	O⁻K⁻99⁻	5.3	4.3	4.3	4.2	4.2	5.3
	O⁻K⁻99⁺	3.0	2.9	4.4	4.8	4.3	4.6
	O⁺K⁻99⁻	5.4	4.6	4.7	4.7	4.0	5.6
	O⁺K⁻99⁺	1.8	4.3	6.4	6.3	5.3	6.0
	O⁺K⁺99⁻	5.4	6.7	8.0	8.3	8.2	8.6
	O⁺K⁺99⁺	6.4	8.3	9.2	9.5	9.2	9.9

Data from Smith and Huggins (1978), with kind permission of the editor of *Journal of Medical Microbiology*.
For other details see Tables 3 and 5.

promoting colonization of the small intestine of these animals by this strain; it was quite equal to that played by the 99 antigen. Loss of the O antigen in addition to the K antigen had little or no additional effect on colonization. Similar results were obtained when these experiments were repeated in two 88S piglets, four 88R piglets and one calf.

The K30 antigen also strongly promoted colonization of the small intestine of an 88R piglet and a calf by two enteropathogenic strains that differed from the O9:K30,99 strain in that their O antigen was 101; they both proliferated to the same extent in the small intestine of the calf and of the piglet despite the fact that one had been isolated originally from a calf and the other from a piglet. Different forms of this calf enteropathogen were also given to twin lambs, one of which unusually, had been given colostrum. Diarrhoea was most severe in the colostrum-deprived lamb. Bacteriological examinations (Table 10) revealed that both the absence of the K30 antigen

Table 10. *The concentration of organisms in different parts of the alimentary tract of twin colostrum-fed and colostrum-deprived lambs given orally a mixture of forms of an O101:K30,99 calf-enteropathogenic strain possessing different combinations of the K and 99 antigens*

Colestral status of lamb	Forms of strain in mixture	stomach contents	\multicolumn{4}{c}{wall scrapings of small intestine, part}	colon contents
			1	3	5	7	
Deprived	K⁻99⁻	3.0	4.3	3.8	4.0	4.0	7.0
	K⁻99⁺	3.5	5.8	9.3	9.5	9.5	10.5
	K⁺99⁻	5.7	5.7	7.0	6.5	6.5	8.3
	K⁺99⁺	6.7	9.3	9.0	9.3	9.5	10.5
Fed	K⁻99⁻	2.5	2.9	3.3	3.6	5.8	6.7
	K⁻99⁺	2.5	3.3	3.7	7.3	9.5	6.3
	K⁺99⁻	4.0	2.0	2.7	4.7	6.0	6.5
	K⁺99⁺	4.0	4.3	6.7	10.0	9.8	8.7

Number of organisms of stated form ($\log_{10}$ per g) in

For other details see Tables 3 and 5.

and the presence of antibody had a restrictive effect on proliferation in the small intestine. This was most clearly seen by comparing the extent to which the K^-99^+ and K^+99^+ forms proliferated in the more anterior regions of the small intestine of both lambs. From the results for the K^-99^+ form in the colostrum-fed lamb it could be erroneously concluded that enteropathogenic strains can proliferate only in the posterior regions of the intestine. From those for the K^+99^+ form in the colostrum-fed lamb and for the K^-99^+ form in the colostrum-deprived lamb the conclusion would be that the middle regions are also susceptible to proliferation. The correct conclusion that proliferation can occur throughout the small intestine was revealed only by the results for the K^+99^+ form in the colostrum-deprived lamb.

In a strain with the same O antigen as the O9:K30,99 strain but with a different K antigen, K35, small intestinal proliferation was again promoted by the K antigen. The concentrations of the $K35^+99^+$ form in the wall scrapings of parts 1 to 7 of the small intestine of an 88R piglet given different forms of this strain were, $\log_{10}$ per gram, 3.6, 4.5, 4.4, 4.5, 5.2, 8.5 and 8.6, respectively, and of a calf 8.5, 10.7, 10.7, 10.8, 10.4, 10.6 and 10.3, respectively. The corresponding figures for the $K35^-99^+$ form were 2.0, 2.3, 2.3, 4.2, 4.2, 4.2 and 4.5 for the piglet and 5.6, 6.3, 6.9, 7.4, 8.0, 10.0 and 9.0 for the calf.

The results of giving another calf mixtures of the $K85^+99^+$ and the $K85^-99^+$ forms of the O8:K85,99 lamb enteropathogenic strain whose $K85^+99^-$ form had previously been shown to be capable of producing diarrhoea in a calf (see Table 7) also emphasized the important part played by the K85 antigen in achieving small intestinal colonization by this strain. In wall scrapings of parts 1 to 7 of the small intestine of this calf, the concentrations, $\log_{10}$ per gram, of the K85$^+$99$^+$ form were 8.6, 9.3, 8.8, 8.8, 9.2, 9.4 and 9.2, respectively, and of the K85$^-$99$^+$ form were 5.3, 5.5, 5.0, 5.2, 5.7, 6.6 and 5.4, respectively.

The Effect of Plasmid-Determined Raffinose Utilization on Colonization of the Alimentary Tract by 88$^+$ Enteropathogenic Organisms

Despite the evidence of molecular studies that the Raf genes and the 88 genes are located on the same plasmid, probably because of instability, spontaneous Raf$^-$ mutants can be obtained from some O141:K85,88 strains without difficulty. However, although most of the *E. coli* that cause diarrhoea in pigs are 88$^+$ and although practically all these strains possess transferable raffinose utilization ability, the administration of mixtures of Raf$^+$ and Raf$^-$ forms of an O141:K85,88 strain to 88S piglets provided no evidence implicating Raf genes in the pathogenesis of *E. coli* diarrhoea. For example, in one experiment equal numbers of organisms of these two forms were given to three 88S piglets. Similar ratios of the Raf$^+$ and Raf$^-$ organisms were found amongst 1200 isolates of the O141:K85,88 strain from contents and wall scrapings of the small intestines and from contents of the stomach and colon of these three piglets when they were killed suffering from severe diarrhoea; a similar result was obtained when the experiment was repeated in two 88R piglets except that they, of course, remained healthy. The role of the Raf genes in *E. coli* diarrhoea, therefore, remains obscure, the position resembling that of the Hly (haemolysin) plasmid which is commonly found in certain serotypes of porcine enteropathogenic *E. coli* but for which no enteropathogenic function can be found (Smith and Linggood, 1971).

The Effect of Giving Piglets *E. coli* Enteropathogenic for Recently-Weaned Pigs

Apart from during the neonatal period, pigs are also susceptible to infection with enteropathogenic strains of *E. coli* during the week or so after weaning, irrespective of their age of weaning; at all other times they are resistant to infection with these strains.

Although under natural conditions some serotypes infect both piglets and recently-weaned pigs, several appear to infect only the latter, the most common of these having the antigenic structure O141:K85, O138:K81 and O139:K82. Despite the fact that adhesive factors have not been discovered in these three serotypes they must surely possess them because they proliferate in the small intestine of recently-weaned pigs (Smith and Halls, 1968) to the same extent as other serotypes known to possess adhesive factors proliferate in the small intestine in piglets, and, in some cases, of recently-weaned pigs. While proliferating there, they can produce toxins additional to enterotoxin which are absorbed and give rise to clinical signs recognizable as oedema disease. One 88S and three 88R piglets given mixtures of an O141:K85 strain, an O138:K81 and an O139:K82 strain developed neither diarrhoea nor signs of oedema disease and only low concentrations of the inoculated organisms were found in their alimentary tracts (Table 11). This implies that *operative* receptors for adhesive factors possessed by these organisms were not present in the small intestines of piglets. It is conceivable, of course, that the piglets used in this experiment might have been

Table 11. *The concentration of organisms in different parts of the alimentary tract of an 88S piglet given a mixture of three strains of* E. coli *enteropathogenic for recently-weaned piglets*

Antigenic structure of strain	Number of organisms of stated strain, $\log_{10}$ per g, in					
	stomach contents	wall scrapings of small intestine, part				colon contents
		1	3	5	7	
O141:K85	5.3	5.0	4.9	5.0	6.3	7.7
O138:K81	4.3	5.6	5.4	5.4	6.3	7.4
O139:K82	5.7	4.8	4.8	5.3	6.4	7.5

For other details see Tables 3 and 5.

genetically resistant to their adhesion as 88R piglets are resistant to 88 antigen adhesion. It is noteworthy in this respect that Smith and Halls (1968) failed to produce clinical disease or small intestinal proliferation in recently-weaned pigs from eight different farms with the O141:K85 strain but they were regularly able to do so in those from another farm, the pigs from all farms being maintained under identical conditions. Their studies also revealed that the physiological state of the small intestine profoundly influenced adhesion by organisms of this strain because both the experimental disease and small intestinal proliferation were prevented simply by restricting the food consumption of inoculated pigs or by replacing their normal diet with a largely indigestible one consisting of barley fibre (Table 12); dietary restriction has no obvious effect in controlling porcine neonatal

Table 12. *The effect of different diets on the response of recently-weaned pigs to oral inoculation with an O141:K85 strain of* E. coli

Diet	Method of administration	No. of pigs	No. that developed		
			diarrhoea	oedema disease and	
				lived	died
Barley meal	*ad libitum*	3	3	0	2
Barley meal + fish meal	*ad libitum*	11	11	2	6
Barley meal + fish meal	150 g twice daily[a]	4	0	0	0
Barley fibre	*ad libitum*	3	0	0	0

Data from Smith and Halls (1968), with kind permission of the editor of *Journal of Medical Microbiology*.
[a] Approximately one-third of the total daily food intake of that of the pigs fed *ad libitum*.
The *E. coli* strain produced heat-stable enterotoxin.

E. coli diarrhoea. The concentration of O141:K85 organisms, $\log_{10}$ per gram, in the contents of parts 1, 3, 5 and 7 of the small intestine of one of the pigs that had been fed on barley meal and fish meal *ad libitum* and that developed diarrhoea was 7.5, 7.4, 8.3 and 9.5 respectively. The corresponding figures for another that had been fed on a restricted diet of this composition and had not developed diarrhoea was 2.7, 2.7, 2.8 and 5.9, respectively. Similar results in a larger experiment have recently been reported by Bertschinger et al (1978/79). Bearing in mind the close similarity between *E. coli* intestinal infections in domestic animals and in human beings, it is interesting to speculate as to whether qualitative and quantitative changes in diet also play a part in the aetiology of some forms of travellers' diarrhoea in human beings and, more importantly, whether restricting food intake might have a preventive effect.

ACKNOWLEDGEMENTS

I am grateful to Miss Debra Pulley for her help with preparation of this manuscript.

REFERENCES

Bertschinger, H.U., Eggenberger, E., Jucker, H. & Pfirter, H.P. (1978/79) Evaluation of low nutrient, high fibre diets for the prevention of porcine *Escherichia coli* enterotoxaemia. *Veterinary Microbiology*, **3**, 281-290.

Isaacson, R.E., Nagy, B. & Moon, H.W. (1977) Colonisation of porcine small intestine by *Escherichia coli*: colonisation and adhesion factors of pig enteropathogens that lack K88. *Journal of Infectious Diseases*, **135**, 531-539.

Jones, G.W. & Rutter, J.M. (1972) Role of the K88 antigen in the pathogenesis of neonatal diarrhoea caused by *Escherichia coli* in piglets. *Infection and Immunity*, **6**, 918-927.

Nagy, B., Moon, H.W. & Isaacson, R.E. (1976) Colonisation of the porcine small intestine by *Escherichia coli*: ileal colonisation and adhesion by pig enteropathogens that lack K88 antigen and by some acapsular mutants. *Infection and Immunity*, **13**, 1214-1220.

Nagy, B., Moon, H.W. & Isaacson, R.E. (1977) Colonisation of porcine intestine by enterotoxigenic *Escherichia coli*: selection of piliated forms *in vivo*, adhesion of piliated forms to epithelial cells *in vitro*, and incidence of a pilus antigen among porcine enteropathogenic *E. coli*. *Infection and Immunity*, **16**, 344-352.

Rutter, J.M., Burrows, M.R., Sellwood, R. & Gibbons, R.A. (1975) A genetic basis for resistance to enteric disease caused by *Escherichia coli*. *Nature* (London), **257**, 135.

Sellwood, R., Gibbons, R.A., Jones, G.W. & Rutter, J.M. (1974) A possible basis for the breeding of pigs relatively resistant to neonatal diarrhoea. *Veterinary Record*, **95**, 574.

Sellwood, R., Gibbons, R.A., Jones, G.W. & Rutter, J.M. (1975) Adhesion of enteropathogenic *Escherichia coli* to pig intestinal brush borders: the existence of two pig phenotypes. *Journal of Medical Microbiology*, **8**, 405-411.

Shipley, P.L., Gyles, C.L. & Falkow, S. (1978) Characterisation of plasmids that encode for the K88 colonisation antigen. *Infection and Immunity*, **20**, 559-566.

Smith, H. Williams & Gyles, C.L. (1970) The relationship between two apparently different enterotoxins produced by enteropathogenic strains of porcine origin. *Journal of Medical Microbiology*, **3**, 387-401.

Smith, H. Williams & Halls, S. (1968) The production of oedema disease and diarrhoea in weaned pigs by the oral administration of *Escherichia coli*: factors that influence the course of the experimental disease. *Journal of Medical Microbiology*, **1**, 45-59.

Smith, H. Williams & Huggins, M.B. (1978) The influence of plasmid-determined and other characteristics of enteropathogenic *Escherichia coli* on their ability to proliferate in the alimentary tracts of piglets, calves and lambs. *Journal of Medical Microbiology*, **11**, 471-492.

Smith, H. Williams & Jones, J.E.T. (1963) Observations on the alimentary tract and its bacterial flora in healthy and diseased pigs. *Journal of Pathology and Bacteriology*, **86**, 387-412.

Smith, H. Williams & Linggood, M.A. (1971) Observations on the pathogenic properties of the K88, Hly and Ent plasmids of *Escherichia coli* with particular reference to porcine diarrhoea. *Journal of Medical Microbiology*, **4**, 467-485.

Smith, H. Williams & Linggood, M.A. (1972) Further observations on *Escherichia coli* enterotoxins with particular regard to those produced by atypical piglet strain and by calf and lamb strains; the transmissible nature of these enterotoxins and of a K antigen possessed by calf and lamb strains. *Journal of Medical Microbiology*, **5**, 243-250.

Smith, H. Williams & Parsell, Z.E. (1975) Transmissible substrate-utilizing ability in enterobacteria. *Journal of General Microbiology*, **87**, 129-140.

10

Pseudomembranous Colitis

ASHLEY B. PRICE

In current clinical practice pseudomembranous colitis (PMC) is seen most often as a complication of antibiotic therapy. The recent discovery of its likely aetiology has come from the interest generated by its association with two particular antibiotics, lincomycin and clindamycin (Cohen, McNeill and Wells, 1973; Scott, Nicholson and Kerr, 1973), though as a consequence the role of other antibiotics may have been underestimated. Good evidence has emerged that PMC, including cases not associated with antibiotics, is due to the proliferation in the intestine of a clostridial organism, *Clostridium difficile*, and the detection of its toxin in the stools of patients now forms the basis of a diagnostic test (Larson et al, 1977; Rifkin, Fekety and Silva, 1977; Bartlett et al, 1978a; George et al, 1978).

CLASSIFICATION AND TERMINOLOGY

PMC is a morphological diagnosis based on identifying the characteristic mucosal plaques or smaller summit lesions (Goulston and McGovern, 1965; Price and Davies, 1977). The closely linked terms 'antibiotic-associated diarrhoea' (AAD) and 'antibiotic-associated colitis' (AAC) have been used less precisely in the literature, but if the relationship between PMC, AAC and AAD is to be understood then these terms need to be carefully defined. The most obvious classification is one based on morphology (Bartlett et al, 1978c). AAC includes all patients with diarrhoea, a recent history of antibiotics and biopsy evidence of a colitis but no pseudomembranes or other diagnostic biopsy picture. AAD is restricted to patients with a similar history but with a normal rectal biopsy. In the light of recent progress these terms must be further qualified by a statement on the presence or absence of *C. difficile* and its specific toxin.

Development of the toxin test (see below) may eventually obviate the need for a classification based on morphology; in particular, the reliance on a rectal biopsy with its inherent sampling error. It is too soon to know if *C. difficile* is the only cause of PMC and therefore premature to exchange the term for '*C. difficile* colitis'.

© 1980 W.B. Saunders Company Ltd.

HISTORICAL PERSPECTIVE

PMC was described well before antibiotics were discovered, with Billroth (1867) and Finney (1893) being rivals for the credit of describing the first case. In the early 1900s the descriptions were indexed under the sonorous titles of 'phlegmonous colitis', 'diphtheric colitis' and even 'grumous colitis' (Newman, 1956). Those early case reports were invariably of autopsy material when the bowel was autolysed and critical detail lost. The description of 40 postoperative cases by Penner and Bernheim (1939) is amongst the earliest published with convincing illustrations. Shock with accompanying vasoconstriction was thought the most likely aetiology and infection was considered to have a secondary role. All the case reports of PMC documented up to and including the 1940s followed surgical procedures (Dixon and Weisman, 1948) but then in 1952 Kleckner, Bargen and Baggenstoss described 14 patients with PMC as a complication of chronic medical illness. The role of shock was again given major importance. About this time the initial accounts of antibiotic-associated PMC appeared accompanied by the suggestion that infection or overgrowth by *Staphylococcus aureus* was the responsible agent (Terplan et al, 1953; Finland, Grigsby and Haight, 1954; Hartman and Angevine, 1956). The pathology described was also on post-mortem material and therefore difficult to evaluate, but in my opinion none of the illustrations depict the classical focal lesions of PMC. In 1960 Dearing, Baggenstoss and Weed showed that antibiotic-associated PMC occurred with or without *S. aureus* present and that *S. aureus* could cause diarrhoea in the absence of any intestinal morphological changes. Furthermore, the organism was present in a significant percentage of patients without any gastrointestinal symptoms. Because there was no consistent pathogen to be found in stool cultures the concept of PMC as an infectious disease lost ground and ischaemia once more assumed importance (Hardway and McKay, 1959; Margaretten and McKay, 1971). Unlike the earlier theories of hypoperfusion and vasoconstriction the observation of fibrin thrombi in mucosal capillaries was given prime significance and believed to explain the initial focal nature of the lesions. McKay et al (1955) produced an enterocolitis in dogs on the basis of capillary microthrombi initiated by an infusion of incompatible blood. Their pictures show haemorrhagic lesions rather than classical pseudomembranes. Capillary microthrombi were a prominent feature in the patients who died of PMC in a series reported by Whitehead (1971). In addition these patients had evidence of more widespread intravascular coagulation with microthrombi in other organs. It was suggested that the precise pathological picture in intestinal ischaemia is determined by the rate of onset of the ischaemic insult and the size of the involved vessels.

The literature contains a confusing number of reports of other varieties of ischaemic bowel disease, for examples haemorrhagic enterocolitis and acute necrotizing enterocolitis (Wilson and Qualheim, 1954; Kay, Richards and Watson, 1958; Killingback and Williams, 1962), which are difficult to separate from PMC. Marston (1977) lumps together 20 such entities, including PMC, into one chapter entitled 'Acute intestinal failure'. Within this group he includes pig-bel and Darmbrand (Fick and Wolken, 1949; Murrell et al, 1966), forms of necrotizing enterocolitis due to infection by *Clostridium welchii* C (or F). The newly discovered clostridial aetiology of PMC raises interesting links with these latter two conditions. Necrotizing enterocolitis of infancy (Kliegman, 1979) may also belong with this group. Its pathology is unlike PMC but clostridial organisms, among others, have been implicated in its aetiology.

None of the conditions mentioned shows the diagnostic focal plaques of PMC but at some stage all may show a mucosal pseudomembrane, either diffuse as in the mucosal necrosis accompanying a vascular occlusion, or focal as seen at a biopsy site. The presence of a membrane does not warrant a diagnosis of PMC unless it is accompanied by other characteristic features. It is a non-specific morphological sign but the one in part responsible for the classification of PMC as of ischaemic aetiology. Although PMC is now considered a clostridial disease some clostridial toxins are vasoconstrictive (Marston, 1977) and an ischaemic mechanism may still have some role in the final pathogenesis of the lesions.

PATHOLOGY

In its typical form the disease has an unmistakable gross and histological picture (Goulston and McGovern, 1965; Price and Davis, 1977). The surgical specimen shows varying numbers of distinct adherent mucosal yellow-white plaques (Figure 1). They may be widely spaced or close together and range in size from pin-point to over 1 cm. Much above this size the plaques become less discrete and cover irregular areas of mucosa (Figure 2). The left side of the colon is more commonly involved than the right side though the rectum is not invariably affected (Kappas et al, 1978; Tedesco, 1979). This limits the value of reports excluding the disease based soley on the sigmoidoscopic findings. Figures for the frequency of involvement at particular sites are not available though in my experience few patients have an entirely normal rectal biopsy throughout the illness. In cases associated with antibiotics the disease usually stops at the ileocaecal valve (Figure 2). An atypical transient right-sided haemorrhagic colitis in which plaques were absent has been described associated with ampicillin (Toffler, Pingoud and Burrell, 1978; Sakurai et al, 1979) but in these studies stools were not examined for *C. difficile* toxin. Small bowel disease occurs but was more common in the pre-antibiotic era. In the small intestine the plaques are less discrete and membranous yellow ridges may be seen running circumferentially over the mucosal folds. The macroscopic diagnosis is less confident as similar gross pathology can occur in primary small bowel ischaemia (Figure 3).

Microscopically the discrete plaque of PMC is a well-defined group of disrupted glands that have 'disgorged' their contents. The epithelial debris, together with mucin, fibrin and polymorphs, sits as a cap over the dilated lower portions of the crypts. This is the 'pseudomembrane' (Figure 4). The adjacent mucosa may be normal or show limited inflammatory changes with

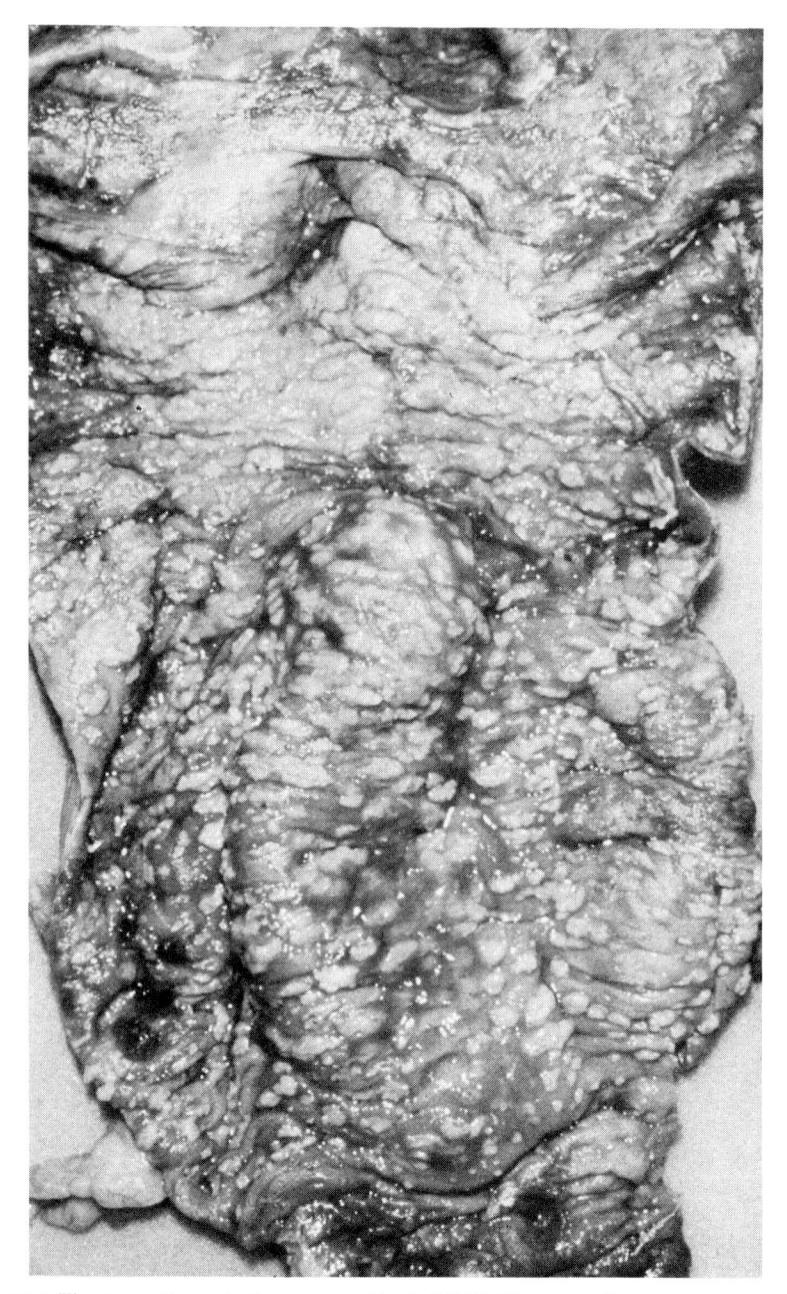

Figure 1. The descending colon from a case of typical PMC. Discrete yellow plaques are seen on the mucosal surface separated by mucosa showing mild hyperaemia.

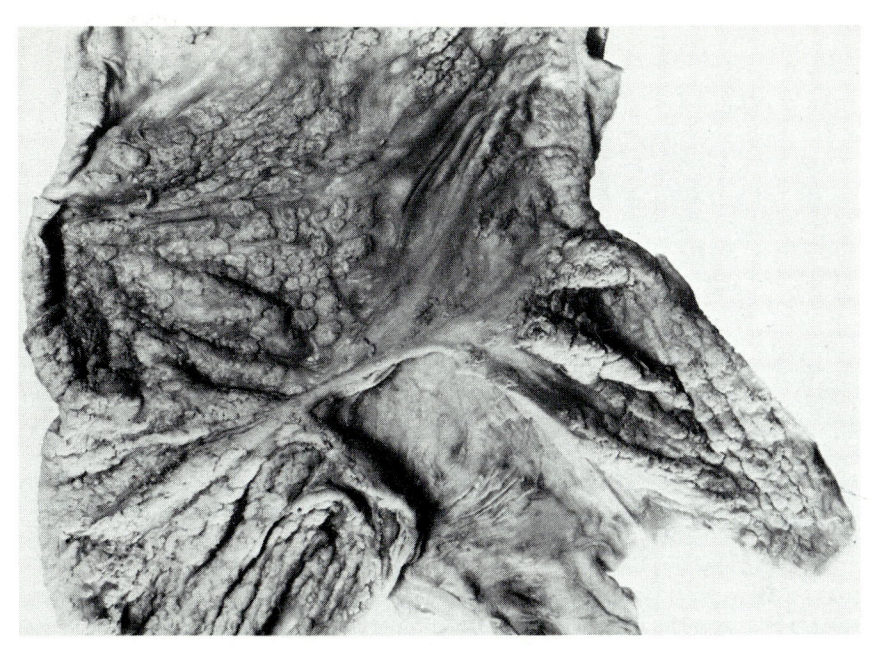

Figure 2. The terminal ileum and caecum from an autopsy on a patient who died of PMC. In the caecum the plaques are beginning to become confluent, particularly in the lower left corner. The ileum is normal. In antibiotic-associated PMC the disease usually stops at the ileocaecal valve.

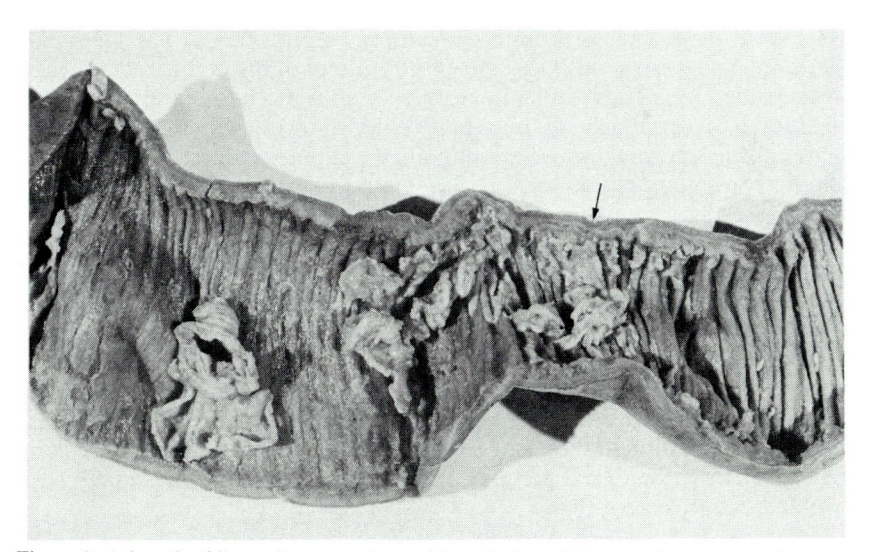

Figure 3. A length of ileum from a patient with occlusion of the superior mesenteric artery. Yellow 'pseudomembranous' material is seen stripped up from the surface, exposing the underlying muscularis propria. The pseudomembrane is still attached to the surface in the area arrowed. The macroscopic distinction of primary ischaemia from pseudomembranous enteritis is less clear cut in the small bowel.

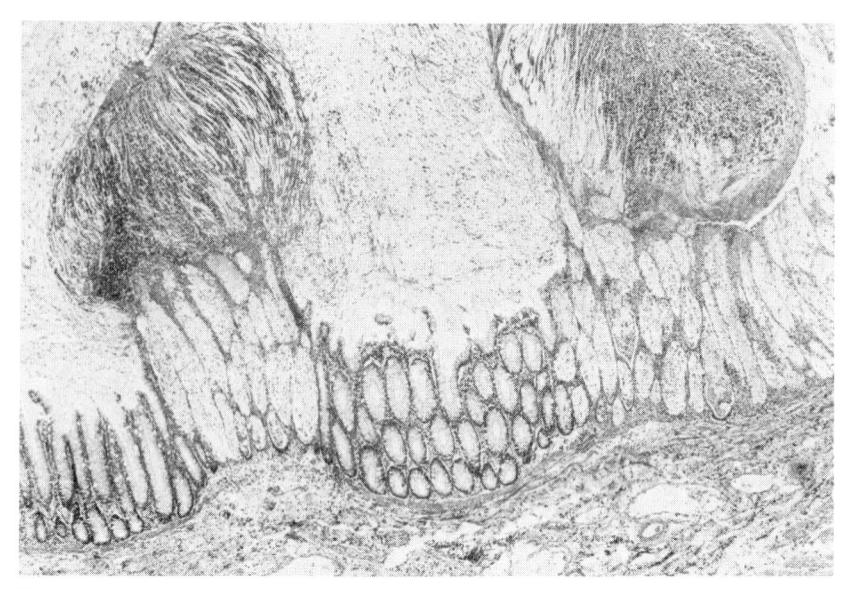

Figure 4. The typical histological picture of PMC. Two groups of disrupted glands are seen covered by a cap of fibrin, epithelial debris, mucin and polymorphs. In between, the surviving mucosa is normal. Haematoxylin and eosin, × 25.

focal collections of polymorphs predominating. The minor inflammatory changes in the adjacent mucosa are an important aid that help to distinguish PMC from other causes of mucosal erosions and necrosis. The glandular disruption progresses until only the ghost outlines of the crypts remain, now accompanied by a heavy inflammatory cell infiltrate in the lamina propria. Finally the involved area of mucosa is replaced by a layer of inflammatory debris, fibrin and mucus. When individual plaques coalesce there may be complete 'pseudomembranous' replacement of large areas of mucosa (Figure 5). At this stage the macroscopic and microscopic appearances are difficult to distinguish from other causes of colitis characterized by extensive mucosal necrosis (Figure 6; Price and Davies, 1977), a point which re-emphasizes that the pseudomembrane per se is not diagnostic of PMC; it simply reflects mucosal necrosis. Deep to the mucosa scattered inflammatory cells may be present but the main infiltrate is limited by the muscularis mucosa. Submucosal oedema is a constant finding. Capillary microthrombi are a variable feature and can no longer be considered of primary aetiological significance, though they may still have some role in the pathogenesis of the complete pathological picture. Toxic megacolon can occasionally be a complication of severe PMC.

Biopsy diagnosis

In a typical case with obvious plaques sigmoidoscopy is diagnostic. A well-taken biopsy should always include a plaque but frequently the clinician's

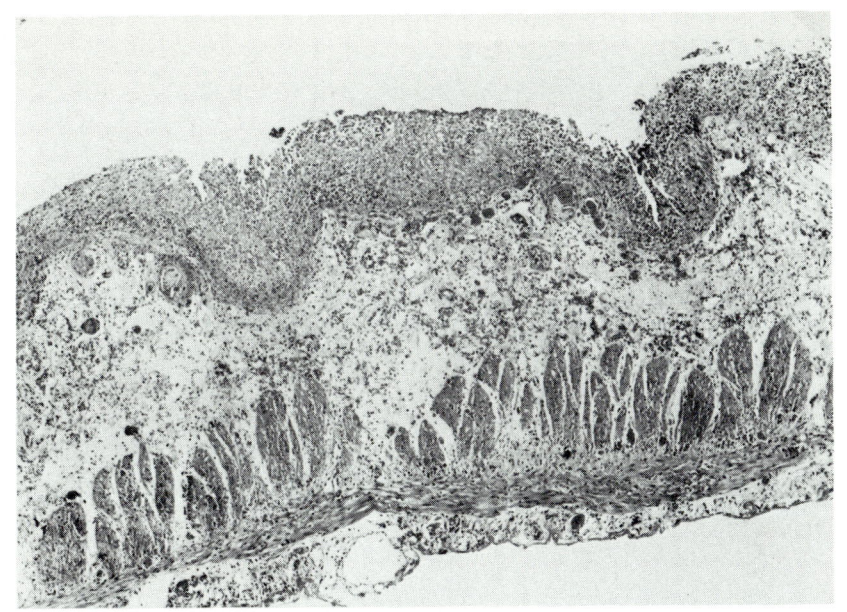

Figure 5. Complete mucosal necrosis produced when the individual plaques seen in Figure 4 become confluent. At this stage, although an inflammatory membrane replaces the mucosa, it is no longer a diagnostic picture. Haematoxylin and eosin, × 40.

view is obscured by fluid faeces and mucopurulent debris. However, even when plaques are not visible a biopsy must be taken as the earliest lesions are too small to be seen at sigmoidoscopy. In theory, because the rectum is not invariably involved colonoscopic examination is required to exclude the disease. This is seldom justified clinically and endoscopy is often contraindicated during an acute attack of colitis. A rectal biopsy and a toxin test (see below) are usually adequate for the clinical management of any individual patient. Repeated examinations may also be necessary (Keighley et al, 1978a) as the lesions can be absent initially.

In a biopsy the focus of disrupted glands, or type 2 lesion (Figure 4), is diagnostic of PMC. Confluent necrosis, or the type 3 lesion, presents more difficulty (Price and Davies, 1977) unless normal mucosa is included at its margin. A biopsy showing only membranous slough can be seen in any severe ulcerative disease (e.g., ulcerative colitis or Crohn's disease) and is of no diagnostic value (Figures 5 and 6).

When plaques are not seen at sigmoidoscopy then the histological summit lesion (type 1) is the earliest pathopneumonic finding (Figure 7). It is often necessary to cut serial sections through the biopsy to detect one of these lesions. It comprises a tiny surface epithelial erosion, accompanied by a luminal shower of polymorphs, fibrin and mucus situated between two crypts (Price and Davies, 1977). In the adjacent superficial mucosa aggregates of polymorphs may be present along with a subepithelial eosinophilic exudate.

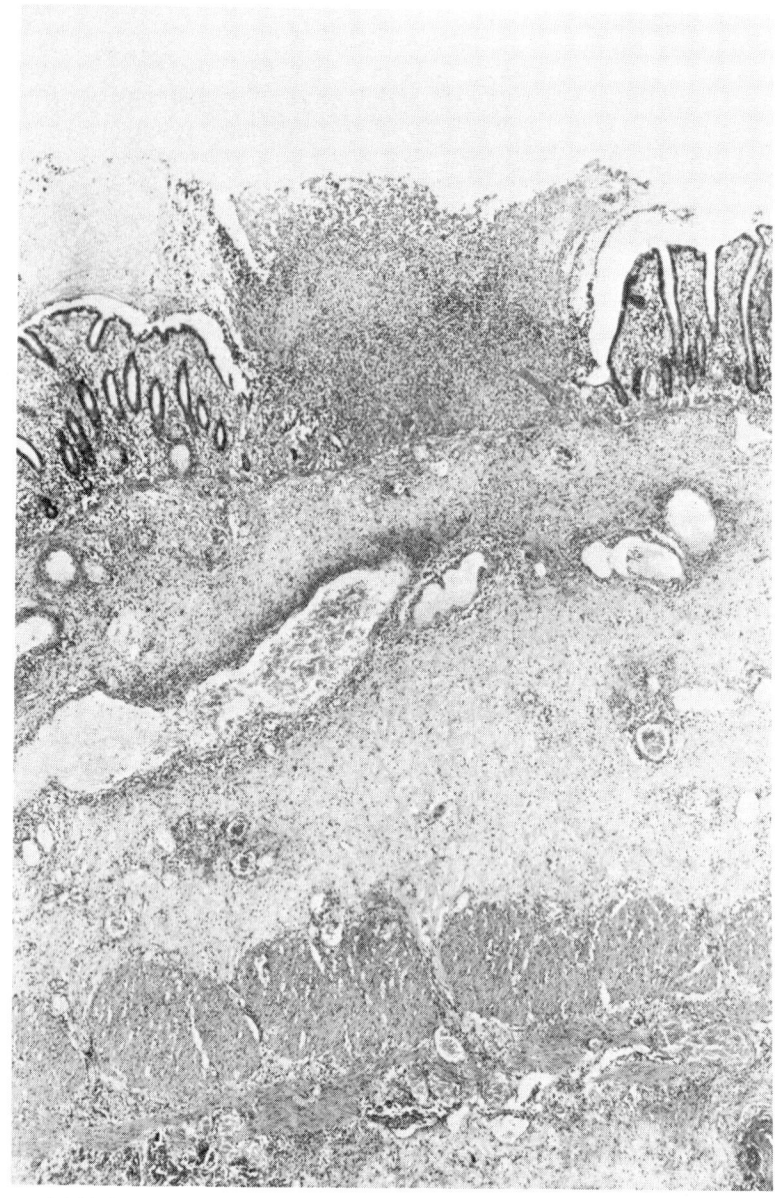

Figure 6. This illustrates a focus of complete mucosal necrosis found adjacent to similar and more extensive mucosal loss from a case of right-sided colonic volvulus. This picture is indistinguishable from PMC at the stage shown in Figure 5. Haematoxylin and eosin, × 35.

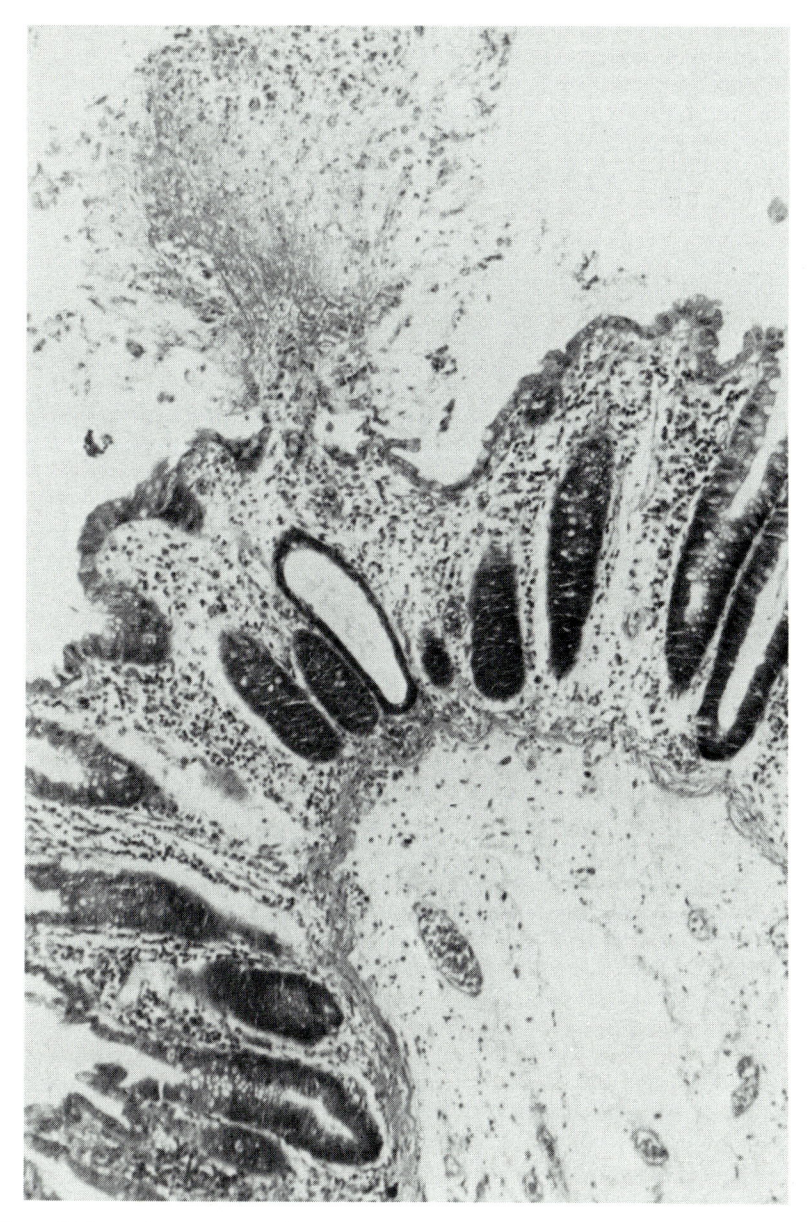

Figure 7. The early type 1 lesion (Price and Davies, 1977) or summit lesion diagnostic of PMC. A luminal spray of fibrin and polymorphs is seen arising from the superficial lamina propria. Haematoxylin and eosin, × 112.

There is also dilatation of capillaries with margination of polymorphs. The surface epithelium between nearby crypts is often infiltrated by polymorphs and nuclear debris. Small tufts of epithelial cells can also be seen imparting a crenated appearance to the mucosal surface, a feature noted by Pitman et al (1977) and observed in hamsters in response to certain antibiotics (Price, Larson and Crow, 1979). Biopsies from patients with AAC, confirmed by the presence of specific faecal toxin, but in whom summit erosions cannot be identified, may simply show the accompanying minor inflammatory pattern (Figure 8). This picture should not be classified under the unhelpful term

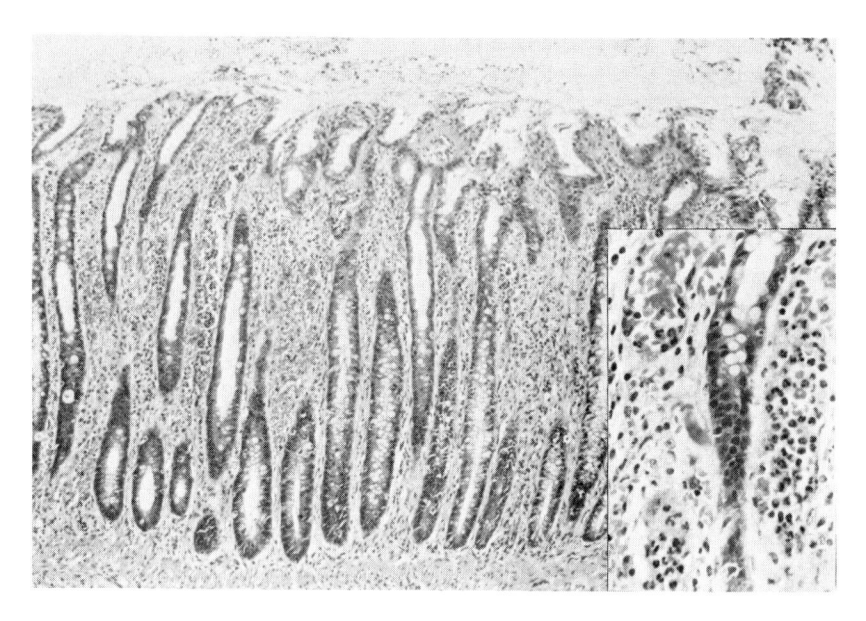

Figure 8. A rectal biopsy from a case of antibiotic-associated colitis with a positive faecal 'toxin' test. The lamina propria contains tiny aggregates of polymorphs (see inset), is slightly oedematous and shows a crenated epithelial surface with epithelial tufts. Some of the features resemble those associated with infectious diarrhoea. Haematoxylin and eosin, × 80.

'non-specific proctitis'. It is my experience that it has a close qualitative resemblance to the changes seen in biopsies from patients with infectious diarrhoea (Price, Jewkes and Sanderson, 1979), a finding of some interest now that PMC has been shown to have a bacterial aetiology.

Differential diagnosis

The type 2 lesions are diagnostic. A biopsy of a type 3 area has to be distinguished from pure ischaemic colitis, and the ulcers of Crohn's disease or ulcerative colitis. Ghost outlines of glands, if still present, suggest PMC but the differential diagnosis is best made by examination of any adjacent mucosa present in the biopsy. If this is normal or has the minor focal abnormalities described above then PMC is likely.

In ulcerative colitis the adjacent mucosa shows glandular irregularity, goblet cell depletion and other typical features (Price and Morson, 1975). Crohn's disease can be more difficult to exclude as mucosa adjacent to areas of ulceration may be normal. However, a chronic inflammatory cell infiltrate of plasma cells and aggregates of lymphocytes is usually present. A granuloma is diagnostic. In ischaemic colitis, depending on the rate of onset, the adjacent mucosa may be frankly haemorrhagic or show signs of glandular atrophy and fibrosis of the lamina propria. In biopsies without plaques or summit lesions but with only focal inflammatory changes (Figure 8), infectious diarrhoea should be excluded (Day, Mandal and Morson, 1978; Price, Jewkes and Sanderson, 1979). In all patients the pathology must be evaluated in conjunction with the clinical and radiological findings. Eventually the role of the biopsy in diagnosis might diminish as the precise relationship between the morphological picture and the presence or absence of the specific faecal toxin becomes known.

RECENT ADVANCES

In 1977 Larson et al noted the presence of a 'toxin' in the stools of five patients with PMC. Faecal suspensions from these patients produced a characteristic cytopathic effect (CPE) on cell culture lines which was absent in control patients or those with other gastrointestinal diseases. It was suggested that this toxic effect might be of bacterial origin. Following on from this Rifkin, Fekety and Silva (1977) showed that the cytopathic effect was neutralized by prior incubation of the stool suspension with gas-gangrene polyvalent antitoxin and in particular with antitoxin to *Clostridium sordellii*. However, attempts to isolate *C. sordellii* from the stools of patients with PMC were unsuccessful (Larson and Price, 1977). Next, Bartlett et al (1978a) showed that rather than *C. sordellii*, *C. difficile* was a constant isolate from patients with PMC and it produced a toxin that cross-reacted with *C. sordellii* antitoxin. This finding was quickly confirmed by others (George et al, 1978; Larson et al, 1978). In parallel with these findings in humans the role of toxigenic *C. difficile* in the aetiology of antibiotic-associated PMC was substantiated by experimental work on the Syrian golden hamster.

The experimental animal model

Small (1968) demonstrated that Syrian golden hamsters developed a fatal enterocolitis when administered lincomycin or clindamycin.

Unlike human PMC, antibiotic-associated colitis in the hamster involves mainly the caecum. Typical pseudomembranous lesions are not seen but the mucosa is either frankly haemorrhagic or shows crypt and epithelial proliferation accompanied by degenerative changes (Figure 9; Humphrey et al,

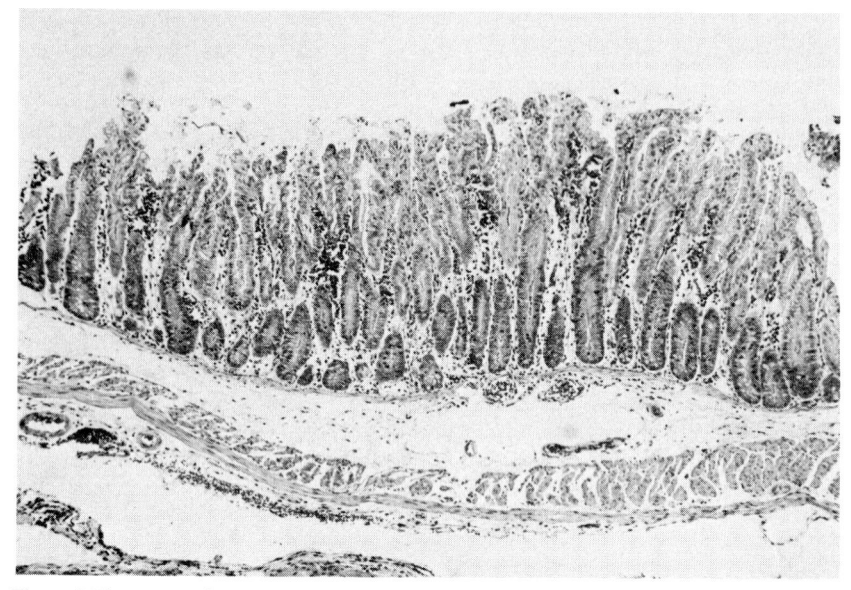

Figure 9. The caecum from a hamster dying with clindamycin-associated caecitis. The mucosa is thickened, with lengthening of the crypts and an irregular tufted surface. Little of the haemorrhagic element is seen in this specimen. No pseudomembrane-like lesions occur. Haematoxylin and eosin, × 65.

1979b; Price, Larson and Crow, 1979). Hamsters may spontaneously develop a morphologically similar picture, confined to the ileum, called 'wet-tail' or 'proliferative ileitis' (Jacoby, 1978), but clostridia have not been implicated.

The caecal contents of hamsters dying with clindamycin-associated caecitis contain a toxin identical to that in the stools of patients with PMC (Bartlett et al, 1977) and *C. difficile* can be isolated (Bartlett et al, 1978b). The organism is not detectable in the faeces of normal hamsters (Price, Larson and Crow, 1979). The caecal contents or extracted cell free filtrates from diseased animals reproduce the disease if inoculated into healthy animals, either directly into the caecum or via an orogastric tube (Rifkin, Silva and Fekety, 1978). Stool suspensions or a cell free filtrate from humans with PMC, when inoculated into hamsters, also give similar results (Larson et al, 1978). Broth cultures of caecal isolates of *C. difficile* from hamsters dying with clindamycin-associated caecitis contain toxin and these too will produce caecitis in healthy animals (Rifkin, Fekety and Silva, 1978). At variance with this, Larson et al (1978) found that if broth cultures of *C. difficile* were first washed free of detectable toxin then administered by orogastric tube to healthy hamsters no disease developed, but when force fed to hamsters who had received antibiotics caecitis developed. As the normal hamster does not carry detectable numbers of *C. difficile* in the gut these results are more akin to those observed in humans. The intestine must first be made susceptible to colonization.

Experiments along other lines support the evidence for the identity of the organism responsible for both human PMC and experimentally induced AAC in the hamster. For example, continual administration of *C. sordellii* antitoxin to hamsters will protect against clindamycin-induced disease (Allo et al, 1979) and incubation of the caecal contents from an affected animal with *C. sordellii* antitoxin (Rifkin, Fekety and Silva, 1978) also prevents disease developing when these contents are subsequently inoculated into a healthy animal.

Like human PMC, enterocaecitis in the hamster can be induced by a wide range of antibiotics (Bartlett et al, 1978b) and animals may be protected by the simultaneous administration of a second antibiotic to which *C. difficile* is susceptible, in particular vancomycin (Bartlett, Onderdonk and Cisneros, 1977). This drug is now used in the treatment of human PMC (Keighley et al, 1978b; Tedesco et al, 1978). However, although vancomycin protects hamsters from antibiotic-induced caecitis, if given alone it lowers the resistance of the gut to subsequent colonization by *C. difficile*. Animals given only vancomycin develop caecitis at intermittent intervals after it has been stopped (Fekety et al, 1979). One explanation for this is that vancomycin promotes spore formation with disease appearing as germination commences (Onderdonk, Cisneros and Bartlett, 1979). However, the animals will survive if caged under sterile conditions (Fekety et al, 1979). Our own current work shows that animals will remain alive after a clindamycin challenge if caged in sterile or non-contaminated conditions (Larson, Price and Borriello, 1979) and the introduction of a contaminated animal, or accidental atmospheric contamination, will then result in an outbreak of caecitis. If these observations are substantiated much of the early experimental work may need re-assessment. It does appear that the environment plays a role in the epidemiology of experimental antibiotic-associated caecitis and that the hamster intestine, like the human, must first be in a 'susceptible' state.

These experimental data show that despite the poor morphological comparison with human PMC the hamster is clearly a useful model for studying the epidemiology and pathogenesis of disease due to *C. difficile* and its toxin.

Clinical studies

Currently the stools of over 90 per cent of patients with PMC have been found to contain *C. difficile* and its toxin (Bartlett, 1979b). The realization of the bacterial aetiology of PMC has provided a rationale for its treatment as well as an explanation for the wide variations in observed incidence of the disease. The specific test for faecal CPE has increased the rate of diagnosis and altered the spectrum of disease presenting to clinicians.

In the past PMC was rarely diagnosed prior to autopsy, and it is still a potentially serious disease in the elderly, especially if there is a delay in diagnosis (Price and Davies, 1977). The mortality figures in patients over 60 years may reach 40 per cent (Mogg et al, 1979). However, the current picture of antibiotic-associated PMC is of a much milder illness, often in a young patient and described by Tedesco, Barton and Alpers (1974) as 'self-limiting and without mortality'. Previously such cases would have passed undiagnosed. The typical hospital in-patient usually has diarrhoea, some abdominal pain, a low-grade fever, a raised white cell count and may develop hypoalbuminaemia (Mogg et al, 1979). Bloody diarrhoea is rare. The onset of diarrhoea in relation to a course of antibiotics is surprisingly variable. It develops in some patients during the course but in many it commences only after the course has finished, often as long as three weeks (Tedesco, 1977). In these circumstances unless a specific inquiry is made the relevance of the drug history may be missed. It must also be remembered that a history of diarrhoea is not an invariable finding (Price and Davies, 1977).

Epidemiology

The unusual temporal and geographical clustering of cases of PMC and the wide disparity in quoted incidence (Miller and Jick, 1977) bear the hallmark of an infectious disease. For example, in prospective series the incidence of clindamycin-associated PMC has varied from 0 per cent up to 10 per cent (Ramirez-Ronda, 1974; Tedesco, Barton and Alpers, 1974; Condon and Anderson, 1978). Even at two hospitals within a short distance of each other a gross disparity in incidence was found. At one, over a short study period, the incidence of AAC rose to 46 per cent among post-surgical patients (Keighley et al, 1978a, 1978b) while at the other hospital no cases of PMC had been seen despite administration of clindamycin to several hundred patients over a period of 10 years (Geddes, 1974). Kabins and Spira (1975) reported AAC in 17 per cent of patients on clindamycin over a two-month period and 8 per cent had PMC. The incidence of PMC in autopsy material was 5 per cent at that time. In the preceding 20 months not a single case had been diagnosed. A similar clustering of cases was noted by Swartzberg, Maresca and Remington (1977) and on a more anecdotal level by Burdon et al (1979). In this instance 12 cases of AAC occurred in one month in one ward. The ward was closed and some patients moved to other wards. Four new cases occurred in one of these wards within two weeks of the transfer of patients. The five cases of PMC reported by Milligan and Kelly (1979) all occurred within an eight-month period yet only one case had been seen in the previous four years. All five occurred in the same ward and disease was concurrent in two pairs of patients. The clustering of cases, resembling small epidemics, supports the concept that PMC is an infectious disease. Although more detailed bacteriological work is still required these observations have important implications in the management of the individual patient.

C. DIFFICILE AND ITS TOXIN; MICROBIOLOGICAL SENSITIVITY AND RATIONALE FOR TREATMENT

The organism, an anaerobic sporing Gram-negative bacillus, was first isolated by Hall and O'Toole (1935) from the stools of neonates. These findings were confirmed by Snyder in 1940 and its presence in the intestinal tract of healthy term and pre-term infants reaffirmed as part of the current interest in PMC. Borriello (1979) found the organism in the stools of 10 of 16 healthy neonates and some also contained toxin. A low titre of exotoxin was also reported in 14 per cent of 121 infants aged from 0 to 5 months by Rietra et al (1978). Seven in this series had diarrhoea but it was not considered to be of clinical significance. Neonates may become colonized from the maternal vagina during delivery as 18 per cent of healthy women attending a family planning clinic were shown to carry the organism (Hafiz et al, 1975).

Part of the evidence that *C. difficile* is a pathogen is that, in contrast to neonates, it is rarely found in the intestine of healthy adults and to my knowledge no symptomless patient has been shown to excrete toxin. George, Sutter and Finegold (1978) isolated *C. difficile* from four of 137 healthy adults but Borriello (1979) was unable to isolate the organism from 100 individuals who were either healthy or had intestinal disorders unrelated to PMC. Transient symptom-free carriage was demonstrated in one volunteer during a course of antibiotics. However, a recent report (Bolton, Sherriff and Read, 1979) suggests *C. difficile* might play a role in the exacerbation of some forms of colitis unrelated to antibiotics. It was found in 16 per cent of patients with diarrhoea in a general medical ward, only one of whom had received antibiotics. Until its association with PMC *C. difficile* was thought to play little part in human disease. Smith and King (1962) isolated it from six patients with diverse infections but concluded it was probably not pathogenic. An isolate from a patient with a perirectal abscess was believed to be pathogenic by Daniellson, Lambe and Persson (1972) on the evidence that changing serum antibodies were demonstrated.

The toxin

Although the isolation of *C. difficile* from stools is difficult identification of the exotoxin by its characteristic cytopathic effect on a variety of cell culture lines is by comparison simple and available as a laboratory result within 24 hours (George, 1979). The toxin is inactivated by heating at 56°C for 30 minutes and by trypsin but survives treatment with RNAse and DNAse. Figures for its molecular weight vary between 240 000 and 700 000 (Aswell et al, 1979; Taylor and Bartlett, 1979). These discrepancies seem to be related to the source of the toxin, whether extracted from human stool, hamster caecal contents or from a broth isolate. Although the toxin has antigenic cross-reactivity in vitro with *C. sordellii* antitoxin the overlap is not a total one. Preparations of crude *C. difficile* antitoxin do not cross-react with *C. sordellii* toxin; furthermore, the latter is rarely cytopathic (Aswell et al, 1979). However, the neutralization of the CPE in a stool from a patient with PMC by *C. sordellii* antitoxin is an essential diagnostic step. Up to 15 per cent of stools from patients with diverse intestinal disorders can show a non-specific CPE (Bartlett, 1979a). When toxin is demonstrated *C. difficile* is invariably found but the organism has been isolated from the stools of patients in the absence of detectable faecal toxin. This undermines the infallibility of the toxin test as a screening procedure for colitis involving *C.*

difficile (Bartlett et al, 1978c; Keighley et al, 1978b). It is still disputed whether in vitro isolates are ever non-toxigenic if optimum conditions prevail (Chang, Gorbach and Bartlett, 1978). Furthermore, if such non-toxigenic strains exist are they still pathogenic? Until the methodology is standardized and made more sensitive it is difficult to interpret the significance of these varying results.

Treatment

Hamsters will survive a clindamycin challenge if given regular *C. sordellii* antitoxin inoculation (Allo et al, 1979), but it has no prophylactic value. This and the difficulties of giving foreign protein rule out the therapeutic value of antitoxin in the treatment of human PMC. *C. difficile*, however, is sensitive to a range of antibiotics and in particular to vancomycin; an interesting observation when it is remembered that this drug was used to treat the outbreaks of staphylococcal enteritis in the 1950s. All strains so far tested have been sensitive to low levels of vancomycin easily obtainable in the stool. Fifteen isolates tested by Fekety et al (1979) were all inhibited or killed at concentrations of less than 2 μg/ml. The 14 tested by George, Sutter and Finegold (1978) had a uniform susceptibility to vancomycin of less than 1 μg/ml. Both papers also showed that the isolates were uniformly sensitive to low concentrations of ampicillin and penicillin; a puzzling fact, as these drugs are often associated with the induction of PMC, in particular ampicillin (Price and Davies, 1977). This has not been true for vancomycin which is therefore the therapeutic drug of choice. In one trial (Keighley et al, 1978b) the toxin titre in patients receiving vancomycin gradually declined over the course of two to seven days, while patients receiving a placebo were still excreting toxin at the end of one week. Metronidazole has been used to treat PMC (Trinh Dinh, Kernbaum and Frottier, 1978) on the same rationale as vancomycin, and cholestyramine has also been tried. This has been shown to act by binding toxin (Humphrey et al, 1979a). There are some reports of relapses after successful vancomycin therapy (W.L. George et al, 1979). As mentioned before disease frequently occurs in the hamster after protection with vancomycin is stopped and the drug may encourage spore formation (Onderdonk, Cisneros and Bartlett, 1979).

GENERAL DISCUSSION

The evidence now suggests that PMC be moved from chapters on bowel ischaemia and appear alongside the causes of infectious diarrhoea. Firstly, an organism, *C. difficile*, which cannot be detected in normals and is pathogenic in the experimental hamster model, has been constantly isolated. Secondly, the geographic and temporal clustering of PMC is characteristic of an infectious disease and environmental contamination has been demonstrated to play a role in the experimental animal model. Attention has already been drawn to the implications of these findings in patient management.

Despite this knowledge of the aetiology of PMC there are few facts about how *C. difficile* is able to colonize the bowel and, once established, how the unique focal mucosal plaques evolve. It is exceptional for a healthy person to develop spontaneous PMC (Jackson and Anders, 1972). Experimental contamination of healthy hamsters with *C. difficile* may also be without effect (Price, Larson and Crow, 1979). It appears that *C. difficile* will only colonize the intestinal tract after an initial change in the gut milieu which results in a state of susceptibility. From the epidemiological data one can postulate that in this state development of the disease now depends on meeting a source of infection. The virulence of this source or an array of host factors might then determine the morphological pattern of disease. Some evidence for this hypothesis exists in that the presence of plaques is associated with the highest toxin titres (Mogg et al, 1979). This is also suggested from one of the few papers classifying antibiotic-associated disease along the lines suggested earlier. Toxin was found in three of 47 (6 per cent) patients classified as AAD, in six of 16 (38 per cent) patients with AAC and in 26 of 27 (97 per cent) patients with biopsy-proven PMC (Bartlett et al, 1978c).

The commonest means of inducing a state of intestinal susceptibility to *C. difficile* is by a course of certain antibiotics and one of the current aims of research is to establish by what mechanism this arises. The simplest theory is that antibiotics select out a resistant organism. This is untenable as isolates of *C. difficile* from patients with PMC are not necessarily resistant to the associated antibiotic. For example, all isolates have been sensitive to ampicillin and some to clindamycin (George, Sutter and Finegold, 1978). This objection would be less significant if disease always began after a course of antibiotics had finished and at a time when stool concentrations of the antibiotic were dropping below inhibitory levels, but it fails to explain the cases which arise during a course. There is some evidence that antibiotics stimulate toxin production and in this manner might enhance the virulence of the organism (Borriello, 1979; R.H. George et al, 1979). This could be a direct effect or via an intermediary mechanism. A second variable in addition to the straightforward presence or absence of *C. difficile* might explain the wide variation in incidence of PMC and why the disease can occur during a course of antibiotics to which *C. difficile* is seemingly sensitive. The most obvious intermediary trigger would be a qualitative alteration in gut flora produced by the antibiotics (Marr, Sans and Tedesco, 1975), allowing *C. difficile* to thrive, or the induction of a single permissive growth factor. This might be of bacterial origin, derived from an endogenous metabolite like the bile acids (Hofman, 1977) or be an actual metabolite of the drug. An alternative view is that 'susceptibility' entails the switching off of an inhibitory mechanism that normally prevents colonization by *C. difficile*. Apart from the mechanisms suggested above the colonic mucosa may be directly involved. The virulence of many intestinal pathogens depends on their ability to adhere to and even penetrate the surface epithelial cells (Smith, 1977). Any change in the physical or chemical properties of the cell surface induced by antibiotics or surgery might be sufficient to allow colonization by an organism which is not normally a gut pathogen.

Once established, it seems probable that the toxin of *C. difficile* causes the initial focus of mucosal necrosis (McDonel and Duncan, 1975) and may be responsible for all the pathological changes. Alternatively, after the initial damage caused by the toxin other agents, previously excluded by the intact mucosa, would have access to the lamina propria and microcirculation. In this way secondary mechanisms like the Shwartzman phenomenon (Hjort and Rapaport, 1965; Berry and Fraser, 1968) or ischaemia might have a role.

CONCLUSIONS

C. difficile and its toxin are one cause, if not the only cause, of PMC. The realization of its bacterial aetiology, the rapidity of the test for faecal CPE and the rationale for the therapeutic use of vancomycin have significantly altered the management and prognosis of the disease. Nowadays the majority of cases are associated with antibiotics. A positive faecal CPE in a patient implies that the diarrhoea is due to *C. difficile* but the associated pathology ranges from no change through a picture of infectious proctitis to PMC and even toxic megacolon. Further clinical research is required, with widespread use of the toxin test and stricter definitions of AAD, AAC and PMC, to delineate the spectrum of disease and the relationships between *C. difficile*, its toxin, antibiotics and the mechanism of intestinal susceptibility. As a specific CPE is found only in some 30 per cent of patients who develop diarrhoea following the administration of antibiotics (Bartlett et al, 1978c) *C. difficile* represents but part of the explanation of a more complex problem. It perhaps defines the group of patients with the potential for developing PMC. Other mechanisms and other organisms (Palton et al, 1978; Knoop, 1979; Lamont, Sonnenblick and Rothman, 1979) as causes for AAD and AAC must still be sought.

ACKNOWLEDGEMENTS

I should like to thank Jillian Jones for the preparation of the manuscript and John Clark for the photography.

REFERENCES

Allo, M., Silva, J. Jr, Fekety, R., Rifkin, G. & Waskin, H. (1979) Prevention of clindamycin-induced colitis in hamsters by *Clostridium sordellii* antitoxin. *Gastroenterology*, **76**, 351-355.

Aswell, J.E., Ehrich, M., Van Tassell, R.L., Tsai, C., Holdeman, L.V. & Wilkins, T. (1979) Characterization and comparison of *Clostridium difficile* and other clostridial toxins. In *Microbiology* (Ed.) Schlessinger, D. pp. 272-275. Washington DC: American Society for Microbiology.

Bartlett, J.G. (1979a) Antimicrobial agent-associated pseudomembranous colitis in patients. In *Microbiology* (Ed.) Schlessinger, D. pp. 264-266. Washington DC: American Society for Microbiology.

Bartlett, J.G. (1979b) Antibiotic-associated colitis. *Clinics in Gastroenterology*, **8**, 783-801.

Bartlett, J.G., Onderdonk, A.B. & Cisneros, R.L. (1977) Clindamycin-associated colitis in hamsters: protection with vancomycin. *Gastroenterology*, **73**, 772-776.

Bartlett, J.G., Onderdonk, A.B., Cisneros, R.L. & Kapser, D.L. (1977) Clindamycin-associated colitis due to toxin producing species of *Clostridium* in hamsters. *Journal of Infectious Diseases*, **136**, 701-705.

Bartlett, J.G., Chang, T.W., Gurwith, M., Gorbach, S.L. & Onderdonk, A.B. (1978a) Antibiotic-associated pseudomembranous colitis due to toxin-producing clostridia. *New England Journal of Medicine*, **298**, 531-534.

Bartlett, J.G., Chang, T.W., Moon, N. & Onderdonk, A.B. (1978b) Antibiotic-induced lethal enterocolitis in hamsters: studies with eleven agents and evidence to support the pathogenic role of toxin producing clostridia. *American Journal of Veterinary Research*, **39**, 1525-1530.

Bartlett, J.G., Moon, N., Chang, T.W., Taylor, N. & Onderdonk, A.B. (1978c) Role of *Clostridium difficile* in antibiotic-associated pseudomembranous colitis. *Gastroenterology*, **75**, 778-782.

Berry, C.L. & Fraser, G.C. (1968) The experimental production of colitis in the rabbit with particular reference to Hirschsprung's disease. *Journal of Pediatric Surgery*, **3**, 36-42.

Billroth, C.A.T. (1867) Ueber duodenalgeschwüre bei septicämie. *Wiener Medizinische Wochenschrift*, **17**, 705-709.

Bolton, R.P., Sherriff, R.J. & Read, A.E. (1979) *Clostridium difficile* associated diarrhoea — a role in inflammatory bowel disease. *Gut*, **20**, A932.

Borriello, S.P. (1979) *Clostridium difficile* and its toxin in the gastrointestinal tract in health and disease. *Research and Clinical Forums*, **1**, 33-35.

Burdon, D.W., Mogg, G.A.G., Alexander-Williams, J., Youngs, D., Johnson, M., George, R.H. & Keighley, M.R.B. (1979) Epidemiology of antibiotic-associated colitis. *11th International Congress of Chemotherapy and 19th Interscience Conference on Antimicrobial Agents and Chemotherapy.* Abstract No. 839.

Chang, T.W., Gorbach, S.L. & Bartlett, J.R. (1978) Neutralization of *Clostridium difficile* toxin by *Clostridium sordellii* antitoxins. *Infection and Immunity*, **22**, 418-422.

Cohen, L.E., McNeill, C.J. & Wells, R.F. (1973) Clindamycin-associated colitis. *Journal of the American Medical Association*, **223**, 1379-1380.

Condon, R.E. & Anderson, M.J. (1978) Diarrhoea and colitis in clindamycin treated surgical patients. *Archives of Surgery*, **113**, 794-797.

Daniellson, D., Lambe, D.W. & Persson, S. (1972) The immune response in a patient to an infection with *Bacteroides fragilis* sub species *fragilis* and *Clostridium difficile*. *Acta Pathologica et Microbiologica Scandinavica B*, **80**, 709-712.

Day, D.W., Mandal, B.K. & Morson, B.C. (1978) The rectal biopsy appearances of *Salmonella* colitis. *Histopathology*, **2**, 117-131.

Dearing, W.H., Baggenstoss, A.H. & Weed, L.A. (1960) Studies on the relationship of *Staphylococcus aureus* to pseudomembranous enteritis and post-antibiotic enteritis. *Gastroenterology*, **38**, 441-451.

Dixon, C.F. & Weisman, R.E. (1948) Acute pseudomembranous enteritis or enterocolitis: a complication following intestinal surgery. *Surgical Clinics of North America*, **28**, 999-1023.

Fekety, R., Silva, J., Toshniwal, R., Allo, M., Armstrong, J., Browne, R., Ebright, J. & Rifkin, G. (1979) Antibiotic-associated colitis: effects of antibiotics on *Clostridium difficile* and the disease in hamsters. *Reviews of Infectious Diseases*, **1**, 386-397.

Fick, K.A. & Wolken, A.P. (1949) Necrotizing jejunitis. *Lancet*, **i**, 519-521.

Finland, M., Grigsby, M.E. & Haight, T.H. (1954) Efficacy and toxicity of oxytetracycline (Terramycin) and chlortetracycline (Aureomycin) with special reference to use of doses of 250 mgms every four to six hours and to occurrence of staphylococcic diarrhoea. *Archives of Internal Medicine*, **93**, 23-43.

Finney, J.M.T. (1893) Gastro-enterostomy for cicatrizing ulcer of the pylorus. *Bulletin of the Johns Hopkins Hospital*, **4**, 53-55.

Geddes, A.M. (1974) Lincomycin and clindamycin colitis. *British Medical Journal*, **iv**, 591.

George, R.H. (1979) A micro-method for detecting toxins in pseudomembranous colitis. *Journal of Clinical Pathology*, **32**, 303-304.

George, R.H., Symonds, J.M., Dimock, F., Brown, J.D., Arabi, Y., Shinagawa, N., Keighley, M.R.B., Alexander-Williams, J. & Burdon, D.W. (1978) Identification of *Clostridium difficile* as a cause of pseudomembranous colitis. *British Medical Journal*, **i**, 695.

George, R.H., Johnson, M., Youngs, D. & Burdon, W. (1979) Induction of *Clostridium difficile* toxin by antibiotics. *11th International Congress of Chemotherapy and 19th Interscience Conference of Antimicrobial Agents and Chemotherapy.* Abstract No. 839.

George, W.L., Sutter, V.L. & Finegold, S.M. (1978) Toxegenicity and antimicrobial susceptibility of *Clostridium difficile*, a cause of antimicrobial agent-associated colitis. *Current Microbiology*, **1**, 55-58.

George, W.L., Sutter, V.L. & Finegold, S.M. (1978) Toxigenicity and antimicrobial suscepti-

Rolfe, R.D. & Finegold, S.M. (1979) Relapse of pseudomembranous colitis after vancomycin therapy. *New England Journal of Medicine*, **301**, 414-415.

Goulston, S.J.M. & McGovern, V.J. (1965) Pseudomembranous colitis. *Gut*, **6**, 207-212.

Hafiz, S., McEntegart, M.G., Morton, R.S. & Watkins, S.A. (1975) *Clostridium difficile* in the urogenital tract of males and females. *Lancet*, **i**, 420-421.

Hall, K. & O'Toole, E. (1935) Intestinal flora in newborn infants with description of a new pathogenic anaerobe, *Bacillus difficilis*. *American Journal of Diseases of Children*, **49**, 390-402.

Hardaway, R.M. & McKay, D.G. (1959) Pseudomembranous enterocolitis; are antibiotics wholly responsible? *Archives of Surgery*, **78**, 446-457.

Hartman, H.A. & Angevine, D.M. (1956) Pseudomembranous colitis complicating prolonged antibiotic therapy. *American Journal of the Medical Sciences*, **232**, 667-673.

Hjort, P.F. & Rapaport, S.I. (1965) The Shwartzman reaction: pathogenetic mechanisms and clinical manifestations. *Annual Review of Medicine*, **16**, 135-168.

Hofman, A.F. (1977) Bile acids, diarrhoea and antibiotics: data, speculation and a unifying hypothesis. *Journal of Infectious Diseases*, **135**, S126-S132.

Humphrey, C.D., Condon, C.W., Cantey, J.R. & Pittman, F.E. (1979a) Partial purification of a toxin found in hamsters with antibiotic-associated colitis. *Gastroenterology*, **76**, 468-476.

Humphrey, C.D., Lushbaugh, W.B., Condon, C.W., Pittman, J.C. & Pittman, F.E. (1979b) Light and electron microscopic studies of antibiotic-associated colitis in the hamster. *Gut*, **20**, 6-15.

Jackson, B.T. & Anders, C.J. (1972) Idiopathic pseudomembranous colitis successfully treated by surgical excision. *British Journal of Surgery*, **59**, 154-156.

Jacoby, R.O. (1978) Transmissible ileal hyperplasia of hamsters. *American Journal of Pathology*, **91**, 433-450.

Kabins, A. & Spira, J.J. (1975) Outbreak of clindamycin-associated colitis. *Annals of Internal Medicine*, **83**, 830-831.

Kappas, A., Shinagawa, N., Arabi, Y., Thompson, H., Burdon, D.W., Dimock, F., George, R.H., Alexander-Williams, J. & Keighley, M.R.B. (1978) Diagnosis of pseudomembranous colitis. *British Medical Journal*, **i**, 675-678.

Kay, A.W., Richards, R.L. & Watson, A.J. (1958) Acute necrotizing (pseudomembranous) enterocolitis. *British Journal of Surgery*, **46**, 45-47.

Keighley, M.R.B., Alexander-Williams, J., Arabi, Y., Youngs, D., Burdon, D.W., Shinagawa, N., Thompson, H., Bentley, S. & George, R.H. (1978a) Diarrhoea and pseudomembranous colitis after gastrointestinal operation. *Lancet*, **ii**, 1165-1168.

Keighley, M.R.B., Burdon, D.W., Arabi, Y., Alexander-Williams, J., Thompson, H., Youngs, D., Johnson, M., Bentley, S., George, R.H. & Mogg, G.A.G. (1978b) Randomised control trial of vancomycin for pseudomembranous colitis and postoperative diarrhoea. *British Medical Journal*, **ii**, 1667-1669.

Killingback, A.J. & Williams, K.L. (1962) Necrotizing colitis. *British Journal of Surgery*, **49**, 175-185.

Kleckner, M.S., Jr, Bargen, J.A. & Baggenstoss, A.H. (1952) Pseudomembranous enterocolitis: clinicopathologic study of fourteen cases in which the disease was not preceded by an operation. *Gastroenterology*, **21**, 212-222.

Kliegman, R.M. (1979) Neonatal necrotizing enterocolitis: implications for an infectious disease. *Pediatric Clinics of North America*, **26**, 327-344.

Knoop, F.C. (1979) Clindamycin-associated enterocolitis in guinea pigs: evidence for a bacterial toxin. *Infection and Immunity*, **23**, 31-33.

Lamont, T.J., Sonnenblick, E.B. & Rothman, S. (1979) Role of clostridial toxin in the pathogenesis of clindamycin colitis in rabbits. *Gastroenterology*, **76**, 356-361.

Larson, H.E. & Price, A.B. (1977) Pseudomembranous colitis: presence of clostridial toxin. *Lancet*, **ii**, 1312-1314.

Larson, H.E., Price, A.B. & Borriello, S.P. (1979) The possible role of environmental *Clostridium difficile* in antibiotic colitis of hamsters and man. *Clinical Research*, **27**, 349A.

Larson, H.E., Parry, J.V., Price, A.B., Davies, D.R., Dolby, J. & Tyrell, D.A.J. (1977) Undescribed toxin in pseudomembranous colitis. *British Medical Journal*, **i**, 1246-1248.

Larson, H.E., Price, A.B., Honour, P. & Borriello, S.P. (1978) *Clostridium difficile* and the aetiology of pseudomembranous colitis. *Lancet*, **i**, 1063-1066.

Margaretten, W. & McKay, D.G. (1971) Thrombotic ulcerations of the gastrointestinal tract. *Archives of Internal Medicine*, **127**, 250-253.

Marr, J.J., Sans, M.D. & Tedesco, F.J. (1975) Bacterial studies of clindamycin-associated colitis. *Gastroenterology*, **69**, 352-358.

Marston, A. (1977) *Intestinal Ischaemia*. 190 pp. London: Edward Arnold.

McDonel, J.L. & Duncan, C.L. (1975) Histopathological effect of *Clostridium perfringens* enterotoxin in the rabbit ileum. *Infection and Immunity*, **12**, 1214-1218.

McKay, D.G., Hardaway, R.M. III, Wahle, G.H. Jr & Hall, R.M. (1955) Experimental pseudomembranous colitis: production by means of thrombosis of intestinal capillaries. *Archives of Internal Medicine*, **95**, 779-787.

Miller, R.R. & Jick, H. (1977) Antibiotic-associated colitis. *Clinical Pharmacology and Therapeutics*, **22**, 1-6.

Milligan, D.W. & Kelly, J.K. (1979) Pseudomembranous colitis in a leukemia unit: a report of five fatal cases. *Journal of Clinical Pathology*, **32**, 1237-1243.

Mogg, G.A.G., Keighley, M.R.B., Burdon, D.W., Alexander-Williams, J., Youngs, D., Johnson, M., Bentley, S. & George, R.H. (1979) Antibiotic-associated colitis — a review of 66 cases. *British Journal of Surgery*, **66**, 738-742.

Murrell, T.G.C., Roth, L., Egerton, J., Samuels, J. & Walker, P.D. (1966) Pig-Bel: enteritis necroticans. *Lancet*, **i**, 217-222.

Newman, C.R. (1956) Pseudomembranous enterocolitis and antibiotics. *Annals of Internal Medicine*, **45**, 409-444.

Onderdonk, A.B., Cisneros, R.L. & Bartlett, J.G. (1979) Effect of vancomycin and clindamycin on *C. difficile* associated gnotobiotic mice. *11th International Congress of Chemotherapy and 19th Interscience Conference on Antimicrobial Agents and Chemotherapy*. Abstract No. 843.

Palton, N.M., Holmes, H.T., Rigg, R.J. & Cheeke, P.R. (1978) Enterotoxaemia in rabbits. *Laboratory Animal Science*, **28**, 536-540.

Penner, A. & Bernheim, A. (1939) Acute post-operative enterocolitis. *Archives of Pathology*, **27**, 966-983.

Pittman, F.E., Norgaard, R.P., Shelley, W.M. & Hennigar, G.R. (1977) The spectrum of sigmoidoscopic and histopathological findings in lincomycin/clindamycin colitis. In *Symposium/Workshop on Epidemiological Issues in Reported Drug-induced Illnesses: SMON and Other Examples*. Ontario: McMaster University Library Press.

Price, A.B. & Davies, D.R. (1977) Pseudomembranous colitis. *Journal of Clinical Pathology*, **30**, 1-12.

Price, A.B. & Morson, B.C. (1975) Inflammatory bowel disease; the surgical pathology of Crohn's disease and ulcerative colitis. *Human Pathology*, **6**, 7-29.

Price, A.B., Jewkes, J. & Sanderson, P.J. (1979) Acute diarrhoea: *Campylobacter* colitis and the role of rectal biopsy. *Journal of Clinical Pathology*, **32**, 990-997.

Price, A.B., Larson, H.E. & Crow, J. (1979) Morphology of experimental antibiotic-associated enterocolitis in the hamster: a model for human pseudomembranous colitis and antibiotic-associated colitis. *Gut*, **20**, 467-475.

Ramirez-Ronda, C.H. (1974) Incidence of clindamycin-associated colitis. Comment and corrections. *Annals of Internal Medicine*, **81**, 860.

Rietra, P.J.G.M., Slaterus, K.W., Zanen, H.C. & Meuwissen, S.G.M. (1978) Clostridial toxin in faeces of healthy infants. *Lancet*, **ii**, 319.

Rifkin, G.D., Fekety, F.R. & Silva, J. Jr (1977) Antibiotic induced colitis, implication of a toxin neutralised by *Clostridium sordellii* antitoxin. *Lancet*, **ii**, 1103-1106.

Rifkin, G.D., Fekety, R. & Silva, J. (1978) Neutralization by *Clostridium sordellii* antitoxin of toxins implicated in clindamycin-induced cecitis in the hamster. *Gastroenterology*, **75**, 422-424.

Rifkin, G.D., Silva, J. & Fekety, R. (1978) Gastrointestinal and systemic toxicity of fecal extracts from hamsters with clindamycin-induced colitis. *Gastroenterology*, **74**, 52-57.

Sakurai, Y., Tsuchiya, H., Ikegami, F., Funatomi, T., Takasu, S. & Uchikoshi, T. (1979) Acute right sided hemorrhagic colitis associated with oral administration of ampicillin. *Digestive Diseases and Sciences*, **24**, 910-915.

Scott, A.J., Nicholson, G.I. & Kerr, A.R. (1973) Lincomycin as a cause of pseudomembranous colitis. *Lancet*, **II**, 1232-1234.

Small, J.D. (1968) Fatal enterocolitis in hamsters given lincomycin hydrochloride. *Laboratory Animal Care*, **18**, 411-420.

Smith, H. (1977) Microbial surfaces in relation to pathogenicity. *Bacteriological Reviews*, **41**, 475-500.

Smith, L.DS. & King, E.O. (1962) Occurrence of *Clostridium difficile* in infections of man. *Journal of Bacteriology*, **84**, 65-67.

Snyder, M.L. (1940) The normal faecal flora of infants between two weeks and one year of age. *Journal of Infectious Diseases*, **66**, 1-16.

Swartzberg, J.E., Maresca, R.M. & Remington, J.S. (1977) Clinical study of gastrointestinal complications associated with clindamycin therapy. *Journal of Infectious Diseases*, **135**, S99-S103.

Taylor, N.S. & Bartlett, J.G. (1979) Partial purification and characterization of a cytotoxin for *Clostridium difficile*. *Reviews of Infectious Diseases*, **1**, 379-385.

Tedesco, F.J. (1977) Clindamycin and colitis: a review. *Journal of Infectious Diseases*, **135**, S95-S98.

Tedesco, F.J. (1979) Antibiotic associated pseudomembranous colitis with negative proctosigmoidoscopy examination. *Gastroenterology*, **77**, 295-297.

Tedesco, F.J., Barton, R.W. & Alpers, D.H. (1974) Clindamycin-associated colitis: a prospective study. *Annals of Internal Medicine*, **81**, 429-433.

Tedesco, F., Markham, R., Gurwith, M., Christie, D. & Bartlett, J.G. (1978) Oral vancomycin for antibioticp-associated pseudomembraneous colitis. *Lancet*, **ii**, 226-228.

Terplan, K., Paine, J.R., Sheffer, J., Egan, R. & Lansky, H. (1953) Fulminating gastroenterocolitis caused by staphylococci; its apparent connection with antibiotic medication. *Gastroenterology*, **24**, 476-509.

Toffler, R.B., Pingoud, E.G. & Burrell, M.I. (1978) Acute colitis related to penicillin and penicillin derivatives. *Lancet*, **ii**, 707-709.

Trinh Dinh, H., Kernbaum, S. & Frottier, J. (1978) Treatment of antibiotic-induced colitis by metronidazole. *Lancet*, **i**, 338-339.

Whitehead, R. (1971) Ischaemic enterocolitis: an expression of the intravascular coagulation syndrome. *Gut*, **12**, 912-917.

Wilson, R. & Qualheim, R.E. (1954) A form of acute haemorrhagic enterocolitis affecting chronically ill individuals. *Gastroenterology*, **27**, 431-444.

11
Crohn's Disease: Definition, Pathogenesis and Aetiology

J.E. LENNARD-JONES

The eponym Crohn's disease is succinct but reveals our inability to define the condition in terms of aetiology or pathogenesis. The patients described in 1932 by Crohn and his colleagues were a small homogeneous group with terminal ileal disease selected from a much larger heterogeneous group of patients with non-specific inflammations of the gut. As time has passed more and more disorders from the heterogeneous group have been included under the general term Crohn's disease so that now inflammations with the histological characteristics associated with the ileal lesion have been described from all parts of the gastrointestinal tract, the lip and mouth, the anus, and also from such diverse sites as the skin, liver, muscle and bone.

DEFINITION AND DIAGNOSIS

Definition

No biochemical, immunological or microbiological technique has so far contributed to definition of the disease and diagnosis is still based on anatomical description. Unfortunately, no defining anatomical feature has been recognized which is present in every patient regarded as suffering from Crohn's disease and absent in all other disorders. Diagnosis depends on recognition of a pattern of abnormalities, some of which are macroscopic and can be observed as well by clinical techniques as in a surgical specimen, and others of which are microscopic. The non-caseating epithelioid granuloma is of particular importance because it is relatively common in Crohn's disease and rare in other conditions. A working definition requires some form of scoring system and the following scheme (Lennard-Jones, 1970) is based on standard pathological texts and on studies involving numerical taxonomy and discriminant analysis:

Macroscopic anatomy
 Discontinuity of inflammation along and around the circumference of the gut anywhere between lip and anus.
 A predilection for involvement of the *terminal ileum* with ulceration of the

© 1980 W.B. Saunders Company Ltd.

mucosa and narrowing of the lumen due to swelling of the mucosa and thickening of the intestinal wall.

A tendency to development of a chronic *anal lesion*, often with ulceration of the anal canal and/or perianal skin, swelling of the skin to form oedematous tags, sepsis and fistula formation.

Cleft-like ulcers or fissures passing perpendicularly from the intestinal lumen into the gut wall.

Fistulae between the inflamed gut and other hollow viscera or the skin surface.

Microscopic anatomy

Epithelioid granulomas, without caseation, and often with Langhans-type giant cells.

Inflammation involving *all layers* of the gut wall (*transmural*).

Fissuring ulceration as already described.

Lymphoid aggregates throughout the thickness of the bowel wall.

Normal epithelial mucus content in the presence of acute inflammation.

This list is not exhaustive but it includes many of the commoner manifestations of Crohn's disease and is summarized in Table 1.

Table 1

	Clinical	X-ray	Biopsy	Specimen
Ileum	+	+		+
Anus	+	+		+
Fistula	+	+		+
Discontinuity	+	+	+	+
Fissure		+·		+
Granuloma			⊕	⊕
Lymphoid			+	+
Mucin			+	+
Transmural				+

Crohn's = +++ or +⊕.

It is suggested that the presence of epithelioid granulomas with one other feature, or the presence of three features in the absence of granulomas, should be regarded as diagnostic of Crohn's disease *provided that specific infection, ischaemia or other recognized cause of tissue damage has been excluded.*

Diagnosis

Table 1 shows that all the macroscopic features can be recognized by clinical examination, endoscopy or x-ray. It is thus possible to make a clinical diagnosis on anatomical grounds without microscopic evidence. However, in most cases biopsy adds greatly to the diagnostic information and the usefulness of biopsy has increased now that specimens can readily be obtained under direct vision from the mouth to the duodenum, and from the anal canal to the distal ileum. The reason why diagnosis is so often based on examination of an operation specimen is apparent because all the anatomical features can be looked for.

Limitation of present diagnostic criteria

Diagnostic schemes of this type limit our concept of Crohn's disease to those patients with major structural lesions. It is possible that by so doing patients with minor inflammation or transient lesions are never recognized so that Crohn's disease is inevitably regarded as a serious, and often chronic or recurring, disorder. The newer techniques of endoscopy with biopsy and double-contrast radiology enable small aphthoid ulcers and other minor mucosal abnormalities to be studied. These techniques may enable us to recognize Crohn's disease at an earlier stage than hitherto, when reversion to normal of the structural changes is a possibility. Efforts must be made to define Crohn's disease in terms of minor abnormalities of structure rather than the major abnormalities which are used at present.

PATHOLOGICAL ANATOMY
The Granuloma

Experimental background

The granuloma tends to be regarded as an anatomical marker whereas it is really a visible manifestation of mononuclear metabolic activity. The following brief account of the granulomatous response as it appears relevant to Crohn's disease is based on the excellent reviews of Spector (1969) and Adams (1976).

Granulomas are largely composed of mononuclear cells derived from the bone marrow which migrate to the site of the lesion. These cells mature with increasing cytoplasmic complexity to become macrophages and, in certain circumstances, epithelioid cells. Scanning microscopy shows that mature macrophages are covered by numerous ridges, flanges and villi; epithelioid cells are larger and interlace with one another by intertwining of the surface processes. The cytoplasm of epithelioid cells is filled by organelles, as is the cytoplasm of Langhans' giant cells, formed by fusion of macrophages or epithelioid cells. Epithelioid cells exhibit less phagocytic activity than macrophages but their structure indicates intense metabolic activity and possibly a secretory function.

Experimental work shows that granulomas tend to form when a foreign substance enters the tissues but for some reason polymorphonuclear leucocytes or mononuclear phagocytes fail to digest and degrade it. Persistence of foreign material may be due to its chemical nature, as with some polymers. A substance normally degraded rapidly may stimulate granuloma formation if it reacts with antibody to form a complex, especially if there is antigen-antibody equivalence or antibody excess. The paradoxical situation may thus occur that a humoral antibody response to an antigen on the part of the host may lead to formation of a complex between the antibody and the antigen and so prevent its degradation, whereas antigen introduced into a non-sensitized animal is rapidly degraded and removed. Radio-autographic labelling of either the antigen or the antibody components of a complex shows that both persist within macrophages, mostly at the centre of the granuloma for at least 20 days (Spector and Heesom, 1969). Under these circumstances, antigen was not demonstrable within epithelioid cells.

These observations suggest that the granuloma in Crohn's disease could be due to entry of a poorly digestible antigen into the gut wall, presumably from the intestinal lumen, or to the formation of antigen-antibody complexes due to a potent humoral antibody response to an antigen which is usually easily degraded.

Observations in Crohn's disease

Electron microscopic observations (Aluwihare, 1971) showed that the epithelioid cells in Crohn's disease contain variable amounts of endoplasmic reticulum and ribosomes, many mitochondria, a Golgi zone, vesicles which are not electron dense, and very little debris. Giant cells have the same structural features as epithelioid cells but contain more debris. Acid phosphatase was found in and around the vesicles, even though they did not contain any visible debris. Proliferation of monocytes in the bone marrow of patients with Crohn's disease, as judged by incubation of bone marrow spicules, was moderately increased, but less than in some other inflammatory disorders without a granulomatous response (Meuret, Bitzi and Hammer, 1978).

Counts of granulomas in sections of diseased tissue from various parts of the gastrointestinal tract showed that the frequency increased progressively from a small number in the ileum, to the largest number at the anus; the colon and rectum showed intermediate values with the same trend towards increase with more distal disease. These observations also suggested that granulomas were more common in patients with a history of up to four years than in those with a longer history (Chambers and Morson, 1979).

Clinical significance of the granuloma

Overall, granulomas are observed in 60 to 70 per cent of cases, but the frequency with which they are found depends on the diligence of the search, the amount of tissue available for study and its origin from different parts of the gut. There is, as would be expected, a spectrum from diffuse histiocytic infiltration, through loose aggregations of histiocytes ('microgranulomas'), to an infiltrate in which granulomas are a dominant feature (Chambers and Morson, 1979).

Earlier observations suggested that liability to recurrence after surgical resection of diseased tissue was independent of the presence or absence of a granulomatous response (Gump et al, 1972). Two recent studies have suggested that a good prognosis is correlated with the presence and number of granulomas (Glass and Baker, 1976; Chambers and Morson, 1979).

Immunofluorescent Studies

Detailed quantitative studies of immunoglobulin-producing cells in the ileal mucosa have been reported by Baklien and Brandtzaeg (1976). In slightly inflamed mucosa the total number of immunoglobulin-containing cells in a defined area were increased threefold compared with normal controls but only minor changes occurred in the relative proportions of cells containing IgA, IgG and IgM. Where the mucosa was severely inflamed but glands persisted, the total immunocyte count rose by a factor of 12 above normal but the predominant increase was among IgG cells which were increased by a factor of 60.9 above normal. Adjacent to a fissure, there was a further increase in the total immunocyte count and here the IgG-producing cells were increased by about 200-fold over the normal value.

There was no significant difference in absolute immunocyte count in severely inflamed mucosa from the ileum or colon. IgD and IgE immunocytes were extremely rare and no consistent increase was found in the inflamed mucosae. The finding of a predominant increase in IgG-producing cells in severely inflamed mucosa accords with the tenfold increase in IgG secretory rate of monuclear cells isolated from intestinal tissue involved in inflammatory bowel disease (mostly Crohn's disease), whereas the IgA secretory rate was normal (Bookman and Bull, 1979).

Mucosa Remote from Obvious Disease

There is doubt as to whether Crohn's disease affects the whole gastrointestinal tract with local manifestations, or whether it is a localized discontinuous process which may have secondary immunological or other effects on the rest of the gut.

Several studies have demonstrated granulomas and other evidence of typical inflammation in macroscopically normal tissue at a distance from the main lesion. For example, such lesions have been demonstrated in biopsies from the stomach, duodenum and rectum in patients with terminal ileal disease.

Subtle changes have become apparent by morphometric methods where there is no obvious histological abnormality. Söltoft (1969) demonstrated an increased number of immunoglobulin-containing cells per unit area in jejunal mucosa in nine patients with terminal ileal disease when the jejunal mucosa showed normal morphology under the dissecting microscope and on section. In 20 patients with Crohn's disease confined to the distal ileum or large bowel, morphometry showed a reduction in jejunal mucosal surface area and an increase in mucosal volume compared with patients suffering from ulcerative colitis or normal controls (Dunne, Cooke and Allan, 1977). Another study revealed an increased plasma cell density in the jejunum regardless of the site of the overt disease (Ferguson, Allan and Cooke, 1975). Significant increases in plasma cell density and volume of the lamina propria were also demonstrated under similar conditions in rectal mucosa which appeared histologically normal (Goodman, Skinner and Truelove, 1976).

Besides these morphological changes, changes in the enzyme content of the mucosa have also been shown. In apparently normal jejunum brush-border disaccharidases were reduced but cytoplasmic dipeptidases were unchanged (Dunne, Cooke and Allan, 1977). In apparently normal rectal mucosa, glucosamine synthetase activity, an epithelial enzyme concerned in the biosynthesis of glycoproteins and a measure of cell regeneration, was increased (Goodman, Skinner and Truelove, 1976). Prolylhydroxylase, an indicator of collagen synthesis, was also found to be increased in rectal mucosa of patients with Crohn's disease, many of whom showed no evidence on biopsy of rectal disease (Farthing et al, 1978).

The 'Early' Lesion

Most descriptions of pathological anatomy refer to advanced disease; clues as to aetiology and pathogenesis are most likely to be found early in the evolution of a lesion. Whether or not the changes found in the plasma cell content and enzyme activity of apparently normal tissue represent 'disease' or a reaction to inflammation elsewhere in the gut is debatable; the latter appears more likely. There are few, if any, reports of repeated biopsies from an accessible site to show the progress or regression of the disease process; such studies are difficult because of the sampling error inherent in the discontinuous nature of the inflammation.

Reports on 'early' lesions are therefore restricted to minor abnormalities adjacent to areas of obvious disease or descriptions of areas with slight evidence of inflammation (Morson, 1972). The significance of the aphthoid ulcer, a characteristic lesion seen on endoscopy and in operation specimens at a distance from the main lesion, is uncertain. Granulomas may be found in areas of mucosa with little structural abnormality and an intact epithelium. Lesions with slight inflammation are associated with an increased number of immunocytes containing IgA, IgG and IgM in normal proportions, suggesting that the great increase in IgG-containing cells in severe inflammation is a secondary phenomenon. Local IgG production in response to entry of antigens and mitogens from the gut lumen due to a break in the epithelium could, in fact, have a deleterious effect (Baklien and Brandtzaeg, 1976).

Electron microscopic studies of colonic mucosa in areas with an intact epithelium 2 to 50 cm distant from ulceration or obvious disease have revealed clusters of bacteria in the mucosa with an increased proportion of lymphocytes and plasma cells in the lamina propria and some oedema. The appearances of the bacteria were not the same in the six cases in which they were found. Organisms were not seen in similar sites of any normal colon, nor in any colon affected by ulcerative colitis and possessing an intact epithelium (Aluwihare, 1971). It is interesting to speculate whether such bacteria are faecal organisms invading the mucosa in a person with a defect in the defence mechanisms, or whether they are specific organisms, peculiar to Crohn's disease, which initiate a granulomatous response by their particular characteristics.

GENETICS

Many studies have shown that about one in ten patients with Crohn's disease have a first-degree relative who also suffers from inflammatory bowel disease. The prevalence of Crohn's disease was 13 times greater than expected among first-degree relatives in a series from Cardiff with almost total ascertainment, a finding most unlikely ($P < 0.0002$) to have occurred by chance (Mayberry, Rhodes and Newcombe, 1980). This prevalence is not high enough to indicate a disease of simple Mendelian inheritance with high penetrance.

The results of this survey from Cardiff agree with all other reports that ulcerative colitis also occurs with unexpectedly high frequency in the same families. Another careful study from Liverpool in which all relatives were examined has confirmed that the two disorders tend to occur in the same families, and also ankylosing spondylitis without apparent bowel disease (McConnell, 1979). No genetic marker associated with inflammatory bowel disease has yet been recognized. However, those patients with ulcerative colitis or Crohn's disease who are of tissue type HLA-B27 appear to have a greater risk of developing ankylosing spondylitis than subjects of this tissue type in the general population.

The familial tendency among patients with Crohn's disease tends to be stronger than among patients with ulcerative colitis. Among the families siblings appear to have a greater risk of developing inflammatory bowel disease than parents, or perhaps children. There is suggestive evidence that a family history of inflammatory bowel disease is particularly common among those who develop one of these conditions in the first two decades of life; a feature suggestive of polygenic inheritance. Several pairs of monozygous twins have been reported, most of whom develop the same type of bowel disease. McConnell (1979) has suggested that all these facts may be explained if several genes contribute to a susceptibility to inflammatory bowel disease. If many of these genes are inherited then Crohn's disease is more likely than ulcerative colitis, so explaining the greater familial tendency in Crohn's disease.

EPIDEMIOLOGY

It is probable that the prevalence of Crohn's disease is greater in Europe and North America than in Africa or the Middle and Far East. All epidemiological studies in Europe tend to show a rising incidence; in England and Wales it is likely that the incidence rose around fivefold during the period 1955 to 1975 (Miller, Keighley and Langman, 1974; Mayberry, Rhodes and Hughes, 1979). These facts suggest that an environmental factor is important in the aetiology of the disorder. Possible factors could be a chemical in the food or water supply, a predisposing effect of diet or an infection.

Chemicals in food or water

It is known that beryllium or zirconium can cause a granulomatous hypersensitivity in the lung or skin, with lesions resembling in some respects those of Crohn's disease. Studies with zirconium have shown that minute quantities can produce a marked granulomatous reaction in sensitive subjects. Elias and Epstein (1968) have estimated that 10 ng of beryllium can elicit a granuloma containing 80 to 90 million cells. No dietary constituent has yet been recognized that can induce a similar reaction in the gut (Carstensen, 1979). The observation that a low molecular weight hydrolysate of one form of carrageenan, a sulphated polygalactose polymer derived from seaweed, can cause caecal and colonic ulceration in animals when given by mouth does not appear relevant to Crohn's disease as this form of carrageenan is not used as a food additive (Abraham and Coulston, 1979). However, induction of colonic ulceration and crypt abscesses, with evidence of uptake of the polymer by macrophages, provides an interesting experimental model of a chemically-induced inflammation.

Diet

Several dietary surveys have shown that patients with Crohn's disease tend to eat more refined sugar, and in one study less raw fruit and vegetables, than matched control groups. The situation is complicated because the change in dietary habit could be a reaction to the disease rather than a predisposing factor. However, this tendency is evident even among patients interviewed within three months of diagnosis, and retrospective inquiry suggested that these patients had not altered their eating habits as a response to their symptoms. Furthermore, patients with ulcerative colitis interviewed in the same way showed no difference from controls in their dietary habits (Thornton, Emmett and Heaton, 1979, 1980).

It seems possible that a diet high in refined carbohydrate could affect the contents of the intestinal lumen, perhaps by altering the bacterial flora. Further research on this topic is needed.

Infection

Crohn's disease has been reported only twice among spouses. However, some factor affecting both patient and spouse is suggested by the finding that lymphocytotoxic antibodies and also antibodies to synthetic polyribonucleotides are not only found more commonly among patients than among matched control subjects, but also found more commonly among the spouses of patients than among the spouses of the control population (Strickland et al, 1977; DeHoratius et al, 1978). The biological significance of lymphocytotoxic antibodies is not clear but they have been observed in virus infections. Similarly, the antibodies to single- or double-stranded RNA could represent a reaction to an RNA virus affecting both patient and spouse. The fact that the spouse has not developed colitis or Crohn's disease might mean that lack of genetic susceptibility, or an environmental factor such as a different dietary habit, determines the reaction to infection.

IMMUNOLOGY

Humoral Immunity

Circulating antibodies to a wide range of dietary and bacterial antigens can be demonstrated in patients with Crohn's disease. Antibodies to bovine serum albumin, casein and lactalbumin, as in many other intestinal disorders, are probably due to abnormal permeability of the mucosa. Antibodies to a wider range of *Escherichia coli* serotypes (mean 13.8) than in patients with ulcerative colitis (mean 7.9) or normal controls (mean 1.5) may reflect exposure to *E. coli* within the diseased tissues (Tabaqchali, O'Donoghue and Bettelheim, 1978). Similarly, antibodies to *Bacteroides vulgatus* were found more commonly in patients with Crohn's disease than in those with ulcerative colitis or normal subjects (Helphinstine et al, 1979). The increased frequency of bacterial antibodies can be made the basis of an indirect diagnostic test for the possibility of Crohn's disease in doubtful cases, and a simple agglutination technique using undiluted serum and killed suspensions of three species of *Eubacterium* and one species of *Peptostreptococcus* has given encouraging results (Van De Merwe, 1980).

Elevated titres to colon antigen from germ-free rats are more common in Crohn's disease than in control sera but no specificity of these antibodies to *E. coli* O:14 was found as in ulcerative colitis (Carlsson, Lagercrantz and Perlmann, 1977). The significance, if any, of anti-colon antibodies in pathogenesis of the disease is unclear.

Cell-Mediated Immunity

The literature on various aspects of cell-mediated immunity is extensive and confusing. Discrepant results may be due to differences in technique and in the types of patients studied, particularly as regards disease severity or treatment. It is hard to distinguish between a primary disorder of cell-mediated immunity and secondary effects. The subject has recently been reviewed by Auer (1979) who gives an extensive bibliography.

T lymphocyte concentrations in blood

Absolute numbers of circulating T lymphocytes were found in one study to be slightly increased in patients with inactive Crohn's disease and a short history, but decreased in patients with inactive disease but a longer history and previous drug treatment (Auer et al, 1979). In another study T lymphocytes were reduced regardless of disease activity (Lyanga, Davis and Thomson, 1979). It is not known whether this decrease is due to luminal loss of cells from the gut, sequestration of lymphocytes in the bowel wall or increased suppressor cell activity.

Primary cell-mediated response

The ability of the immune system to mount an immune response to a new antigen, such as dinitrochlorobenzene, is probably unaltered in the absence of malnutrition or other non-specific depression of immune function (Bolton et al, 1974).

Anamnestic response

Skin responses or in vitro mitogenic responses of lymphocytes to antigens previously encountered give conflicting results; some reports show depression, even in patients with inactive disease (Meuwissen et al, 1975), whereas others ascribe any depression found to severity of the disease (Bolton et al, 1974).

Mitogen-induced lymphocyte proliferation

There is conflicting evidence concerning stimulation of lymphocytes by phytohaemagglutinin A, concanavalin A, Varidase and Poke Weed mitogen (Bolton et al, 1974; Auer, 1979; Lyanga, Davis and Thomson, 1979).

Gut-Associated Lymphocytes

High rates of DNA synthesis and blast transformation of lymphocytes cultured from small bowel mucosa involved in Crohn's disease have been observed in comparison with lymphocytes cultured from normal intestinal mucosa (Clancy, 1976). Most of the cells isolated are macrophages or B lymphocytes (Bookman and Bull, 1979).

Antibody-Dependent Cell-Mediated Cytotoxicity

Circulating K lymphocytes isolated from patients with Crohn's disease or ulcerative colitis exhibit cytotoxicity against colonic epithelial cells but not against gastric or duodenal epithelium (Stobo et al, 1976). Normal lymphocytes can be rendered cytotoxic to colonic epithelium by incubation with an immunoglobulin fraction of molecular weight greater than 200 000 from a patient with inflammatory bowel disease (Shorter et al, 1971) or by incubation with enterobacterial antigen for several days. It has thus been suggested that enterobacterial antigen or perhaps a circulating antigen-antibody complex may initiate cytotoxicity to colonic epithelium. The evidence for such a mechanism in vitro is strong but its importance in vivo, especially in Crohn's disease where the major lesion often affects the small intestine, is uncertain. Recent observations have failed to demonstrate the presence of K cells or antibody-dependent cytotoxicity among mucosal cells isolated from diseased tissue (Bookman and Bull, 1979). Observations on circulating K cell levels have shown normal or raised levels (Eckhardt et al, 1977; Lyanga, Davis and Thomson, 1979).

Phagocytic Function

Polymorphonuclear and mononuclear phagocytes both exhibit mobility, chemotaxis, adherence, phagocytosis and intracellular microbial killing and degradation. The polymorph kills and degrades phagocytosed organisms rapidly and completely. The macrophage appears to have an additional role in association with lymphocytes of developing an immune response to ingested antigen. Ward (1977, 1979) has suggested that there is a primary macrophage defect in patients with Crohn's disease but at present there is no direct evidence to support this hypothesis. It has been shown that the production and release of two acid hydrolases by peripheral blood monocytes is markedly increased in patients with inflammatory bowel disease (Ganguly et al, 1978).

Migration of polymorphonuclear leucocytes from abraded skin is reduced in patients with Crohn's disease (Segal and Loewi, 1976) and the leucocytes also show a reduced capacity to phagocytose yeast particles as compared with normal (Krause, Michaëlsson and Juhlin, 1978).

MICROBIOLOGY

Microbiological agents could play a primary role in the aetiology of Crohn's disease, either by tissue invasion and damage or by the induction of an immunological or tissue reaction to some chemical constituent of the organism. Alternatively, secondary invasion of tissue initially damaged by some other mechanism could be a feature of the pathogenesis of the disease.

Transmission and Passage

The demonstration that a granulomatous reaction developed after inoculation of the foot pad of the mouse with diseased tissue from patients with Crohn's disease, and that this lesion could be passaged to other mice, appeared to be a major advance (Mitchell and Rees, 1970). Subsequently, a lesion transmissible to the ileum of rabbits was described (Cave et al, 1973). Subsequent work has tended to confuse rather than clarify the issues and the subject has been well reviewed by Sachar and Auslander (1978). These authors draw attention to the lack of reproducibility of findings in different laboratories; some of which, despite extensive work and apparently similar techniques, can detect no evidence of a transmissible lesion (Heatley et al, 1975). Other laboratories report a different time-scale or frequency of the granulomatous response. Lack of uniformity of histological interpretation complicates the issue and independent review of experimentally produced lesions showed that some, at least, were due to parasites or other artefacts. In some studies normal bowel homogenates have produced a transient granulomatous response.

From all this work it seems reasonably certain that a lesion can develop in mouse foot pad or rabbit ileum after injection of Crohn's disease tissue filtered through a 0.2 μm filter. The development of granulomatous inflammation is inconstant and the pathology of any gut lesion bears no obvious resemblance to Crohn's disease. The results are consistent with the introduction of a cell-wall deficient bacterium, a virus or a chemotactic tissue component into the host animal. At present the significance of this research is difficult to assess but it has given great impetus to the microbiological study of Crohn's disease.

Virus Studies

Findings of a positive cytopathic effect of tissue extracts from patients with Crohn's disease on various cell lines in culture have been reported and the literature is reviewed by Beeken (1979). Some studies have suggested the presence of a small RNA virus in tissue from patients with Crohn's disease, but also various other gastrointestinal disorders. This virus was always present in low titre (maximum 10^3), which has precluded detailed study. Other workers have failed to find any evidence of a virus in Crohn's disease tissue (Phillpotts, Hermon-Taylor and Brooke, 1979). The situation is complicated by the possibility that the cytopathic effect in some studies was due to a contaminating *Mycoplasma* (Kapikian et al, 1979).

Chlamydia

An initial serological study suggested the possibility of increased frequency of antibodies against chlamydia of the lymphogranuloma venereum type in Crohn's disease (Schuller et al, 1979). This organism is an intracellular parasite and can induce a granulomatous response. Three other studies have since failed to confirm this result; it has also proved impossible to demonstrate chlamydia in cell culture or by immunofluorescence in tissue (Swarbrick et al, 1979; Taylor-Robinson et al, 1979; Elliott et al, 1980).

Cell-Wall Deficient Bacteria

Experimental observations have shown that cell-wall deficient bacteria may provoke a persistent granuloma on injection, unlike the acute inflammation induced by the same organism with a cell wall (Spector, 1969). These observations and the fact that transmission of a lesion may follow injection of Crohn's tissue filtered through a 0.2 μm filter, which would remove normal bacteria, have aroused interest in the possible role of cell-wall deficient organisms in Crohn's disease.

Filtrates of homogenized tissues grown in hypertonic media yielded cellwall deficient variants of *Pseudomonas*-like bacteria (group Va) from all of 8 patients with Crohn's disease but not from patients with ulcerative colitis or other gastrointestinal disorders (Parent and Mitchell, 1978). A serological response to this organism was demonstrable in the blood of patients with Crohn's disease and the titres fell after surgical treatment (Mitchell and Parent, 1979). So far, it has not been possible for other workers to repeat this finding (Drasar, Elliott and Lennard-Jones, 1980) and immunofluorescence to the organisms has not been detected in tissue sections (Whorwell et al, 1978).

Culture for mycobacteria of lymph nodes obtained at operation from patients with Crohn's disease has yielded an unidentified organism in many cases, possibly a cell-wall deficient form (Burnham et al, 1978). It has not yet proved possible to characterize the nature of this growth which is more common on culture of lymph nodes from patients with Crohn's disease than from those with ulcerative colitis or other disorders (Stanford et al, 1979).

Quantitative Culture of Bacteria

Bacterial population of the intestinal lumen and faeces

The faecal flora of patients with Crohn's disease has shown a small increase of anaerobic Gram-negative rods ($P < 0.02$) and a larger increase of anaerobic Gram-positive coccoid rods ($P < 0.02$) of the genus *Eubacterium*, as compared with normal subjects (Wensinck, 1976).

Culture of bacteria within the intestinal lumen at operation, or in the stool in a few patients, has shown an increase in numbers of *Escherichia coli* ($P < 0.001$) and *Bacteroides fragilis* ($P < 0.001$) in the ileum and of *E. coli* ($P < 0.001$) and lactobacilli ($P < 0.01$) in the colon compared with control subjects. The abnormal flora in the ileum was unrelated to disease activity, narrowing of the lumen or excision of the ileocaecal valve; the abnormal colonic flora was not related to the presence of macroscopic colitis (Keighley et al, 1978).

Bacterial population of diseased tissue

Culture of the whole thickness of the bowel wall from diseased segments, apparently uninvolved bowel and a control group without Crohn's disease has shown that among the bacterial isolates aerobic bacteria predominated in Crohn's tissue whereas in control tissue aerobes and anaerobes were present in approximately equal proportions (Peach et al, 1978). Greater numbers of bacteria were associated with colonic tissue than tissue from the jejunum; samples from the ileum were intermediate. There was no statistical difference in the numbers of bacteria associated with Crohn's tissue compared with histologically normal tissue from the same patients and from the control group of patients.

Interaction Between Intestinal Bacteria and Intestinal Defence Mechanisms

There have been few studies of the biological properties of bacteria isolated from the gut of patients with Crohn's disease and of the interaction between the bacteria and antibodies from the blood of the host. In one such study (Van De Merwe, 1980) three species of *Eubacteria* showed different properties. Two of three bacterial species were readily phagocytized by leucocytes. Antibodies from patients to two species, but not the third, showed opsonizing properties; phagocytosis of the third species was potentiated by complement. Two of the three species activated complement by the alternative pathway and could thus initiate an inflammatory response.

CONCLUSIONS

The nature of Crohn's disease, its aetiology and pathogenesis so far elude definition despite much research. Several promising lines of investigation have proved frustrating: for example, the study of cell-mediated immunity, the transmission experiments, observations on circulating antibodies to possible infective agents, viral culture and attempts to isolate cell-wall deficient bacteria. Promising clues that await further study are the granulomatous tissue response, the high concentration of IgG-producing cells in severely inflamed mucosa, the genetic susceptibility, the possible role of diet, and the studies on intestinal and mucosal bacterial flora.

The following avenues of research deserve exploration:

1. The definition of Crohn's disease is based on anatomical changes, some of which are seen only in advanced disease. Efforts should be made to characterize those anatomical features which precede severe changes or may be reversible. Earlier diagnosis, the recognition of mild or reversible forms of the disorder, and increased understanding of pathogenesis may result.
2. The granulomatous response in gut mucosa deserves experimental study, particularly the identification of antigens, or antigen-antibody complexes, capable of inducing this response.
3. The antigen(s) associated with the marked IgG response in diseased mucosa need identification.
4. Further experimental observations are indicated on the interaction between intestinal bacteria and the defence mechanisms of the host such as phagocytosis, the interaction with antibody and the liberation of chemical mediators of inflammation.
5. A relationship should be sought between high dietary consumption of refined carbohydrate and the intestinal bacterial flora.
6. A possible role of food additives or deficiencies in subjects taking a high refined-carbohydrate, low-fibre diet deserves study.
7. The increased susceptibility of close relatives, particularly siblings, to Crohn's disease awaits further immunological and epidemiological investigation.

REFERENCES

Abraham, R. & Coulston, F. (1979) Ulcerative lesions due to carrageenan. *Zeitschrift für Gastroenterologie*, **17** (Suppl.), 154-158.

Adams, D.O. (1976) The granulomatous inflammatory response. *American Journal of Pathology*, **84**, 164-191.

Aluwihare, A.P.R. (1971) Electron microscopy in Crohn's disease. *Gut*, **12**, 509-518.

Auer, I.O. (1979) Immunology in Crohn's disease. *Zeitschrift für Gastroenterologie*, **17** (Suppl.), 83-93.

Auer, I.O., Gotz, S., Ziemer, E., Malchow, H. & Ehms, H. (1979) Immune status in Crohn's disease. 3. Peripheral blood B lymphocytes enumerated by means of $F(ab)_2$-antibody fragments, Null and T lymphocytes. *Gut*, **20**, 261-268.

Baklien, K. & Brandtzaeg, P. (1976) Immunohistochemical characterization of local immunoglobulin formation in Crohn's disease of the ileum. *Scandinavian Journal of Gastroenterology*, **11**, 447-457.

Beeken, W.L. (1979) Evidence of virus infection as a cause of Crohn's disease. *Zeitschrift für Gastroenterologie*, **17** (Suppl.), 101-104.

Bolton, P.M., James, S.L., Newcombe, R.G., Whitehead, R.H. & Hughes, L.E. (1974) The immune competence of patients with inflammatory bowel disease. *Gut*, **15**, 213-219.

Bookman, M.A. & Bull, D.M. (1979) Characteristics of isolated intestinal mucosal lymphoid cells in inflammatory bowel disease. *Gastroenterology*, **77**, 503-510.

Burnham, W.R., Lennard-Jones, J.E., Stanford, J.L. & Bird, R.G. (1978) Mycobacteria as a possible cause of inflammatory bowel disease. *Lancet*, **ii**, 693-696.

Carlsson, H.E., Lagercrantz, R. & Perlmann, P. (1977) Immunological studies in ulcerative colitis. VIII. Antibodies to colon antigen in patients with ulcerative colitis, Crohn's disease and other diseases. *Scandinavian Journal of Gastroenterology*, **12**, 707-714.

Carstensen, J. (1979) Food additives and their possible role in Crohn's disease. *Zeitschrift für Gastroenterologie*, **17** (Suppl.), 145-153.

Cave, D.R., Mitchell, D.N., Kane, S.P. & Brooke, B.N. (1973) Further animal evidence of a transmissible agent in Crohn's disease. *Lancet*, **ii**, 1120-1122.

Chambers, T.G. & Morson, B.C. (1979) The granuloma in Crohn's disease. *Gut*, **20**, 269-274.

Clancy, R. (1976) Isolation and kinetic characteristics of mucosal lymphocytes in Crohn's disease. *Gastroenterology*, **70**, 177-180.

DeHoratius, R.J., Strickland, R.G., Miller, W.C., Volpicelli, N.A., Gaeke, R.F., Kirsner, J.B. & Williams, R.C. Jr (1978) *Lancet*, **i**, 1116-1119.

Drasar, F., Elliott, P.R. & Lennard-Jones, J.E. (1980) in preparation.

Dunne, W.T., Cooke, W.T. & Allan, R.N. (1977) Enzymatic and morphometric evidence for Crohn's disease as a diffuse lesion of the gastrointestinal tract. *Gut*, **18**, 290-294.

Eckhardt, R., Kloos, P., Dierich, M.P. & Meyer Zum Büschenfelde, K.H. (1977) K-lymphocytes (killer-cells) in Crohn's disease and acute virus B-hepatitis. *Gut*, **18**, 1010-1016.

Elias, P.M. & Epstein, W.L. (1968) Ultrastructural observations on experimentally induced foreign-body and organised epithelioid-cell granulomas in man. *American Journal of Pathology*, **52**, 1207-1223.

Elliott, P.R., Forsey, T., Darougar, S., Treharne, J.D. & Lennard-Jones, J.E. (1980) Chlamydia and inflammatory bowel disease. In course of publication.

Farthing, M.J.G., Dick, A.P., Heslop, G. & Levene, C.I. (1978) Prolyl hydroxylase activity in serum and rectal mucosa in inflammatory bowel disease. *Gut*, **19**, 743-747.

Ferguson, R., Allan, R.N. & Cooke, W.T. (1975) A study of the cellular infiltrate of the proximal jejunal mucosa in ulcerative colitis and Crohn's disease. *Gut*, **16**, 205-208.

Ganguly, N.K., Kingham, J.G.C., Lloyd, B., Lloyd, R.S., Price, C.P., Triger, D.R. & Wright, R. (1978) Acid hydrolases in monocytes from patients with inflammatory bowel disease, chronic liver disease, and rheumatoid arthritis. *Lancet*, **i**, 1073-1075.

Glass, R.E. & Baker, W.N.W. (1976) Role of the granuloma in recurrent Crohn's disease. *Gut*, **17**, 75-77.

Goodman, M.J., Skinner, J.M. & Truelove, S.C. (1976) Abnormalities in the apparently normal bowel mucosa in Crohn's disease. *Lancet*, **i**, 275-278.

Gump, F.E., Sakellariadis, P., Wolff, M. & Broell, J.R. (1972) Clinical-pathological investigation of regional enteritis as a guide to prognosis. *Annals of Surgery*, **176**, 233-242.

Heatley, R.V., Bolton, P.M., Owen, E., Jones Williams, W. & Hughes, L.E. (1975) A search for a transmissible agent in Crohn's disease. *Gut*, **16**, 528-532.

Helphingstine, C.J., Hentges, D.J., Campbell, B.J., Butt, J. & Barrett, T. (1979) Antibodies detectable by counter-immunoelectrophoresis against bacteroides antigens in serum of patients with inflammatory bowel disease. *Journal of Clinical Microbiology*, **9**, 373-378.

Kapikian, A.Z., Barile, M.F., Wyatt, R.G., Yolken, R.H., Tully, J.G., Greenberg, H.B., Kalica, A.R. & Chanock, R.M. (1979) Mycoplasma contamination in cell culture of Crohn's disease material. *Lancet*, **ii**, 466-467.

Keighley, M.R.B., Arabi, Y., Dimock, F., Burdon, D.W., Allan, R.N. & Alexander-Williams, J. (1978) Influence of inflammatory bowel disease on intestinal microflora. *Gut*, **19**, 1099-1104.

Krause, U., Michaëlsson, G. & Juhlin, L. (1978) Skin reactivity and phagocytic function of neutrophil leucocytes in Crohn's disease and ulcerative colitis. *Scandinavian Journal of Gastroenterology*, **13**, 71-75.

Lennard-Jones, J.E. (1970) Crohn's disease: definition and diagnosis. *Skandia International Symposia—Regional Enteritis (Crohn's Disease) 1971*. pp. 105-112. Stockholm: Nordiska Bokhandelns Förlag.

Lyanga, J.J., Davis, P. & Thomson, A.B.R. (1979) In vitro testing of immunoresponsiveness in patients with inflammatory bowel disease: prevalence and relationship to disease activity immunoresponsiveness in IBD. *Clinical and Experimental Immunology*, 37, 120-125.

Mayberry, J.F., Rhodes, J. & Hughes, L.E. (1979) Incidence of Crohn's disease in Cardiff between 1934 and 1977. *Gut*, 20, 602-608.

Mayberry, J.F., Rhodes, J. & Newcombe, R.G. (1980) Familial prevalence of inflammatory bowel disease in relatives of patients with Crohn's disease. *British Medical Journal*, 280, 84.

McConnell, R.B. (1979) Genetics in Crohn's disease. *Zeitschrift für Gastroenterologie*, 17 (Suppl.), 61-65.

Meuret, G., Bitzi, A. & Hammer, B. (1978) Macrophage turnover in Crohn's disease and ulcerative colitis. *Gastroenterology*, 74, 501-503.

Meuwissen, S.G.M., Schellekens, P.Th.A., Huismans, L. & Tytgat, G.N. (1975) Impaired anamnestic cellular immune response in patients with Crohn's disease. *Gut*, 16, 854-860.

Miller, D.S., Keighley, A.C. & Langman, M.J.S. (1974) Changing patterns in epidemiology of Crohn's disease. *Lancet*, ii, 691-693.

Mitchell, D.N. & Rees, R.J.W. (1970) Agent transmissible from Crohn's disease tissue. *Lancet*, ii, 168-171.

Mitchell, P.D. & Parent, K. (1979) Cell wall-defective *Pseudomonas*-like bacteria: their possible significance in the etiology of Crohn's disease. *Zeitschrift für Gastroenterologie*, 17 (Suppl.), 109-112.

Morson, B.C. (1972) The early histological lesion of Crohn's disease. *Proceedings of the Royal Society of Medicine*, 65, 71-72.

Parent, K. & Mitchell, P. (1978) Cell wall-defective variants of *Pseudomonas*-like (Group Va) bacteria in Crohn's disease. *Gastroenterology*, 75, 368-372.

Peach, S., Lock, M.R., Katz, D., Todd, I.P & Tabaqchali, S. (1978) Mucosal-associated bacterial flora of the intestine in patients with Crohn's disease and in a control group. *Gut*, 19, 1034-1042.

Phillpotts, R.J., Hermon-Taylor, J. & Brooke, B.N. (1979) Virus isolation studies in Crohn's disease: a negative report. *Gut*, 20, 1057-1062.

Sachar, D.B. & Auslander, M.O. (1978) Missing pieces in the puzzle of Crohn's disease. *Gastroenterology*, 75, 745-748.

Schuller, J.L., Piket-Van Ulsen, J., Veeken, I.V.D., Michel, M.F. & Stolz, E. (1979) Antibodies against chlamydia of lymphogranuloma-venereum type in Crohn's disease. *Lancet*, i, 19-20.

Segal, A.W. & Loewi, G. (1976) Neutrophil dysfunction in Crohn's disease. *Lancet*, ii, 219-221.

Shorter, R.G., Huizenga, K.A., Spencer, R.J., Aas, J. & Guy, S.K. (1971) Inflammatory bowel disease: cytophilic antibody and the cytotoxicity of lymphocytes for colonic cells in vitro. *American Journal of Digestive Diseases*, 16, 673-690.

Söltoft, J. (1969) Immunoglobulin-containing cells in normal jejunal mucosa and in ulcerative colitis and regional enteritis. *Scandinavian Journal of Gastroenterology*, 4, 353-360.

Spector, W.G. (1969) The granulomatous inflammatory exudate. *International Review of Experimental Pathology*, 8, 1-55.

Spector, W.G. & Heesom, N. (1969) The production of granulomata by antigen-antibody complexes. *Journal of Pathology*, 98, 31-39.

Stanford, J.L., White, S.A., Burnham, W.R., Lennard-Jones, J.E. & Bird, R.G. (1979) Mycobacteria and inflammatory bowel disease. *Lancet*, i, 444.

Stobo, J.D., Tomasi, T.B., Huizenga, K.A., Spencer, R.J. & Shorter, R.G. (1976) In vitro studies of inflammatory bowel disease. Surface receptors of the mononuclear cell required to lyse allogeneic colonic epithelial cells. *Gastroenterology*, 70, 171-176.

Strickland, R.G., Miller, W.C., Volpicelli, N.A., Gaeke, R.F., Wilson, I.D., Kirsner, J.B. & Williams, R.C. (1977) Lymphocytotoxic antibodies in patients with inflammatory bowel disease and their spouses—evidence for a transmissible agent. *Clinical and Experimental Immunology*, 30, 188-192.

Swarbrick, E.T., Kingham, J.G.C., Price, H.L., Blackshaw, A.J., Griffiths, P.D., Darougar, S. & Buckell, N.A. (1979) Chlamydia, cytomegalovirus and yersinia in inflammatory bowel disease. *Lancet*, **ii**, 11-12.

Tabaqchali, S., O'Donoghue, D.P. & Bettelheim, K.A. (1978) *Escherichia coli* antibodies in patients with inflammatory bowel disease. *Gut*, **19**, 108-113.

Taylor-Robinson, D., O'Morain, C.A., Thomas, B.J. & Levi, A.J. (1979) Low frequency of chlamydial antibodies in patients with Crohn's disease and ulcerative colitis. *Lancet*, **i**, 1162-1163.

Thornton, J.R., Emmett, P.M. & Heaton, K.W. (1979) Diet and Crohn's disease: characteristics of the pre-illness diet. *British Medical Journal*, **ii**, 762-764.

Thornton, J.R., Emmett, P.M. & Heaton, K.W. (1980) Diet and ulcerative colitis. *British Medical Journal*, **280**, 293-294.

Van De Merwe, J. (1980) *Serum Antibodies to Anaerobic Coccoid Rods in Crohn's disease*. Rotterdam: Bronder-Offset B.V.

Ward, M. (1977) The pathogenesis of Crohn's disease. *Lancet*, **ii**, 903-905.

Ward, M. (1979) Phagocytic function in Crohn's disease. *Zeitschrift für Gastroenterologie*, **17** (Suppl.), 116-124.

Wensinck, F. (1976) Faecal flora of Crohn's patients. Serological differentiation between Crohn's disease and ulcerative colitis. In *The Management of Crohn's Disease* (Ed.) Weterman, I.T., Pēna, A.S. & Booth, C.C. pp. 103-107. Amsterdam, Oxford: Excerpta Medica.

Whorwell, P.J., Davidson, I.W., Beeken, W.L. & Wright, R. (1978) Search by immunofluorescence for antigens of rotavirus, *Pseudomonas maltophilia*, and *Mycobacterium kansasii* in Crohn's disease. *Lancet*, **ii**, 697-698.

PART THREE

Gastrointestinal Malignancy

12
Malabsorption and Intestinal Lymphomas

PETER ISAACSON
D.H. WRIGHT

An association between malabsorption and the development of intestinal lymphoma was first noted in 1937 (Fairley and Mackie). As reports of this association accumulated (Sleisenger, Almy and Barr, 1953) the accepted view came to be that the lymphoma was somehow responsible for the malabsorption. Later, as case reports appeared describing patients in whom long histories of malabsorption preceded the development of lymphoma (Scudamore, 1961) doubt was raised as to the malabsorption being secondary to lymphoma and finally, following the development of the peroral jejunal biopsy, Gough, Read and Naish (1962) firmly established the opposite view with the publication of their paper entitled 'Intestinal reticulosis as a complication of idiopathic steatorrhoea'. That intestinal lymphoma occurs as a complication of malabsorption is now generally accepted. There is, however, still some debate as to the cause of the malabsorption. The histological lesion in the intestine is identical to that found in coeliac disease and in an increasing number of cases histological response of this lesion to a gluten-free diet has been demonstrated (Freeman et al, 1977). Thus it appears likely, although by no means proven, that the malabsorption that is associated with intestinal lymphoma is due to coeliac disease. This, of course, applies only to those cases of malabsorption-associated intestinal lymphoma occurring in temperate countries where coeliac disease is the principal cause of malabsorption. A second type of malabsorption associated with intestinal lymphoma was first noted by Frand and Ramot (1963) in Israel. This form of lymphoma is known by a variety of names, most notably Mediterranean lymphoma, and is sometimes associated with α-heavy-chain disease (Al-Saleem and Zardawi, 1979). The intestinal lesion responsible for malabsorption is morphologically quite different from coeliac disease which is rare in the countries where Mediterranean lymphoma commonly occurs (Eidelman, Parkins and Rubin, 1966). The issue may be confused, however, by the concurrence of cases of intestinal lymphoma with tropical enteropathy or tropical sprue (Isaacson, 1979b), the lesion of which resembles coeliac disease.

This report will confine itself to a discussion of intestinal lymphoma that

© 1980 W.B. Saunders Company Ltd.

occurs in association with coeliac disease. Criteria for the diagnosis of coeliac disease (Cooke and Asquith, 1974) vary from the simple demonstration of a flat jejunal mucosa to morphological demonstration of gluten sensitivity requiring three jejunal biopsies (before and after a gluten-free diet and following a gluten challenge). The cases of intestinal lymphoma on which this report is based were selected on the basis of the presence in non-tumorous mucosa of changes histologically indistinguishable from those of coeliac disease. In addition to 18 cases initially described, a further 21 cases have been reviewed (Isaacson and Wright, 1978a, 1978b). A detailed analysis of the histological features of the tumour using a variety of techniques including plastic sections, ultrastructural studies, histochemistry and immunohistochemistry has shown that the lymphoma is uniformly of true histiocytic derivation. The pattern of dissemination is identical to that described in malignant histiocytosis (Byrne and Rappaport, 1973), also known as histiocytic medullary reticulosis (Scott and Robb-Smith, 1939). Accordingly, it is felt that the most appropriate name for this tumour is malignant histiocytosis of the intestine (MHI).

CLINICAL FEATURES

Malignant histiocytosis of the intestine occurs predominantly in the fifth to seventh decade with occasional cases in younger patients. The incidence is equal in males and females. In those patients in whom coeliac disease has been diagnosed the disease may manifest with return of steatorrhoea which no longer responds to a gluten-free diet. Sudden onset of weight loss, abdominal pain and diarrhoea may occur in patients with coeliac disease and is the commonest presentation in patients without a history of coeliac disease. Other significant features may include pyrexia, finger clubbing and an ichthyotic skin rash (Hodges et al, 1979). Perforation of the tumour with peritonitis occurs commonly and may be the initial mode of presentation. Characteristically, following surgical resection of the tumour, there is further intestinal perforation or haemorrhage which proves fatal. Less commonly the tumour causes intestinal obstruction rather than perforation. Cases may present with peripheral adenopathy due to disseminated tumour, the true nature of the disease becoming apparent only later.

GROSS APPEARANCES

The tumour may occur in any part of the small intestine but more commonly involves the jejunum. It is often multifocal and may occur in the form of multiple ulcers (Figure 1) or strictures (Figure 2) which appear inflammatory rather than neoplastic. Small ulcers are often concealed by mucosal folds and may easily be missed. Alternatively, larger plaques or nodules are sometimes formed or there may be diffuse thickening of a segment of bowel. The mesentery is often thickened and mesenteric lymph nodes are conspicuously enlarged. In a few cases no macroscopic lesion can be found even when the entire small intestine is examined post-mortem.

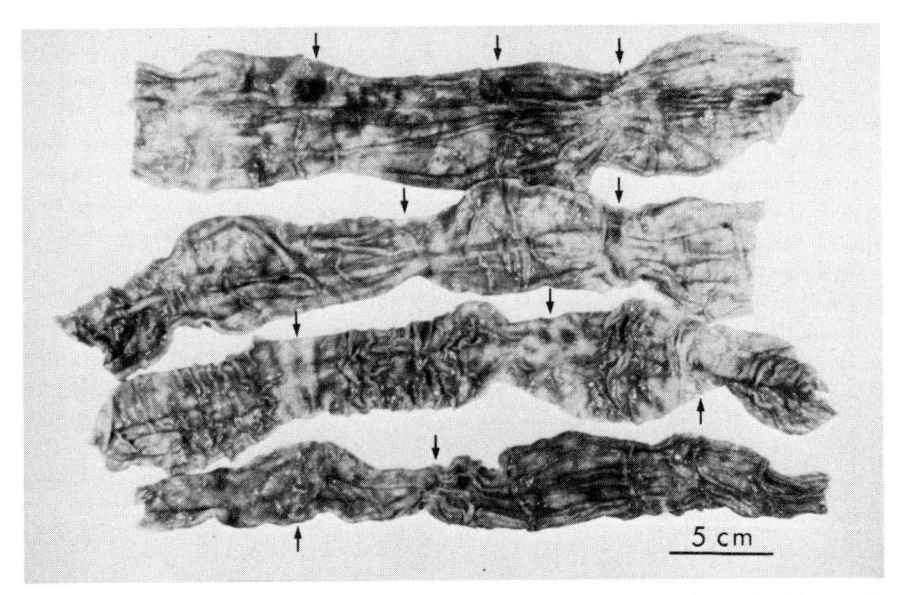

Figure 1. Post-mortem specimens showing multiple ulcers and strictures (arrows) of the small intestine from a 57-year-old man with MHI.

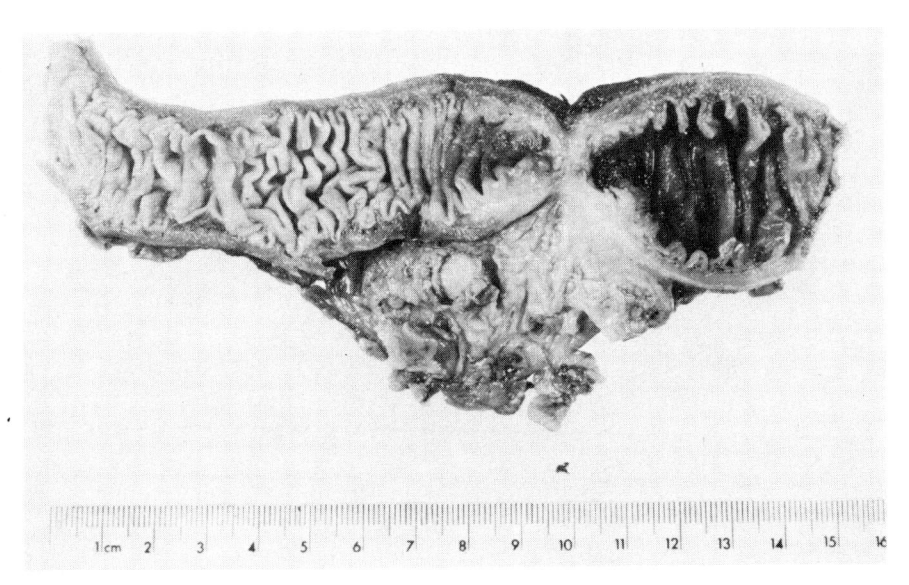

Figure 2. Surgical resection specimen of jejunum from a 60-year-old woman showing an isolated stricture which appears inflammatory rather than neoplastic. Histologically both stricture and enlarged mesenteric node showed MHI. From Hodges et al (1979), with kind permission of the editor of *Digestive Diseases and Sciences*.

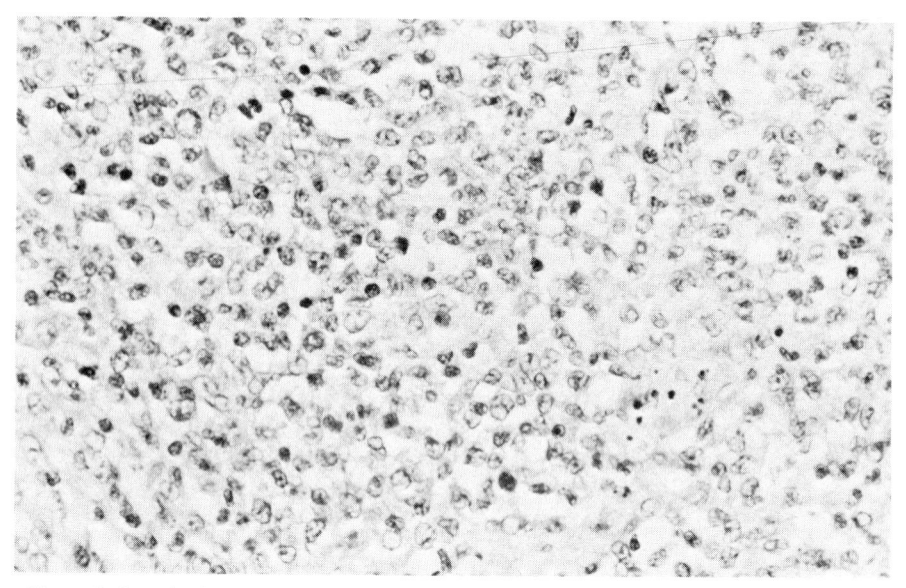

Figure 3. Intestinal tumour from a case of MHI consisting of sheets of well-differentiated malignant histiocytes. The nuclei show coarsening and peripheral condensation of chromatin with prominence of nucleoli.

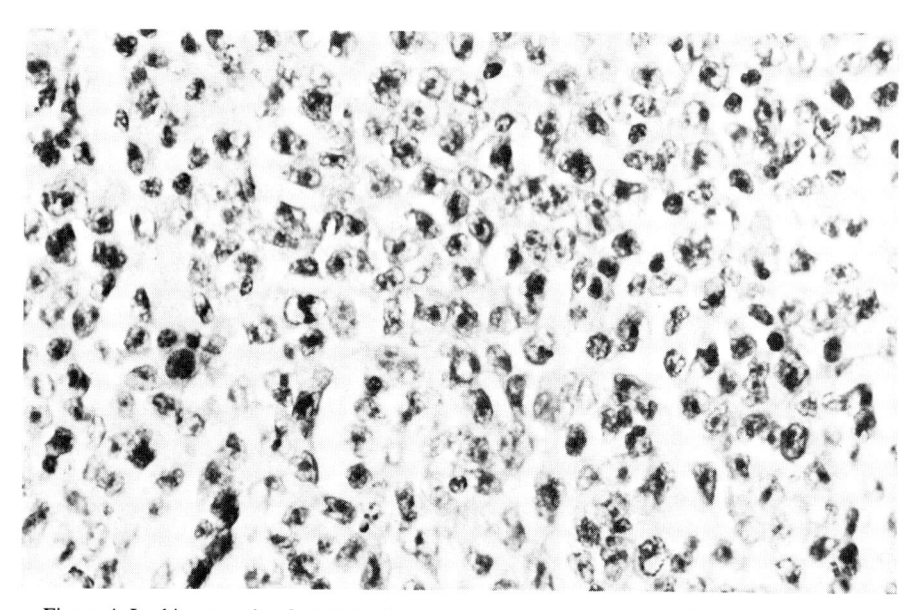

Figure 4. In this example of MHI the histiocytes show clear malignant characteristics but the tumour is relatively monomorphic. Differentiation from other large cell lymphomas is difficult; the cells stained strongly for α-1-antitrypsin as illustrated in Figure 21.

HISTOLOGY

Histological appearances vary markedly, both between cases and between different sites of tumour in the same patient. Thus, the infiltrate may consist of well-differentiated histiocytes showing only marginal atypia in the form of enlarged nuclei with slight coarsening of chromatin and prominence of nucleoli (Figure 3). Monomorphic infiltrates of immature cells may occur, resembling poorly-differentiated lymphoid malignancy (Figure 4), and in some instances the tumour is highly pleomorphic with an abundance of multinucleated giant cells (Figure 5). A heavy inflammatory infiltrate of lymphocytes and plasma cells and eosinophils is often present which may almost obscure the malignant histiocytes which occur as isolated cells amidst the infiltrate. Eosinophils may be especially prominent (Figure 6). Associated features commonly present include invasion of blood vessels and lymphatics (Figure 7) and infiltration of blood vessel walls producing a vasculitis-like lesion (Figure 8). The malignant cells are occasionally organized into fairly well-defined granulomas (Figure 9) which may cause confusion with Crohn's disease. In some of the ulcerating lesions it may be impossible to identify tumour cells and multiple sections of the bowel may be required before malignant cells are identified. In this type of case examination of mesenteric nodes, liver, spleen or bone marrow is sometimes more fruitful than searching for malignant cells amidst the heavy reactive inflammation in the ulcer bases.

Villous atrophy and crypt hyperplasia with a heavy plasmacytic infiltrate are invariably present in the uninvolved jejunal mucosa (Figure 10). This lesion, which is typical of coeliac disease, improves distally until a virtually normal mucosal architecture may be present in the terminal ileum. This must be borne in mind when the tumour involves more distal regions of the small intestine, and if there is any doubt a peroral jejunal biopsy should be done to confirm jejunal villous atrophy.

DISSEMINATION

In the majority of cases the tumour is disseminated when the diagnosis is made. Even when the lesion in the intestine may not be visible macroscopically mesenteric lymph nodes are often enlarged. Histologically they show marked follicular hyperplasia together with sinusoidal infiltration by malignant histiocytes (Figure 11). The infiltrate later extends into medullary cords and eventually replaces the lymph node. As the malignant histiocytes invade they are accompanied by fibrosis and frequently plasmacytosis. Involvement of spleen, liver and bone marrow is extremely common but the subtle nature of the infiltrate in malignant histiocytosis means that these organs must be examined with the greatest care before involvement is excluded. The spleen is characteristically not enlarged in MHI and indeed is often smaller than normal (40 to 50 g), reflecting splenic atrophy that is a feature of coeliac disease (Figure 12). Malignant histiocytes are present primarily in the red

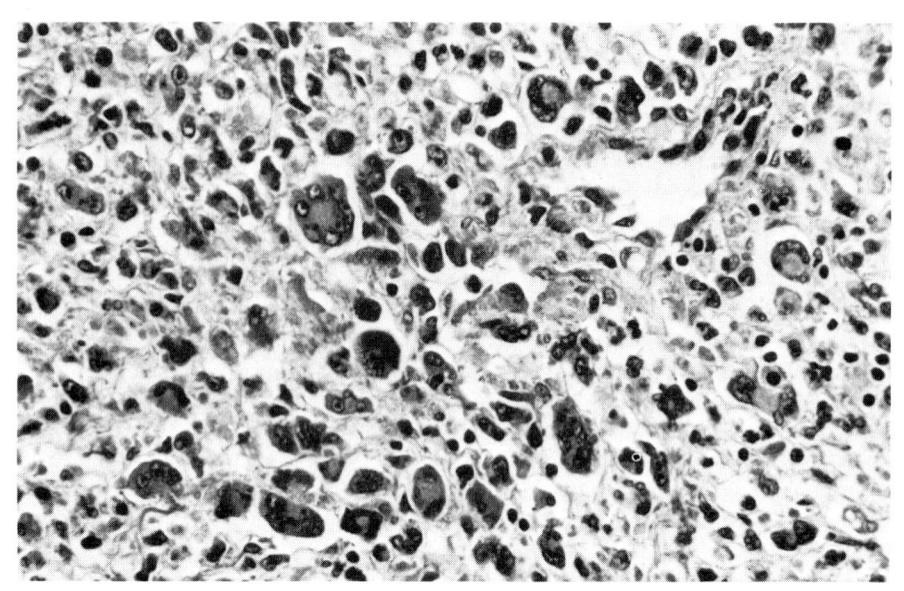

Figure 5. Highly pleomorphic variety of MHI with characteristic multinucleate giant cells. From Isaacson and Wright (1978b), with kind permission of W.B. Saunders, Philadelphia.

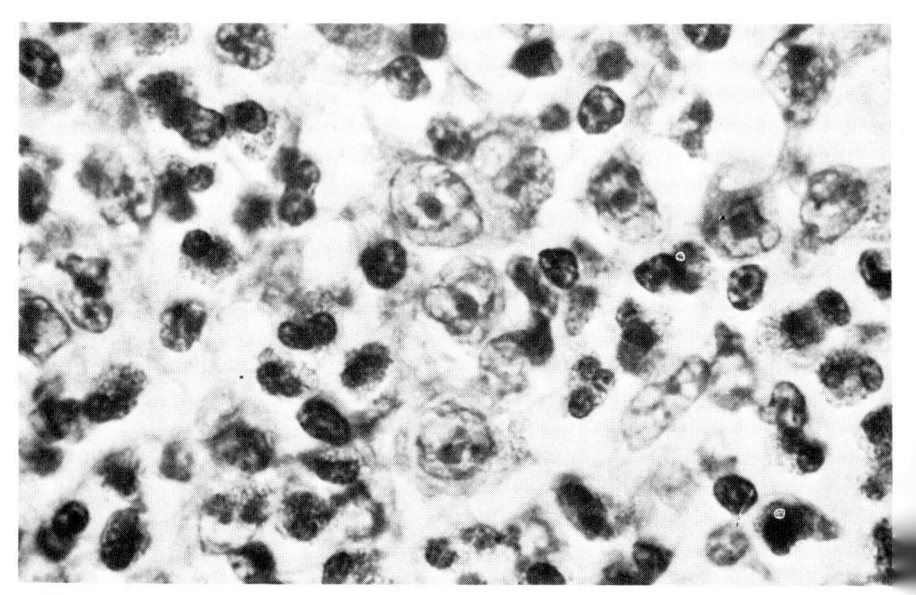

Figure 6. The malignant histiocytes are almost obscured by a heavy infiltrate of eosinophils.

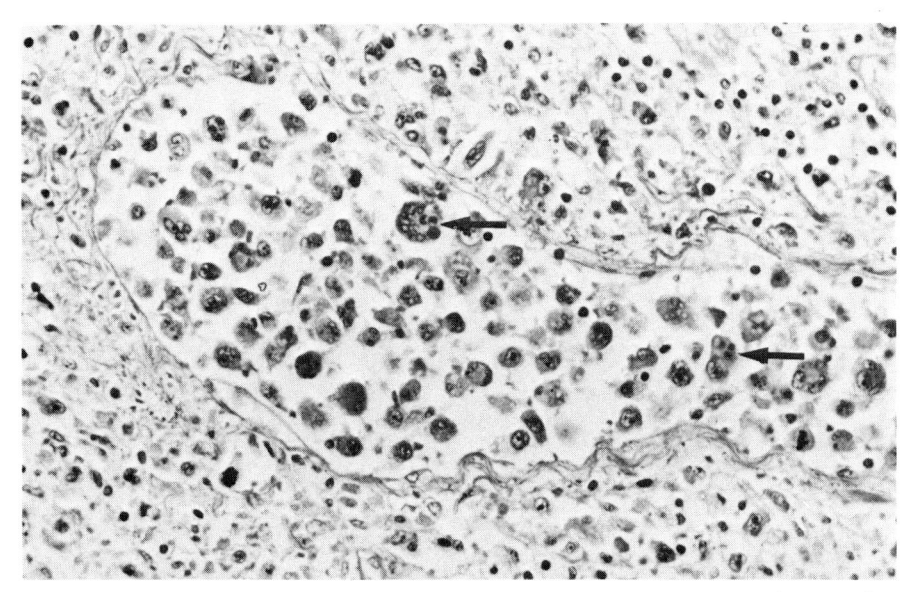

Figure 7. Vascular invasion by bizarre malignant histiocytes. Note the erythrophagocytosis (arrows).

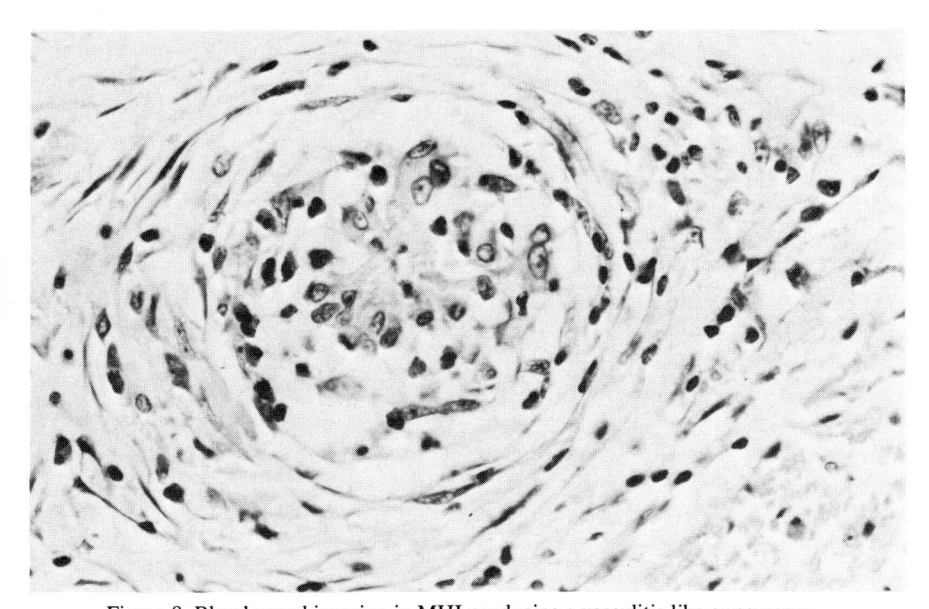

Figure 8. Blood vessel invasion in MHI producing a vasculitis-like appearance.

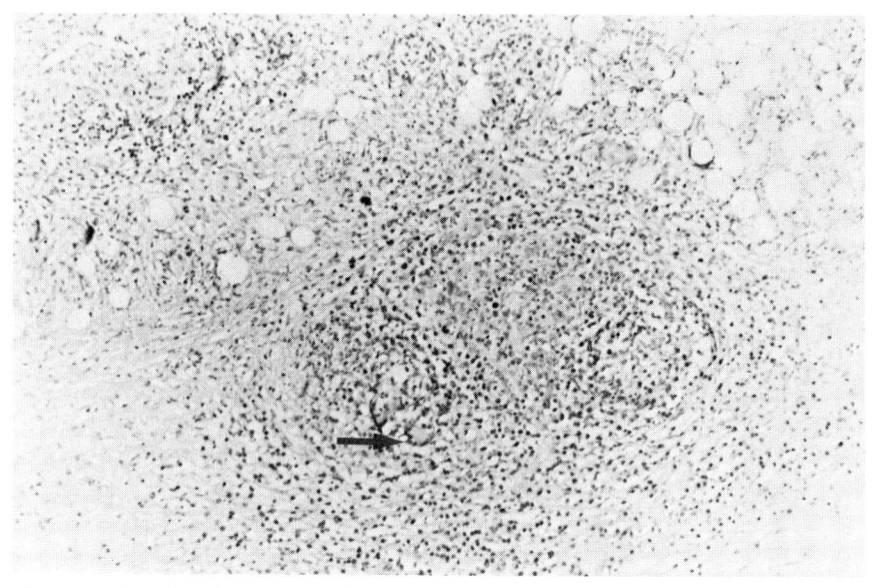

Figure 9. Invasion of mesenteric fat by malignant histiocytes which are organized into granulomas. Note the multinucleate giant cells (arrow).

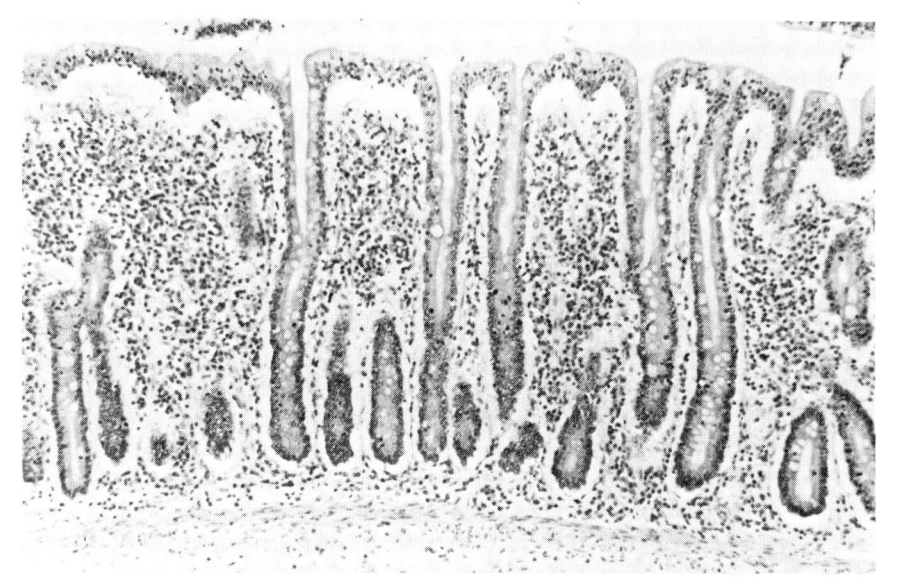

Figure 10. Jejunal mucosa from a case of MHI showing villous atrophy, crypt hyperplasia with plasmacytosis of the lamina propria and increased intra-epithelial lymphocytes. From Isaacson and Wright (1978b), with kind permission of W.B. Saunders, Philadelphia.

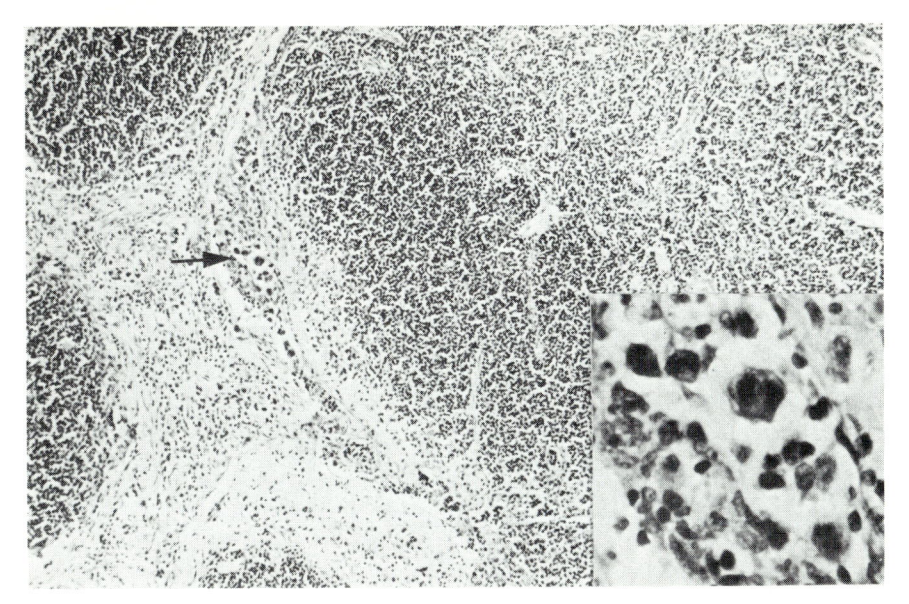

Figure 11. Mesenteric lymph node showing subtle early involvement. The malignant histiocytes in the sinus (arrow) are shown in greater detail in the inset.

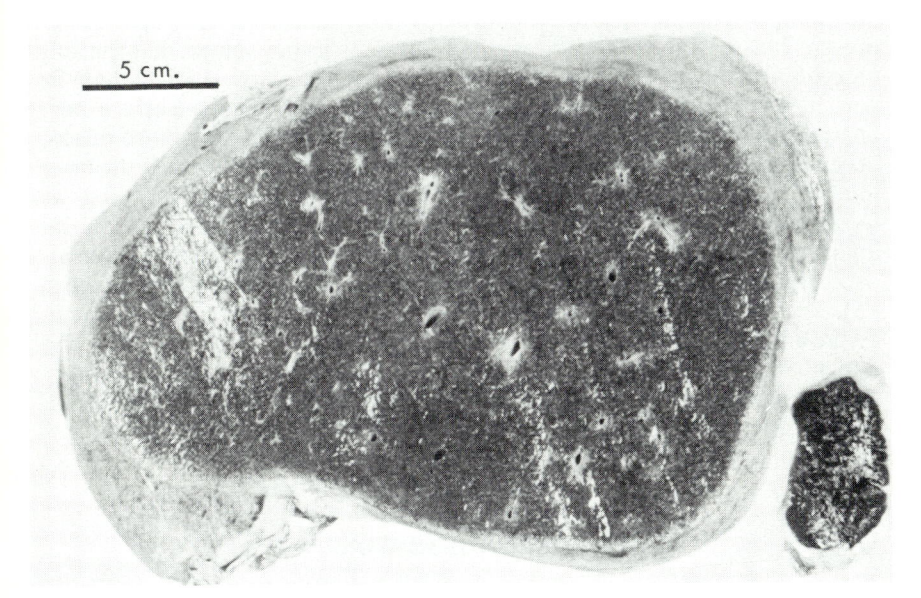

Figure 12. Liver and spleen from a 57-year-old man with MHI. The liver weighed 3000 g and the spleen 40 g. Both showed diffuse involvement.

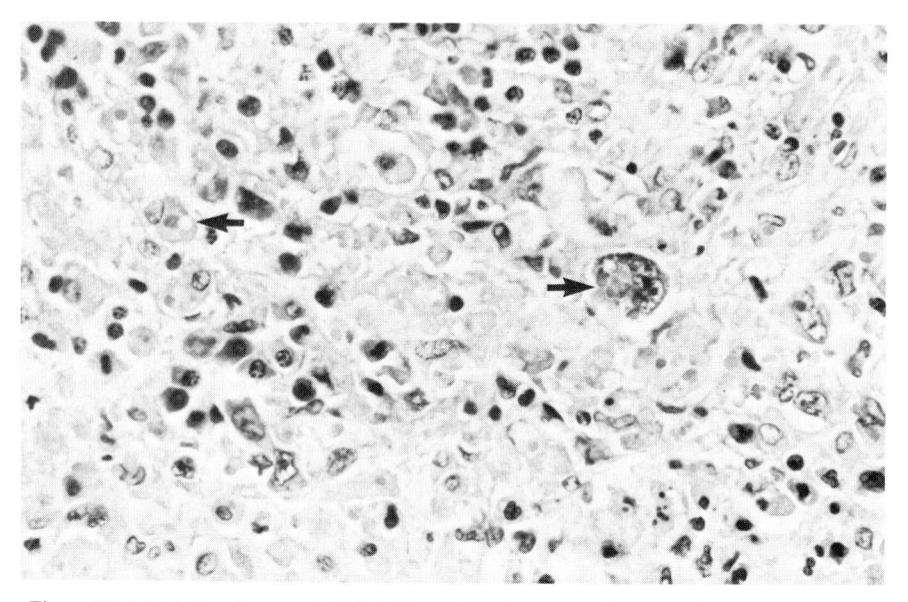

Figure 13. Splenic involvement in MHI. There is replacement of normal tissue by histiocytes showing varying degrees of atypia and erythrophagocytosis by both benign-appearing and clearly malignant cells (arrows).

pulp where erythrophagocystosis is often prominent (Figure 13). In more advanced cases the white pulp, too, is infiltrated by the cells which may show only marginal atypia. Scattered, more obviously malignant cells are usually present but these have to be searched out. It is in the spleen that the full morphological range of the malignant histiocytes is best appreciated. In particular, the striking plasmacytoid appearance of some of the cells is best appreciated here (Figure 14). The liver is often enlarged and, more rarely, may contain nodules of tumour. Needle biopsies of liver are very difficult to interpret and may appear negative where wedge biopsies taken at laparotomy or post-mortem sections of liver show clear involvement. The infiltrate involves portal triads and characteristically spreads intrasinusoidally into the parenchyma which often also shows sinusoidal ectasia (Figure 15). Here again, interpretation can be difficult in the face of marginally atypical histiocytes and differentiation from Kupffer cell hyperplasia can be difficult. The bone marrow is best examined in the form of an aspirate smear rather than a trephine. Characteristically bizarre phagocytic histiocytes are often present (Figure 16) but in some cases the atypical mononuclear cells are not phagocytic.

HISTOCHEMISTRY

If fresh tissues are available histochemistry on imprints or frozen sections can be performed. Stains for acid phosphatase and non-specific esterase are

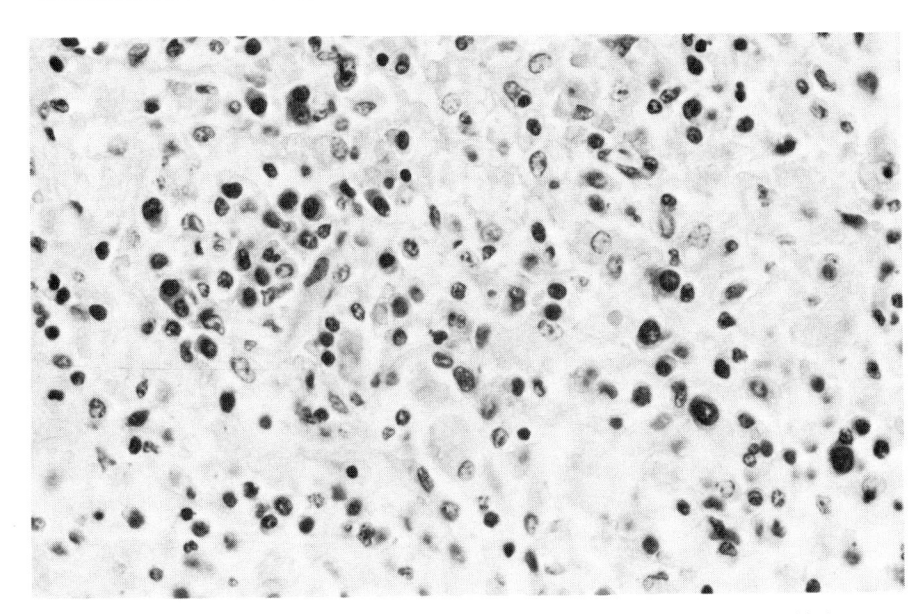

Figure 14. Another area of the spleen illustrated in Figure 13. Here the malignant histiocytes show a resemblance to plasma cells.

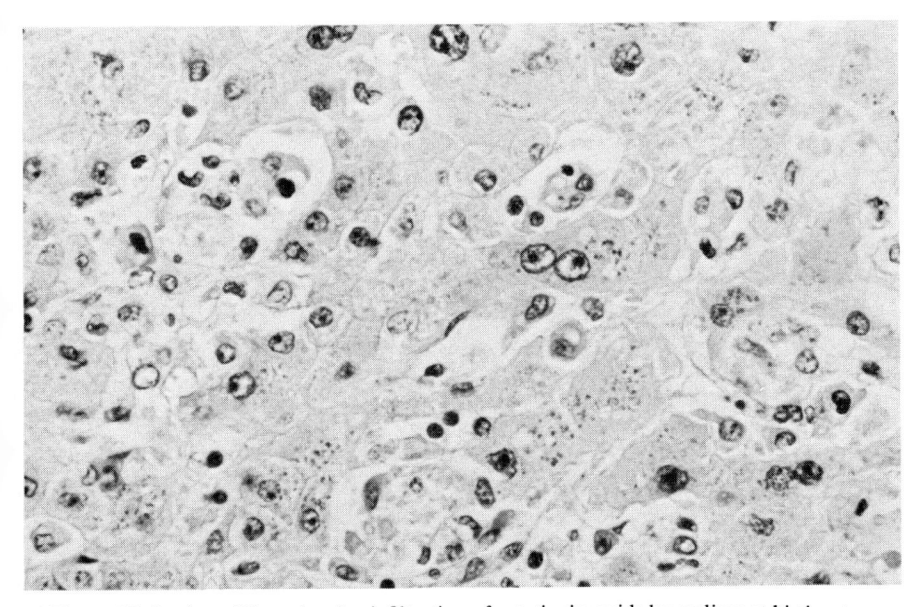

Figure 15. Section of liver showing infiltration of ectatic sinusoids by malignant histiocytes.

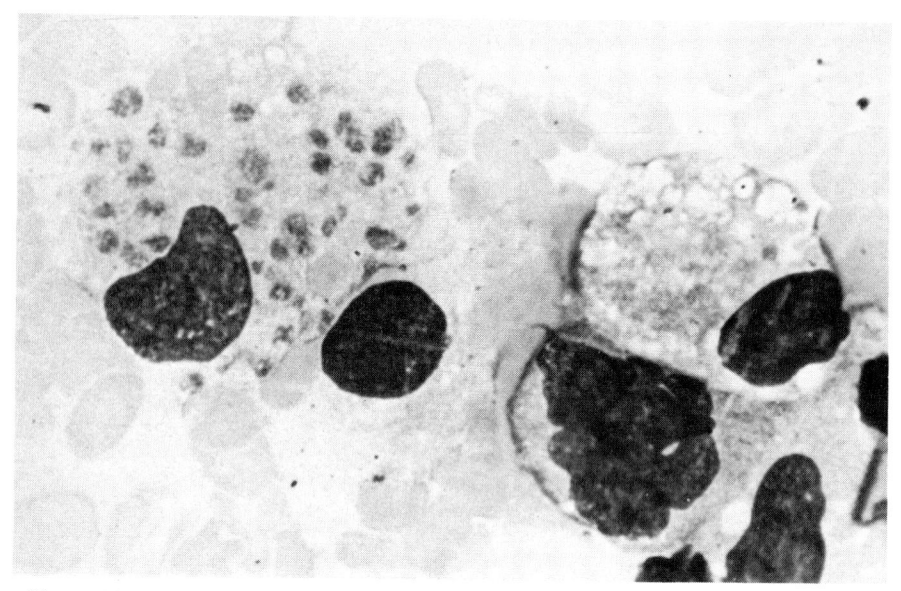

Figure 16. Bone marrow aspirate containing malignant histiocytes, some of which have phagocytosed platelets, red blood cells, and other material. From Isaacson and Wright (1978b), with kind permission of W.B. Saunders, Philadelphia.

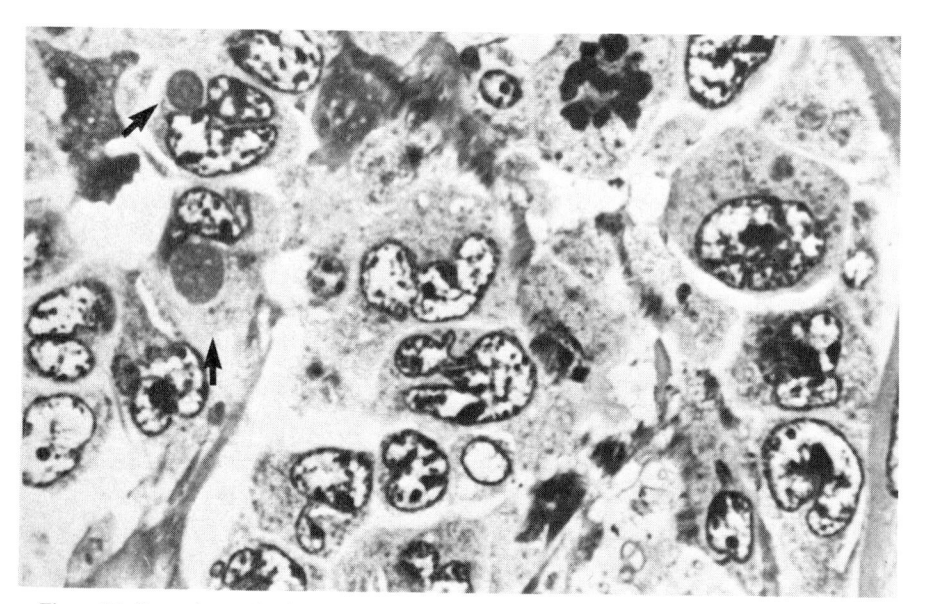

Figure 17. One-micron plastic-embedded sections from an intestinal tumour. The complexity of the nuclei is well shown, as is phagocytosis by the malignant cells (arrows).

characteristically positive, although this might not be the case in very immature tumour cells.

PLASTIC SECTIONS AND ELECTRON MICROSCOPY

As with all lymphoreticular tumours 1 μm plastic sections are invaluable in assessing detailed cell morphology. Good formalin fixation is adequate (as it is for electron microscopy). These sections in MHI often highlight the coarse chromatin and complexity of the nucleus and, by rendering a much better definition of the cytoplasm, demonstrate phagocytic activity which cannot be appreciated in paraffin sections (Figure 17). Differentiation of the more immature infiltrates from large cell lymphomas of lymphoid origin (centroblastic lymphomas, immunoblastic sarcomas) is also better appreciated in plastic sections. The nuclei of the malignant histiocytes are often slightly indented, with coarse chromatin and multiple large nucleoli variously sited. The ultrastructural appearances of the malignant histiocytes vary with their maturity. The immature tumour cell (Figure 18) has a large nucleus with a

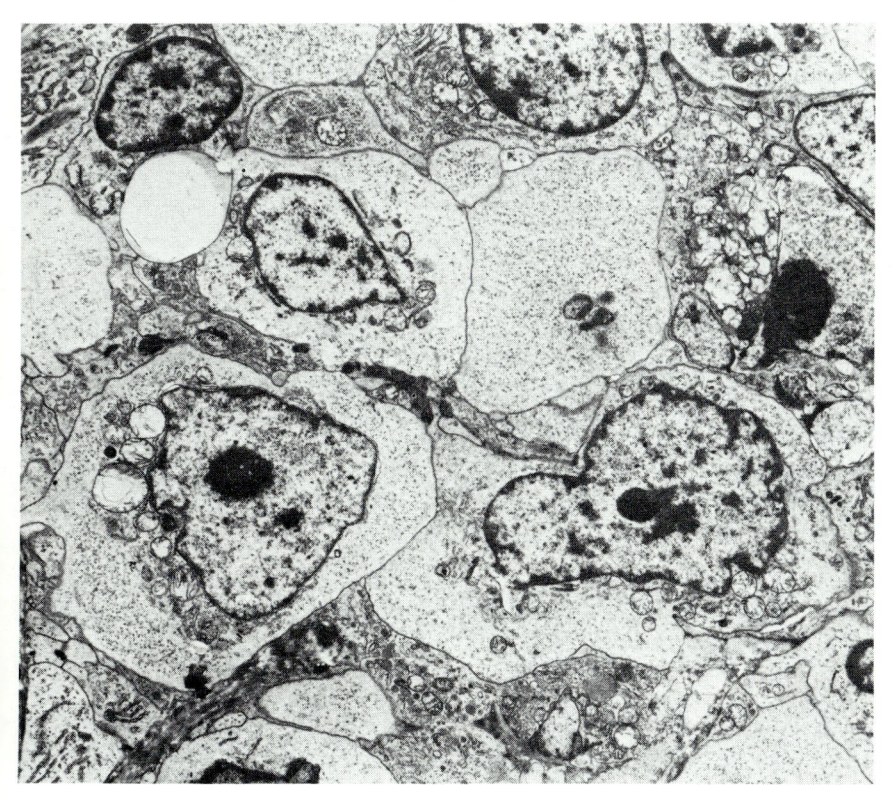

Figure 18. Electron micrograph of intestinal tumour (same case as Figures 4 and 21) showing undifferentiated cells containing numerous polyribosomes, little rough endoplasmic reticulum and occasional lysosomes. × 4000.

prominent nucleolus, abundant polyribosomes in the cytoplasm and scattered lysosomes. In contrast, the more mature cells may show a denser nucleus with abundant mitochondria and lysosomes together with a variable amount of rough endoplasmic reticulum (Figure 19).

IMMUNOPEROXIDASE STUDIES

Using an indirect immunoperoxidase (PAP) technique with prior trypsin digestion (Mepham, Frater and Mitchell, 1979), immunoglobulin, particularly IgG, can be detected in the malignant histiocytes in some cases. The immunoglobulin is found predominantly in multinucleated giant cells where it is present polytypically, that is, both κ- and λ-light chains are present in the same cell. This polytypia, together with other findings (Isaacson, 1979a; Isaacson and Wright, 1979), indicates that the immunoglobulin is not synthesized by the cells but, rather, taken up from the environment. Muramidase (lysozyme) can be detected in the malignant cells of some cases (Figure 20)

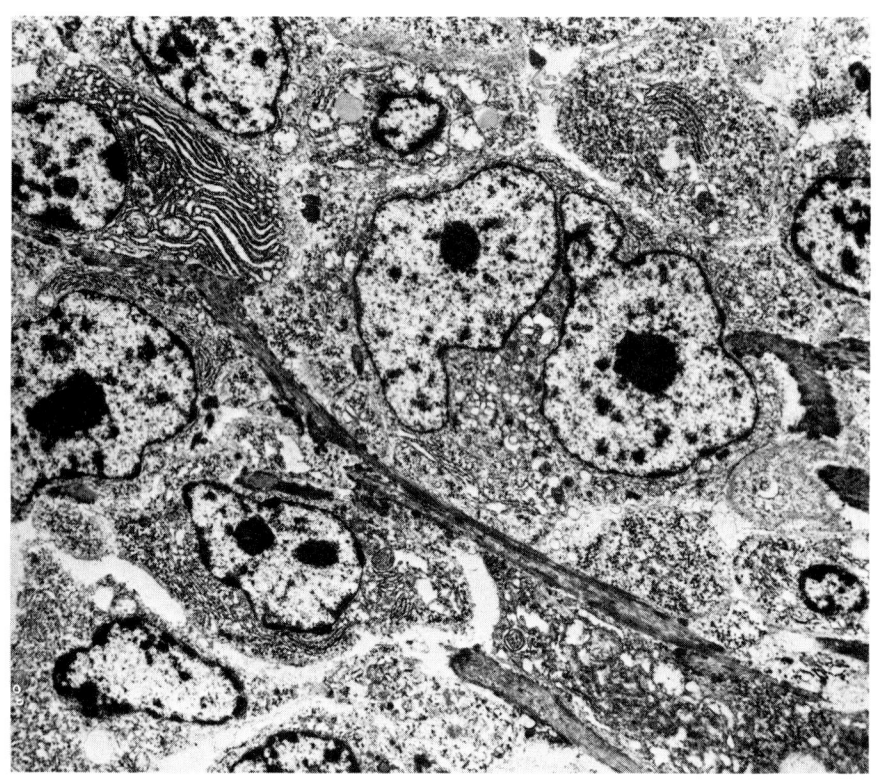

Figure 19. Electron micrograph showing a group of better-differentiated malignant histiocytes (same case as Figure 3). Note abundance of rough endoplasmic reticulum and lysosomes. Compare with the plasma cell at upper left. × 4000.

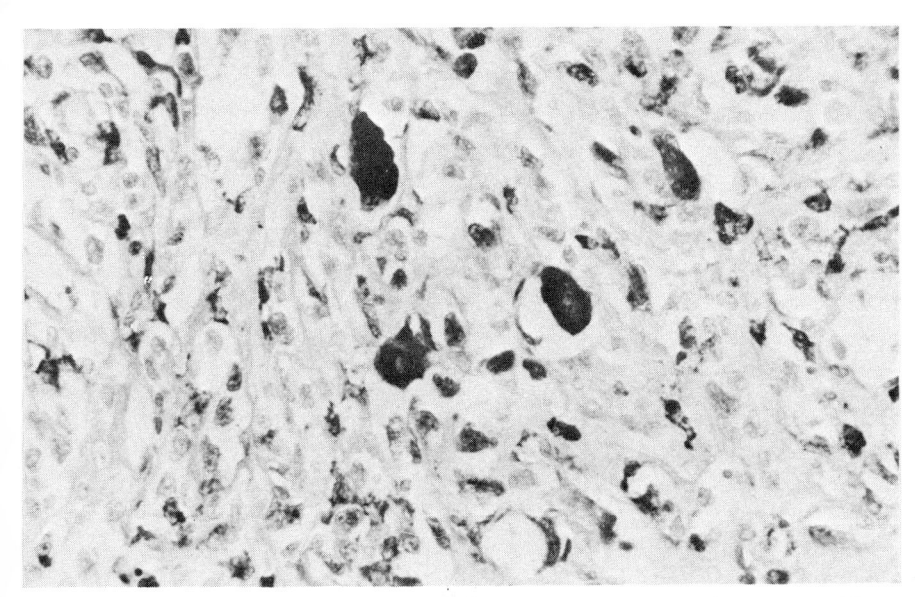

Figure 20. Section of pleomorphic variety of MHI stained for lysozyme by immunoperoxidase technique. Both bizarre large cells and smaller tumour cells show coarse granular staining.

but its presence is variable even within an individual section. A far more reliable marker is α-1-antitrypsin (Isaacson et al, 1979). This powerful protease inhibitor appears to be synthesized by cells of the monocyte macrophage system (Isaacson, Jones and Judd, 1979) and is visualized as fine intracellular granules (Figure 21) or in more primitive tumour cells as a single large granule in the region of the Golgi apparatus. Alpha-1-antitrypsin is not present in lymphoid cells.

THE EARLY LESION OF MHI

Small histiocytic aggregates are sometimes seen in 'uninvolved' mucosa well separated from sites of obvious tumour. These are also sometimes seen in peroral biopsies of patients with MHI or in whom MHI develops at a later date (Isaacson, 1980). The histiocytes show minimal atypia and tend to collect beneath the surface epithelium (Figure 22). They also surround crypts and invade and destroy the crypt epithelium with resultant histiocytic 'crypt abscesses' (Figure 23). Similarly, there may be invasion of surface epithelium with subsequent ulceration. These lesions may be seen in peroral biopsies many years prior to the development of overt disease and their presence supports the suggestion that there is a prolonged latent phase in MHI analogous to that in mycosis fungoides (Isaacson and Wright, 1978b).

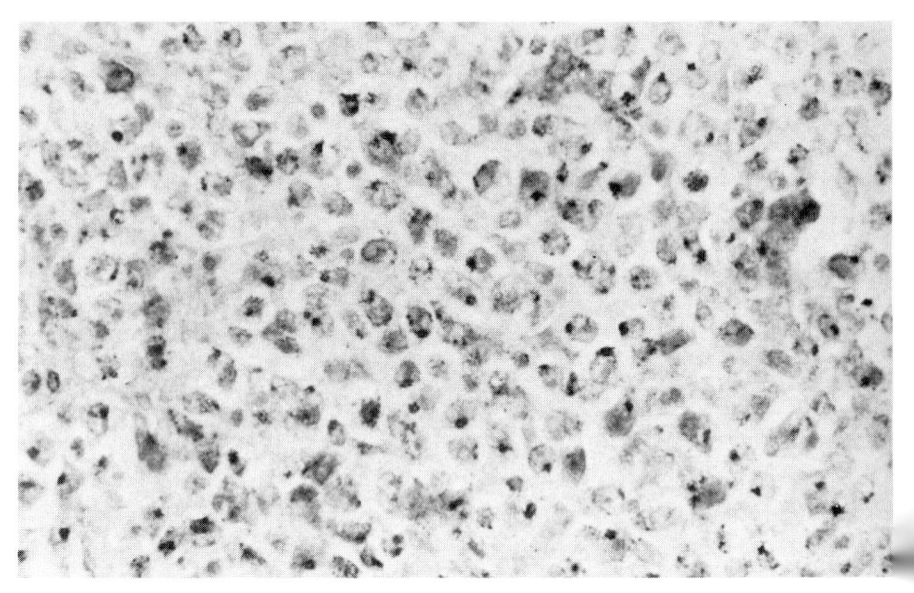

Figure 21. Immunoperoxidase stain for α-1-antitrypsin showing characteristic granular staining within monomorphic tumour cells (same case as Figure 4).

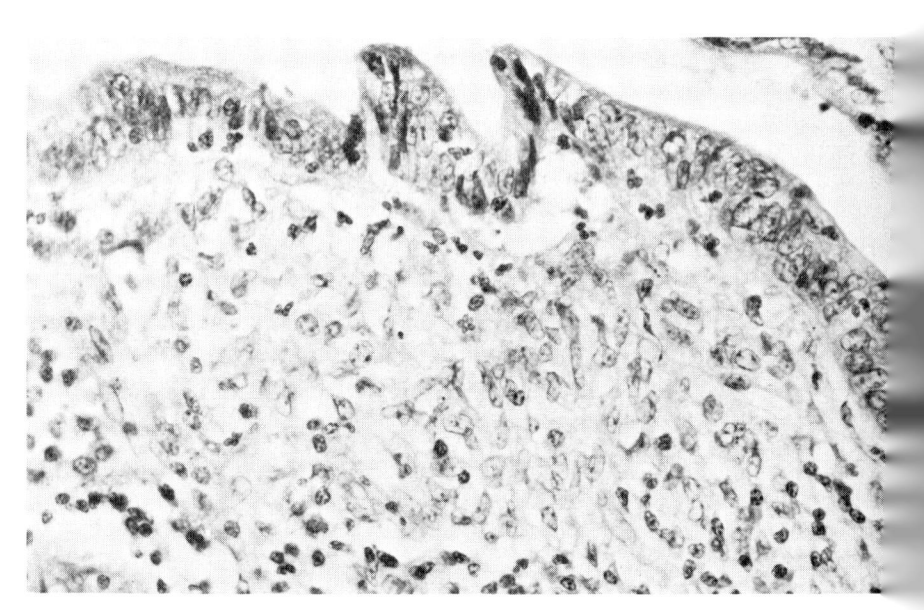

Figure 22. 'Early lesion' of MHI in the form of sheets of histiocytes beneath the mucosal surface.

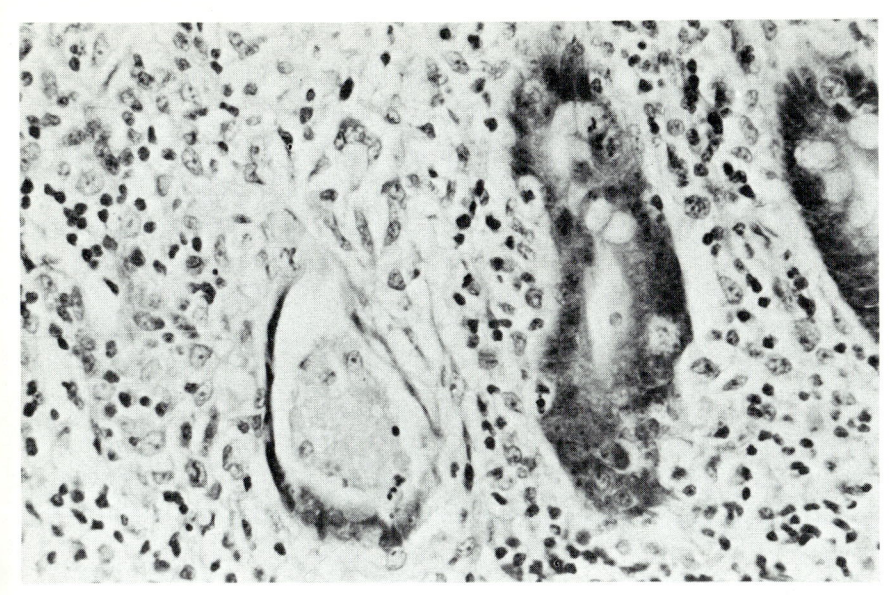

Figure 23. Collection of histiocytes in the jejunal mucosa from a case of MHI with invasion and destruction of an isolated crypt.

ULCERATIVE JEJUNITIS AND MHI

The relationship of ulcerative jejunitis (non-granulomatous jejunoileitis) to coeliac disease is very similar to that of intestinal lymphoma (Bayless et al, 1967). In this condition, which is highly lethal, there are multiple ulcers of the small intestine, one or more of which may perforate. The inflammatory infiltrate in the base of these ulcers has been described as non-specific. Multiple 'benign' ulcers are also found in MHI (Figure 24). In some cases these are the predominant lesion and foci of obvious malignancy may be impossible to detect in the intestine itself without taking multiple sections. Examination of mesenteric lymph nodes, liver, spleen and bone marrow may, however, reveal malignant histiocytes and sometimes a very careful examination of the ulcers will reveal occasional bizarre histiocytes. Recognition of the early lesion of MHI (see above) does much to explain the pathogenesis of these 'benign' ulcers since it can be appreciated that the inflammatory reaction which follows the early ulceration may totally obscure the invasive collections of histiocytes. Given that the malignant cells in malignant histiocytosis may be deceptively benign in appearance it is understandable how they may be obscured by inflammation. It is in our opinion highly likely that ulcerative jejunitis is but a manifestation of MHI.

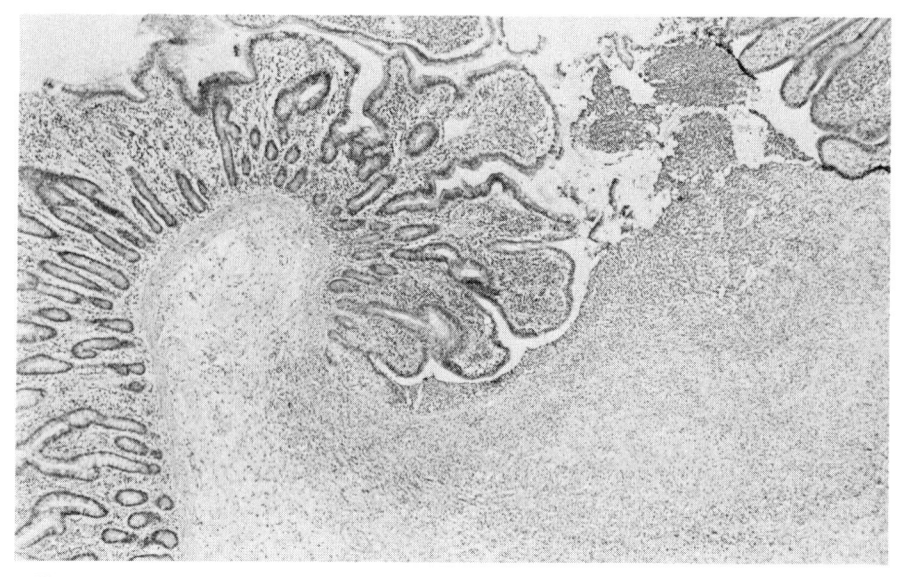

Figure 24. One of multiple 'benign' ulcers in a case of MHI; a single focus of malignancy was found only after taking numerous sections.

THE RELATIONSHIP OF MHI TO COELIAC DISEASE

The exact relationship of MHI to coeliac disease remains a vexed question. The jejunal lesion present in these patients is identical to that found in coeliac disease and in an increasing proportion of patients this lesion can be shown to be responsive to gluten withdrawal (Freeman et al, 1977). HLA typing has been performed in a few cases (Freeman et al, 1977) and found to conform to the types characteristically found in coeliac disease. The presence of splenic atrophy in many of the cases is further corroborative evidence since this is a well-described finding in coeliac disease. None of the patients with MHI has had a firm diagnosis of childhood coeliac disease which is, perhaps, not surprising since peroral jejunal biopsies were not introduced until 1957 (Crosby and Kugler). Thus, it will be many years before the first group of childhood coeliacs diagnosed by objective methods (biopsy response to a gluten-free diet) enters the age group in which MHI occurs. Although some patients with MHI have histories going back to childhood most have presented as adults either with coeliac disease or with MHI. That coeliac disease can present in adult life is now well established and it is likely, but not certain, that these patients have had subclinical disease since childhood. The latent phase of MHI, however, may be prolonged and the possibility cannot be excluded that the onset of this strange malignant disease may itself alter the sensitivity of the mucosa to gluten. This argument is, of course, a return to the very first thoughts on the association of malabsorption and coeliac disease and can only be fully refuted in time. It is not an unimportant argument, however, for while we label patients with MHI as coeliacs as much for convenience as anything else, it is of small comfort to the patient with childhood coeliac disease or his parents to be aware of the relationship of the disease with intestinal lymphoma.

CONCLUSION

Malignant histiocytosis of the intestine is not a rare disease in the United Kingdom. Most pathologists will encounter cases from time to time and it is important to make an accurate diagnosis if effective forms of therapy are to evolve. The recognition of the histiocytic nature of this malignant disease raises, too, some basic questions as to aetiology, the role of the histiocyte in the immune response, and the nature of other lymphoreticular malignancies associated with hyperstimulation of the immune system.

REFERENCES

Al-Saleem, T. & Zardawi, I.M. (1979) Primary lymphomas of the small intestine in Iraq. *Histopathology*, 3, 89-106.

Bayless, T.M., Kapelowitz, R.F., Shelley, W.M., Balliner, II. W.F. & Hendrix, T.R. (1967) Intestinal ulceration — a complication of celiac diseases. *New England Journal of Medicine*, 276, 996-1002.

Byrne, G.E. & Rappaport, H. (1973) *Malignant Histiocytosis in Malignant Diseases of the Hematopoietic System* (Gann Monograph on Cancer Research, Vol. 15) (Ed.) Akazaki, T., Rappaport, H., Berard, C.W. et al. Baltimore, MD: University Park Press.

Cooke, W.T. & Asquith, P. (1974) Introduction and definition of coeliac disease. *Clinics in Gastroenterology*, 3, 3-10.

Crosby, W.H. & Kugler, H.W. (1957) Intraluminal biopsy of the small intestine. *American Journal of Digestive Diseases*, 2, 236-241.

Eidelman, S., Parkins, A. & Rubin, C.E. (1966) Abdominal lymphoma presenting as malabsorption. A clinico-pathological study of nine cases in Israel and a review of the literature. *Medicine*, 45, 111-137.

Fairley, N.H. & Mackie, F.P. (1937) The clinical and biochemical syndrome in lymphadenoma and allied diseases involving the mesenteric lymph glands. *British Medical Journal*, i, 3972-3980.

Frand, V. & Ramot, B. (1963) Malignant lymphoma: an epidemiological study. *Harefuah*, 65, 83-86.

Freeman, H.J., Weinstein, W.M., Shnitka, T.K., Piercey, J.R.A. & Wensel, R.H. (1977) Primary abdominal lymphoma. Presenting manifestation of celiac sprue or complicating dermatitis herpetiformis. *American Journal of Medicine*, 63, 585-594.

Gough, K.R., Read, A.E. & Naish, J.M. (1962) Intestinal reticulosis as a complication of idiopathic steatorrhoea. *Gut*, 3, 232-239.

Hodges, J.R., Isaacson, P., Smith, C.L. & Sworn, M.J. (1979) Malignant histiocytosis of the intestine. *Digestive Diseases and Sciences*, 24, 631-638.

Isaacson, P. (1979a) Immunohistochemical demonstration of J chain: a marker of B-cell malignancy. *Journal of Clinical Pathology*, 32, 802-807.

Isaacson, P. (1979b) Middle East lymphoma and α-chain disease: an immunohistochemical study. *American Journal of Surgical Pathology*, 3, 431-441.

Isaacson, P. (1980) Malignant histiocytosis of the intestine: the early histological lesion. *Gut*, in press.

Isaacson, P. & Wright, D.H. (1978a) Intestinal lymphoma associated with malabsorption. *Lancet*, i, 67-70.

Isaacson, P. & Wright, D.H. (1978b) Malignant histiocytosis of the intestine: its relationship to malabsorption and ulcerative jejunitis. *Human Pathology*, **9**, 661-677.

Isaacson, P. & Wright, D.H. (1979) Anomalous staining patterns in immunohistologic studies of malignant lymphoma. *Journal of Histochemistry and Cytochemistry*, **27**, 1197-1199.

Isaacson, P., Jones, D.B. & Judd, M.A. (1979) Alpha l-antitrypsin in human macrophages. *Lancet*, **ii**, 964-965.

Isaacson, P., Wright, D.H., Judd, M.A. & Mepham. B.L. (1979) Primary gastrointestinal lymphomas: a classification of 66 cases. *Cancer*, **43**, 1805-1819.

Mepham, B.L., Frater, W. & Mitchell, B.S. (1979) The use of proteolytic enzymes to improve Ig staining by the PAP technique. *Journal of Histochemistry*, **11**, 345-357.

Scott, R.B. & Robb-Smith, A.H.T. (1939) Histiocytic medullary reticulosis. *Lancet*, **ii**, 194-198.

Scudamore, H.H. (1961) Observations on secondary malabsorption syndromes of intestinal origin. Regional enteritis, lymphoma, jejunal diverticulosis, gastrojejunocolic fistula. *Annals of Internal Medicine*, **55**, 433-447.

Sleisenger, M.H., Almy, T.P. & Barr, D.P. (1953) The sprue syndrome secondary to lymphoma of the small bowel. *American Journal of Medicine*, **15**, 666-674.

13
Non-Hodgkin's Lymphomas of the Gut

A.J. BLACKSHAW

Recent investigations into the pathology of gut lymphomas have concentrated mainly on cellular morphology and the controversial topic of tumour classification. Other aspects of these uncommon but increasingly important diseases have regrettably received less attention. It is difficult to make an accurate assessment of the incidence of lymphoma with a primary origin in the gut. A figure of 1.6/100 000 persons per year in the United Kingdom will serve as a rough estimate of the frequency of such tumours in a Western society (Green et al, 1979). The Registrar General's mortality statistics for 1977 give 2569 deaths from malignant lymphoma of all types, including Hodgkin's disease, at all sites. Only a small proportion of these represent primary diseases of the gut, but again this proportion is difficult to estimate with any accuracy. By and large most gut tumours present as surgical problems whereas nodal lymphomas are managed by medical oncologists or radiotherapists. For this reason, series from oncology or radiotherapy centres probably underestimate the proportion of all lymphomas which originate in the gut. Green et al (1979) have found that primary gastrointestinal lymphomas constitute some 15 per cent of all non-Hodgkin's lymphomas in the Grampian region.

Various aspects of the pathology of gut lymphoma will be discussed in comparison with similar aspects of a much commoner malignancy — adenocarcinoma of the large bowel. A great deal of detailed information is available about the genesis, staging, typing and prognosis of colorectal cancer and it is hoped that such a comparison will serve to emphasize the gaps, which urgently require closure, in current knowledge of gut lymphomas. By analogy, this may also serve as a guide to a more rational approach to management of patients with gut lymphomas and those at risk of their development.

Classification of non-Hodgkin's lymphomas will only be mentioned here insofar as labels are required for the various examples given. The Kiel classification is preferred by the author, but wherever possible the alternative terminology in other classifications will be given.

© 1980 W.B. Saunders Company Ltd.

CRITERIA FOR PRIMARY GUT LYMPHOMAS

The literature on lymphoma in the gut prior to 1961 is confusing because few authors made a clear distinction between tumours originating within the gut and those that secondarily involved the gut during the dissemination of primarily nodal disease. The latter situation is very much more frequent than the former and consequently many of the larger series of gut lymphomas published from single institutions were heavily 'contaminated' from the point of view of information on primary gut tumours. Dawson, Cornes and Morson (1961) studied 38 cases of lymphoma which they believed had a primary origin in the gut. Their criteria for acceptance of a primary tumour in the gut were carefully stated and are reproduced here.

1. No palpable superficial lymphadenopathy at presentation.
2. Chest x-ray shows no enlargement of mediastinal nodes.
3. Normal WBC (total and differential).
4. At laparotomy the bowel lesion predominates, the only obviously affected lymph nodes being those immediately related.
5. The liver and spleen appear free of tumour.

These five criteria have been almost universally adopted in subsequent publications on this subject. This uniformity of criteria has the major advantage of allowing some comparison between published series.

In recent years new investigative techniques have enabled the medical profession to detect increasingly more subtle evidence of disease in many sites of the body. Lymphangiography of retroperitoneal nodes, bone marrow aspiration and computerized axial tomography are examples of investigations in increasing use in the staging of lymphomas. In these circumstances it is quite reasonable to question whether the criteria given above require expansion or modification. There is no guarantee, however, that any modification would command the widespread acceptance which makes these criteria so useful. Perhaps the best attitude to adopt is that the criteria of Dawson, Cornes and Morson (1961) should be taken as the minimal essential criteria to be satisfied for inclusion in a series of primary gut lymphomas. Additional information from more sophisticated techniques could then be used for the further exclusion of certain cases.

STAGING

The Dukes' staging of carcinoma of the colon and rectum takes account of the known manner of spread of colorectal carcinoma and can be clearly related to prognosis. Above all it is simple in its concept and in its application to surgically resected tumours. No comparable system of staging of gut lymphomas has found acceptance, and yet a simple and suitable staging is urgently required.

The Ann Arbor staging enjoys widespread usage for malignant lymphoma of all types and sites, although it was originally designed for use only in Hodgkin's disease. The assumption that Ann Arbor staging is appropriate for (a) non-Hodgkin lymphomas and (b) extranodal tumours has been questioned by serveral authors (Jaffe et al, 1977; Rosenberg, 1977; Blackledge et al, 1979). Adherence to Ann Arbor staging for extranodal lymphoma is prompted no doubt by a desire for a uniform approach to the lymphomas as a whole. It is certainly true that the same histological types of lymphoma can be identified both in primary nodal and primary gut tumours, although the relative proportions differ. Although superficially it would seem advantageous to adopt a uniform staging system, it is in fact unnecessary to stage nodal and gut lymphoma in the same way. Localized tumours at each site are treated entirely differently. The primary mode of treatment for gut tumours is attempted radical surgical excision. Radical lymphadenectomy has long since been abandoned for nodal lymphomas and the primary treatments here are radiotherapy and chemotherapy. Thus groups of nodal and gut tumours are not comparable stage for stage.

A staging system akin to those used for carcinomas would be more appropriate for primary gut lymphomas. The manner of spread of many types of lymphoma in the gut is similar to that of carcinoma, with infiltration progressively from the mucosal surface towards the serosa or mesenteric fatty tissue. Like carcinomas, lymphomas permeate lymphatic channels, invade veins on occasion and involve regional lymph nodes in a progressive fashion along the line of lymphatic drainage. Metastatic lymphoma in mesenteric nodes often even shows partial nodal replacement, a pattern more often associated with carcinoma than with primary nodal lymphoma. The Ann Arbor staging takes no account of the depth of invasion of tumour in the wall of the bowel, of the detailed distribution of regional nodal involvement, of perforation into the peritoneal cavity or of the distinct tendency for *primary* gut lymphomas to be multifocal. All these factors are likely to have a profound effect on prognosis (Friedman, 1959; Lim et al, 1977; Blackledge et al, 1979).

Alternatives to the Ann Arbor staging have been proposed by some authors. The Tumour-Node-Metastasis (TNM) system used for gastric carcinoma was modified for 50 cases of gastric lymphoma (Lim et al, 1977; Table 1). Unfortunately, the detailed nature of the TNM system and the number of its various combinations or categories may limit its usefulness for uncommon tumours for which large series cannot be accumulated. In addition, the influence of multifocal primary tumours is not taken into account. Multiplicity may be of less importance in the stomach than in the small and large intestine, but an ideal staging system for lymphoma at all sites in the gut should encompass this factor. Blackledge et al (1979), dissatisfied with Ann Arbor staging, have devised an alternative system of staging for gut lymphoma at all sites (Table 2). This has the advantage of relative simplicity and takes into account both perforation and multiplicity of tumours. However, depth of penetration in the wall of the bowel is not considered apart from perforation, which implies serosal involvement. One possible disadvantage is the use of roman numerals for the different stages so that confusion with the Ann Arbor system may result.

Both the above groups have shown a relationship between their staging and the prognosis for the patients.

Table 1. *Modification of TNM staging applied to gastric lymphoma*

Stage I. No metastasis in regional lymph nodes and no distant metastasis
   A. Carcinoma confined to the mucosa
      No metastasis in regional lymph nodes
      No distant metastasis
      T1, N0, M0
   B. Carcinoma involving the submucosa or serosa but not penetrating through the serosa
      No metastasis in regional lymph nodes
      No distant metastasis
      T2, N0, M0
   C. Carcinoma with penetration through the serosa with or without invasion of contiguous structures
      No metastasis in regional lymph nodes
      No distant metastasis
      T3, N0 M0

Stage II. Diffuse involvement of the stomach wall
   No lymph nodes involved
   No distant metastasis
      T4, N0, M0
      or
   Any involvement of the stomach wall as defined by T1 to T4 and including involvement of the perigastric lymph nodes in the immediate vicinity of the primary tumour; no distant metastasis
      T1-4, N1, M0

Stage III. Tumour involving the stomach wall in any classification of T1-4, but including involvement of the perigastric regional nodes at a distance from the primary tumour or on both curvatures of the stomach; no distant metastasis
      T1-4, N2, M0

Stage IV. Any T or N classification but with distant metastasis
      M1

From Lim et al (1977), with kind permission of the authors and the editor of *Cancer*.

Table 2. *Staging of gastrointestinal lymphoma*

Stage	
I.	A. Tumour confined to gastrointestinal tract.
	B. Multiple tumours confined to gastrointestinal tract.
II.	A. Tumour with local nodal involvement.
	B. Tumour with perforation and adherence to adjacent structures.
	C. Tumour with perforation and peritonitis.
III.	Tumour with widespread nodal involvement (para-aortic or more distant nodes).
IV.	Tumour with disseminated disease (e.g., liver, bone marrow involvement).

From Blackledge et al (1979), with kind permission of the authors and the editor of *Clinical Oncology*.

None of the several proposed methods of staging accommodate one particular distinctive variety of lymphoma in the gut. Several names have been applied to this condition which is currently known as multiple lymphomatous polyposis (Cornes, 1961; Sheahan et al, 1971; Figures 1 and 2).

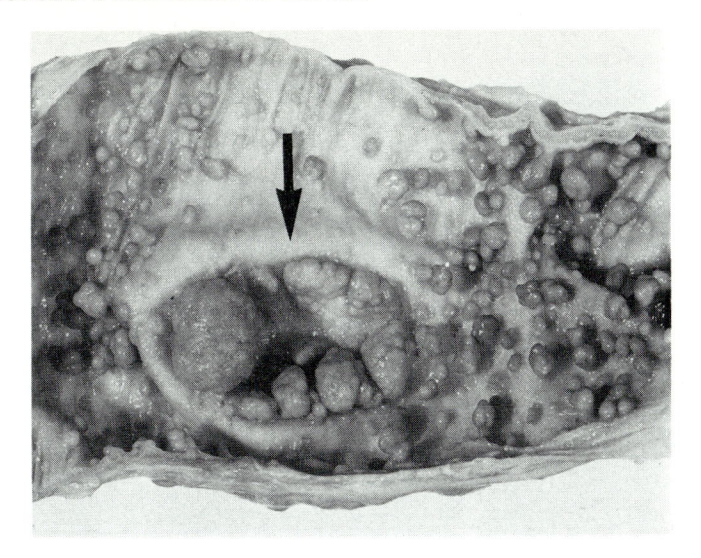

Figure 1. Multiple lymphomatous polyposis in terminal ileum. (Arrow indicates enlarged infiltrated Peyer's patch.) Natural size.

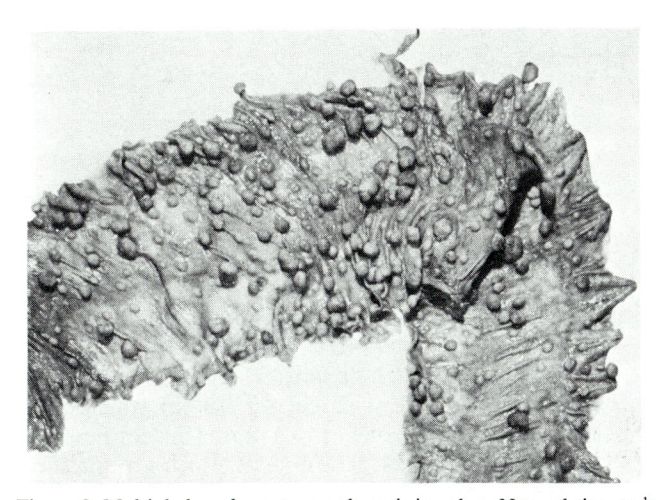

Figure 2. Multiple lymphomatous polyposis in colon. Natural size, × ⅕.

Characteristically this form of lymphoma produces an extensive, often confluent, but mainly superficial infiltrate in mucosa and submucosa (Figure 3). Considerable lengths of small or large intestine are involved and sometimes the entire gastrointestinal tract is affected. Despite this considerable extent of disease the tumour rarely penetrates into the muscularis propria even at a late stage when marked tumorous expansion of mucosa and submucosa has occurred. It would be greatly misleading in any staging to compare this type of multiple tumour formation (Figures 1 and 2) with the

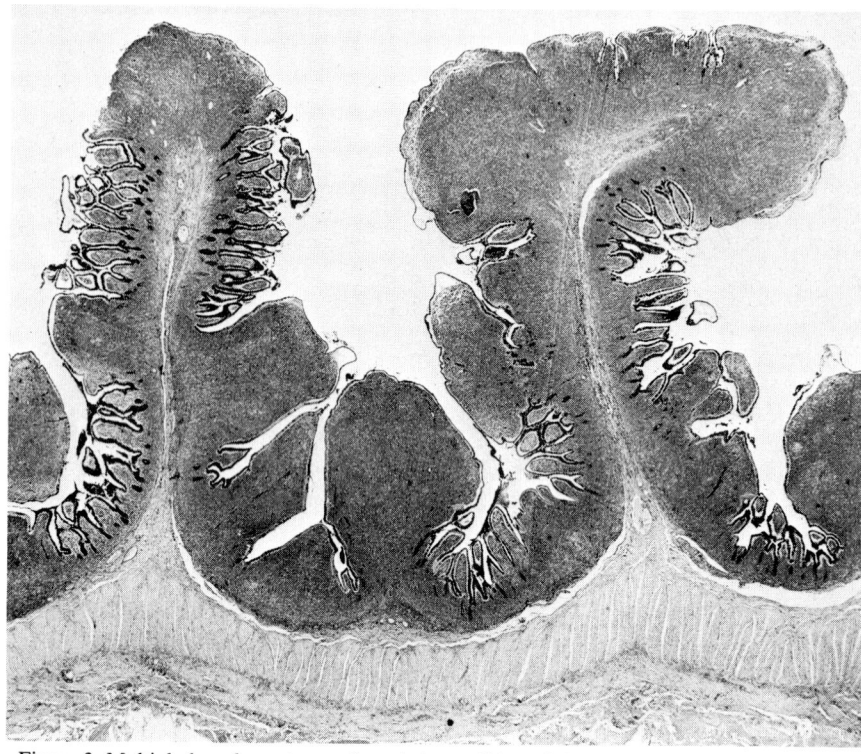

Figure 3. Multiple lymphomatous polyposis in small bowel. Note preservation of muscularis propria. PAS × 8.

more localized lymphomas even when the latter are multifocal (Figure 4). Multiple lymphomatous polyposis is, because of extent, probably not eradicable by surgery. Multiple focal primary lymphomas are at least potentially so curable.

Although the direction in which proposed staging for gut lymphomas is moving can be discerned, there is as yet no system which can be given unqualified approval. Any final conclusions in this matter must result from discussion between clinicians and pathologists. Both groups should avoid imposing a unilateral solution.

HISTOLOGICAL GRADING

An analogy between primary gut lymphoma and colorectal carcinoma does not hold good in one important respect. Adenocarcinoma of the colorectum is regarded as a single disease entity which can be arbitrarily divided into three histological grades, or degrees of differentiation. These grades indicate differing degrees of aggressiveness and relate to different survival rates but are essentially sections of a continuous spectrum of appearances.

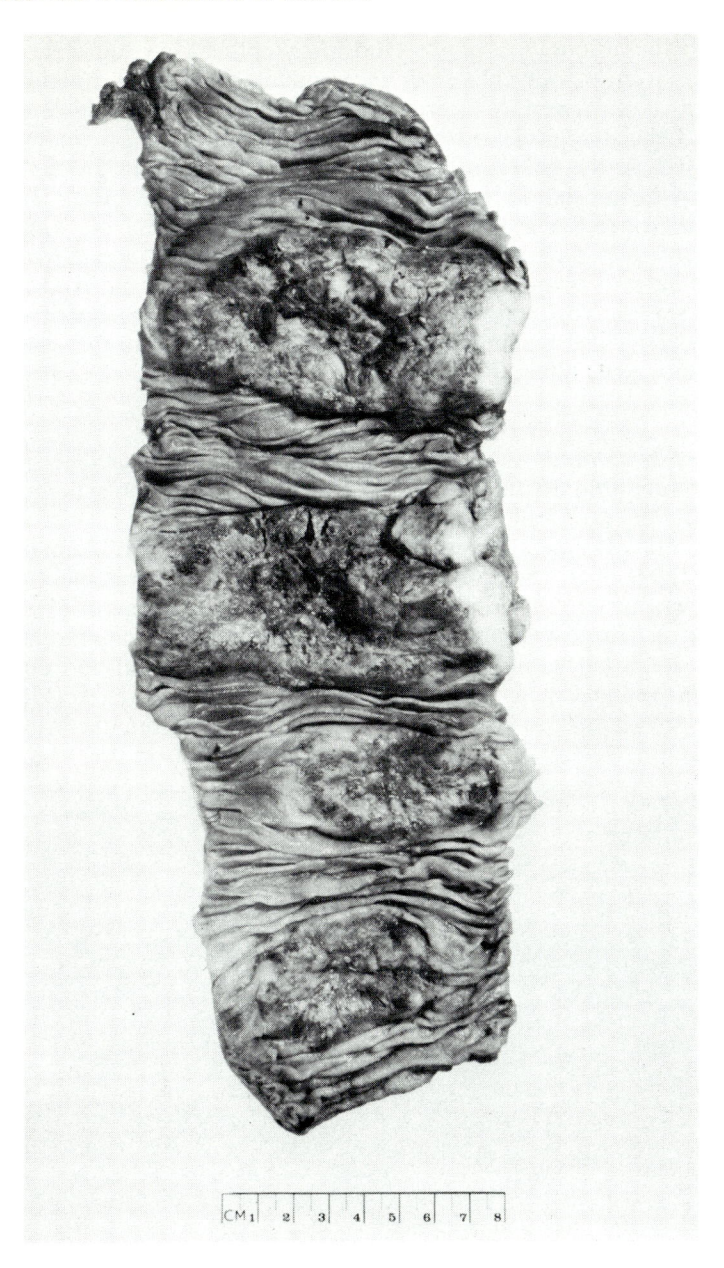

Figure 4. Multifocal primary lymphomas of small bowel. Compare with Figure 1. Natural size, × ½.

Certainly the various types of non-Hodgkin lymphoma have differing degrees of aggressiveness, but unlike adenocarcinoma these types should not be regarded as representing degrees of differentiation of a single type of tumour. On histological grounds the varieties of lymphoma are more clearly separable than the grades of adenocarcinoma. The various groups of lymphoma of the gut should properly be regarded as discrete entities, although transition from a low-grade type of tumour to a high-grade one is occasionally observed, as in nodal lymphoma. Each type of non-Hodgkin lymphoma tends to have its own characteristic mode of behaviour, and the following examples will serve to support the contention that each represents a separate disease entity. The manner in which lymphomas infiltrate the wall of the bowel and spread to other tissues differs according to the histological categories.

Malignant lymphoma — immunoblastic (Kiel): diffuse histiocytic (Rappaport); undifferentiated large cell (NLI)*; immunoblastic sarcoma (Lukes).

This tumour is typically found in adults and is histologically a high-grade type of malignancy. The cytological appearances are illustrated in Figure 5. The pattern of infiltration of the muscularis propria is one of effacement over a broad front with a relatively well-defined advancing margin to the tumour. Fissuring within the tumour is commonly noted and doubtless underlies the high frequency of perforation of this type of tumour (Figure 6). Metastasis to lymph nodes produces a discrete focus of tumour with loss of

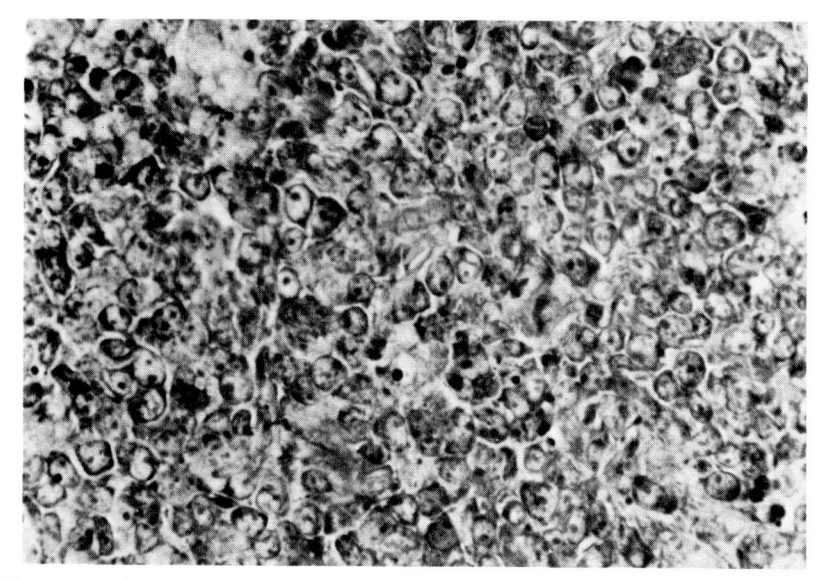

Figure 5. Malignant lymphoma of immunoblastic type from small bowel. Haematoxylin and eosin, × 550.

*NLI = National Lymphoma Investigation.

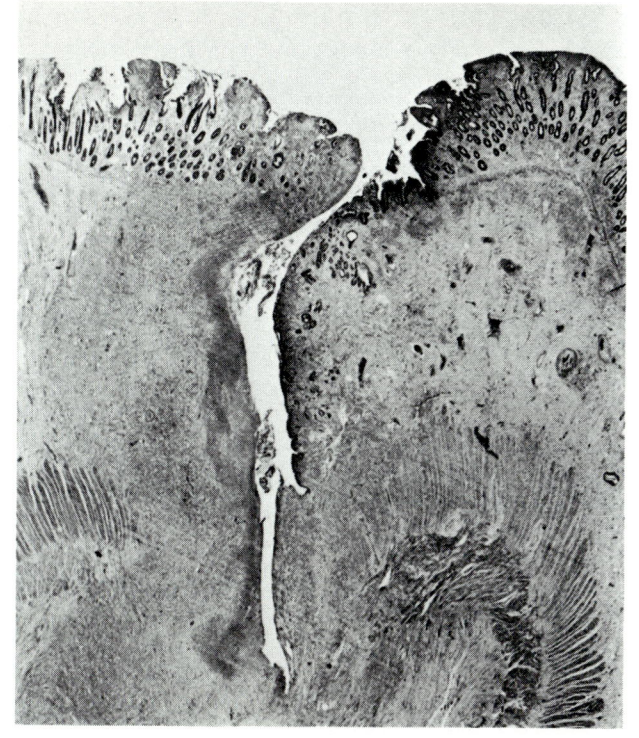

Figure 6. Fissuring ulceration in malignant lymphoma. The muscularis propria is disrupted. Haematoxylin and eosin, × 8.5.

nodal architecture and not a subtle infiltration of the pulp. Immunoblastic lymphoma in mesenteric nodes often shows a partial involvement akin to carcinomatous deposits (Figure 7).

Malignant lymphoma — lymphoblastic (Kiel): undifferentiated or poorly differentiated lymphocytic (Rappaport); poorly differentiated lymphocytic (NLI); large non-cleaved follicular centre cell (Lukes).

This is the typical high-grade lymphoma of the bowel in children but it may occasionally be seen in adults. In children it is almost exclusively confined to the ileocaecal region when a primary tumour. In contrast to immunoblastic lymphoma, the muscularis propria is spared to a remarkable degree even when much tumour has reached the serosa (Figure 8). Fissuring ulceration is rarely seen and this pattern of spread explains the very low frequency of perforation of this variety. Intussusception and obstruction are the most frequent modes of presentation. This variety of lymphoblastic lymphoma is remarkable also for its apparent reluctance to invade lymph nodes, which may be seen sometimes intact but encircled by massive tumorous infiltration of mesenteric fat. Intra-abdominal recurrence after radical surgical resection is a common problem in the absence of adjuvant

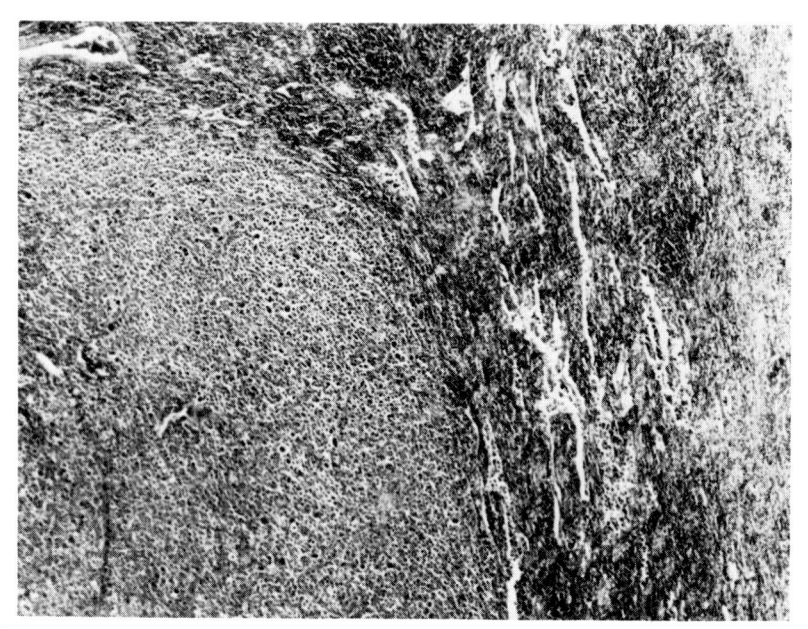

Figure 7. Partial involvement of mesenteric lymph node by immunoblastic lymphoma. Haematoxylin and eosin, × 35.

treatment, and there is a distinct tendency to early widespread dissemination.

Multiple lymphomatous polyposis — centrocytic (Kiel): intermediate differentiated lymphocytic (NLI); small cleaved follicular centre cell — diffuse (Lukes); no clearly corresponding category in Rappaport classification.

The pattern of infiltration in this condition has already been mentioned (see Figures 1, 2 and 3). The literature on this subject suggests that any variety of lymphoma, including Hodgkin's disease, may be the histological basis of lymphomatous polyposis. However, the author, in a study of more than 40 such cases, has found a very high degree of correlation between this pattern of infiltration and one particular histological type of low-grade lymphoma — centrocytic lymphoma (Figure 9). Lymph nodes, even when partially involved, do not show the mode of invasion seen for instance in immunoblastic lymphoma (Figure 10). The high frequency of evolution of a leukaemia and of peripheral lymphadenopathy in this condition suggests that it may not truly be localized to the gut, despite meeting the required criteria initially (Halkin et al, 1973; Fromke and Weber, 1974; Blackshaw, 1980, unpublished observations).

Which particular system of classification is used for gut lymphoma is clearly less important than to appreciate what any given label implies in terms of the correlations mentioned above. Unfortunately, the attention given to cellular morphology has distracted investigators from studies of the patterns of infiltration by lymphoma in such an architecturally complex organ as the gut.

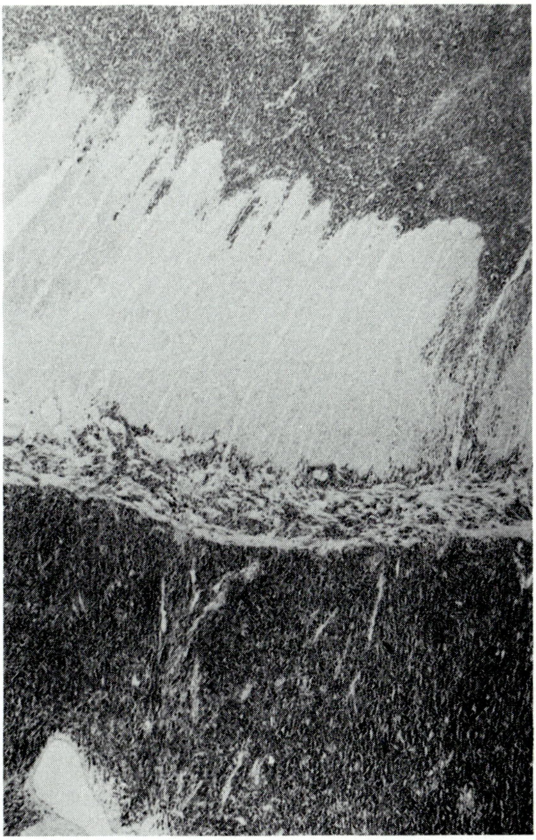

Figure 8. Malignant lymphoma of lymphoblastic type from terminal ileum of a child. Note the preservation of muscularis propria despite massive tumorous involvement of serosa in lower half of Figure. Giemsa, × 63.

These patterns of infiltration have important correlations with the clinical behaviour of the varieties of gut lymphoma.

SURVIVAL

In published discussions of prognosis in gut lymphoma survival is often given in the form of five- or ten-year survival rates. The concept that the types of lymphoma are separate diseases has implications for the manner in which data on survival are presented. It may be quite misleading simply to compare five-year survival rates, for instance. Survival curves probably provide a clearer indication of the biological behaviour of types of lymphoma and the effect of treatment. As an example the crude survival rates at varying periods of time for a low-grade and a high-grade type of lymphoma in the rectum are given in Table 3.

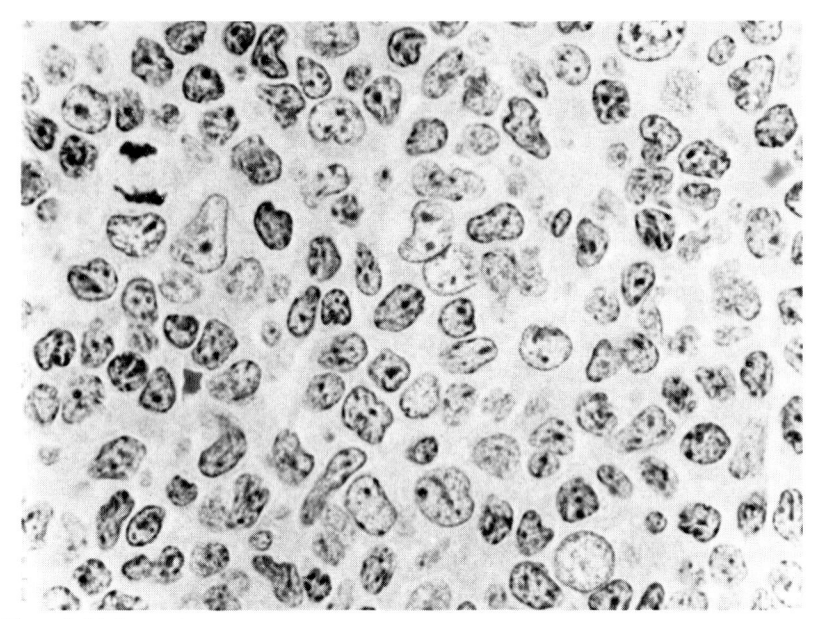

Figure 9. Malignant lymphoma of centrocytic type. Same case as Figures 1 and 2. Haematoxylin and eosin, × 900.

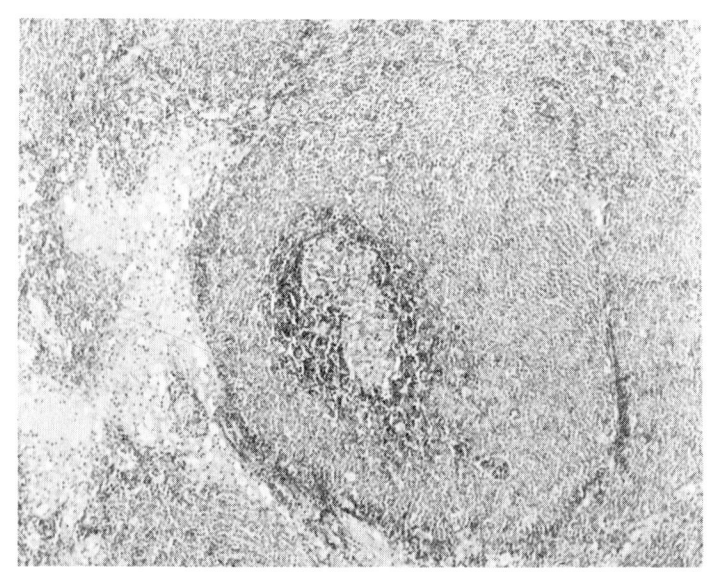

Figure 10. Interfollicular infiltration of lymph node by centrocytic lymphoma without disruption of architecture in this instance. Haematoxylin and eosin, × 85.

lymphoid polyposis testifies to the rarity of this possible evolution (Kahn and Novis, 1974). For practical purposes, therefore, this association is not considered to represent the usual mode of genesis of malignant lymphoma, even if it is more than just a fortuitous association in this particular instance. Malignant lymphomatous polyposis would appear to arise by a diffuse replacement of pre-existing lymphoid tissue in a manner reminiscent of leukaemic infiltration (hence the older terminology of 'pseudoleukaemia gastrointestinalis'). No relationship is claimed between this condition and benign lymphoid polyposis, and mixtures of benign and malignant lymphoid polyps are not seen.

Chronic ulcerative colitis

Adenocarcinoma is a known complication of chronic ulcerative colitis and is the culmination of a process of progressive epithelial atypia probably beginning as a simple regenerative hyperplasia. Malignant lymphoma of the colorectum is also a complication of chronic ulcerative colitis. Like carcinoma it tends to occur in patients with extensive disease and a long history, and to be multifocal. Approximately one lymphoma of the large bowel will be seen for every ten carcinomas in the context of chronic ulcerative colitis (Renton and Blackshaw, 1976). However, an origin in this setting cannot account for most primary lymphomas of the large bowel. It is disappointing that no histological changes which might reasonably be described as prelymphomatous have been detected in intact mucosa at a distance from primary lymphomas in ulcerative colitis.

α-Heavy-chain disease

In this condition the characteristic lymphoplasmacytic infiltrate in the small intestinal mucosa can justifiably be regarded as the morphological expression of a premalignant condition. The evolution of infiltrating primary lymphomas in this setting has been studied by several groups (Lewin, Kahn and Novis, 1976; Skinner et al, 1976; Galian et al, 1977; Ramot et al, 1977; Al-Saleem and Zardawi, 1979). Such studies of α-heavy-chain disease in Middle-Eastern populations probably have only limited relevance to the genesis of gut lymphomas in Western populations. They do serve to focus attention, however, on the diffuse lymphoreticular tissue of the lamina propria rather than the organized lymphoid tissue of the gut (solitary lymphoid follicles and Peyer's patches).

Coeliac disease

Malignancy in coeliac disease is discussed elsewhere in this issue. It is sufficient here to note that the expansion of the diffuse chronic inflammatory infiltrate in the lamina propria in this disease provides the substrate for the development of lymphoreticular malignancy according to current thinking. Some success has already been achieved in the definition of premalignant lymphoreticular atypia in coeliac disease. The significance for patient management of finding such changes in jejunal biopsies has yet to be determined. Useful comparisons might be made between the management of coeliac disease and of ulcerative colitis in respect of premalignant changes in mucosal biopsies.

Chronic gastritis

Considering that the stomach is the commonest of the sites within the gut for primary lymphomas, it is surprising that the mode of genesis of gastric lymphoma has never been considered in the literature. The relationship between chronic gastritis and adenocarcinoma of the stomach is well studied. It is tempting to speculate that the mucosal lymphocytic and plasmacytic infiltrate of chronic gastritis is potentially the source of malignant lymphomas. Organized lymphoid tissue is sparse in the normal stomach but well-formed lymphoid follicles are seen often in chronic gastritis and in the vicinity of chronic benign peptic ulcers.

The epithelium at the margin of peptic ulcers is thought by many to undergo malignant change on occasion. The same may be true of the chronic inflammatory infiltrate associated with gastric ulcers. The same histological criteria as apply to carcinoma should also apply when making the decision about possible development of lymphoma in pre-existing benign ulcers.

A study of the relationship between chronic inflammation and lymphoma development in the stomach could well prove fruitful.

What to Look For?

Histological descriptions of lymphoreticular atypia in the mucosa of the bowel are very sparse in the literature, apart from accounts of 'Mediterranean' lymphoma. Most concern patients with coeliac disease (Whitehead, 1968). The details of the microscopic changes are the subject of another paper but some unresolved issues will be mentioned here.

If coeliac disease provides an appropriate model for the development of most primary gut lymphomas then the tumours originate in the mucosa and not in submucosa as repeatedly stated until recently (McGovern, 1977). This presumption of submucosal origin, for which there is a total lack of evidence, probably results from the twin fallacies that, (a) solitary lymphoid follicles and Peyer's patches constitute the only lymphoid tissue of the gut and must perforce be the site of origin of lymphoma, and that (b) these structures are indeed submucosal. Microscopy clearly shows that lymphoid follicles have at least half their bulk within the mucosa in any case. This is not to say that some lymphomas do not have their genesis in the organized lymphoid tissue but all primary lymphomas of the gut probably have an intramucosal component even if this is secondarily lost by ulceration. Relevant to this point about the exact site of genesis is the fact that follicular lymphoma is rarely represented as a primary gut tumour, in contrast to the primary nodal non-Hodgkin's lymphomas. It must be remembered that the lamina propria contains not only lymphocytes and plasmacytes which belong to a single cellular system, but also histiocytes which belong to the separate mononuclear phagocyte system.

The question remains unresolved whether nuclear and cytoplasmic atypia per se are sufficient to define premalignancy in lymphoreticular populations. Should evidence be sought in addition of epithelial invasion or crypt destruction? Does breaching of the muscularis mucosae by an atypical lymphoreticular infiltrate constitute evidence of established malignancy? (Figures 13 and 14.) What exactly constitutes nuclear atypia, particularly in histiocytes? These questions must be resolved before histopathologists can contribute to the management of gut lymphoma in general and coeliac disease in particular.

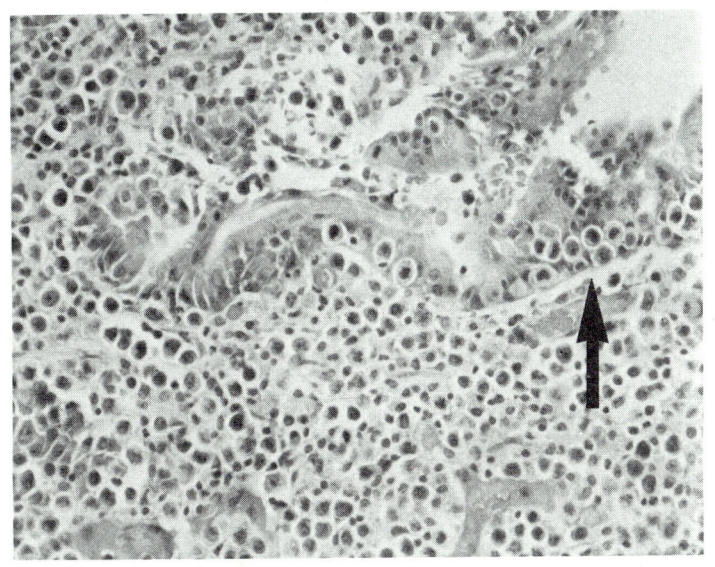

Figure 13. Intramucosal lymphoreticular atypia with invasion of epithelium. Arrow indicates intra-epithelial atypical cells. Haematoxylin and eosin, × 220.

NEW TECHNIQUES

One of the recent advances in the study of lymphomas in general has been the application of new experimental techniques. Many of these techniques such as enzyme staining (Figure 15) require either fresh tissue to be available or else rapid fixation in special fixatives. For obvious reasons these requirements are not often met in cases of gut tumours which are surgically removed at infrequent intervals, often at inconvenient times, and without a prior definitive diagnosis. The necessity for fresh tissue excludes retrospective analysis of such properties of gut lymphomas as surface markers, enzyme content and also to a large extent electron microscopy. Analysis of gut lymphomas must rely heavily on histological assessment of conventional light microscopic preparations. There are three special techniques which can be applied to formalin-fixed tissue and are therefore of potential value.

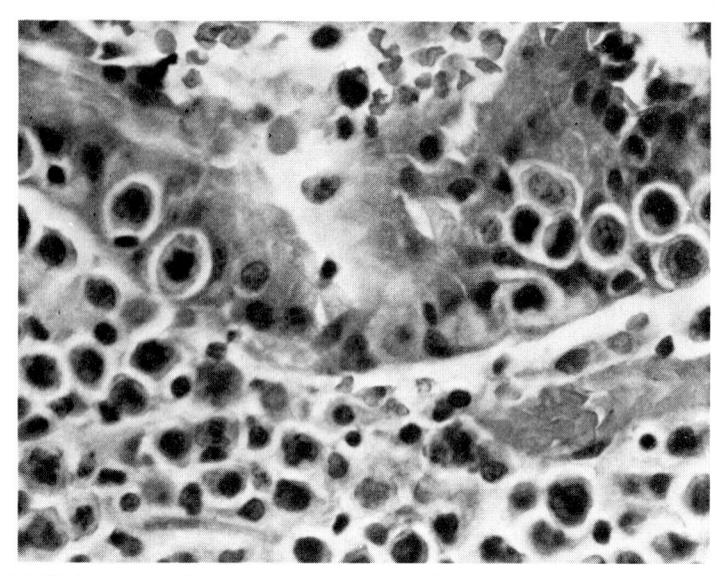

Figure 14. Higher power of Figure 13 to show atypical intra-epithelial cells. Haematoxylin and eosin, × 550.

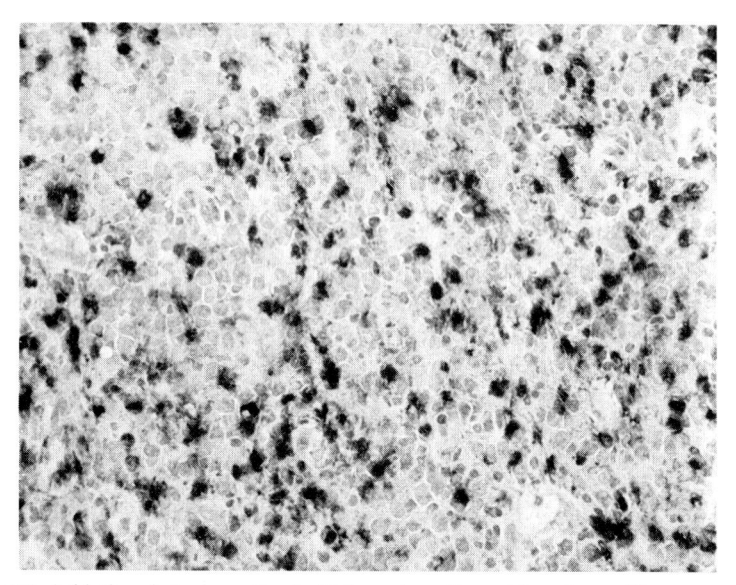

Figure 15. Acid phosphatase reaction in high-grade malignant lymphoma. Numerous darkly staining cells are reactive histiocytes. This pattern of staining should not be interpreted as evidence of histiocytic origin of the tumour. Neoplastic cells are negative. × 220.

Immunoperoxidase Staining

Details of this technique are available elsewhere (Taylor, 1978; Heyderman, 1979). It can be adapted to the demonstration of a great number of antigens within tissues, including intracellular immunoglobulin. A major advantage is that sections can subsequently be counterstained with a variety of conventional methods, thus making possible an assessment of the overall context in which a particular antigen is demonstrated. The immunoperoxidase staining technique in gut lymphomas has not yet fulfilled its early promise. Some complicating factors are the necessity to distinguish intracellular immunoglobulin synthesized by cells of the plasmacyte series from that ingested by histiocytes; and the presence of a reactive inflammatory overlay in so many gut tumours.

It is probably fair to say that immunoperoxidase staining has provided useful additional information in tumours which are clearly plasmacytoid in nature as judged by conventional morphology (Skinner et al, 1976; Scott, Dupont and Webb, 1978). However, this technique has largely left unresolved the vexing question of the nature of the large cell lymphomas, of which there is a preponderance amongst gut tumours. Such at least has been the experience of the author.

The demonstration of a monoclonal population of immunoglobulin-containing cells is extremely good presumptive evidence of their neoplastic nature. The reverse, that polyclonal staining indicates a reactive non-neoplastic proliferation, is not necessarily true and here caution must be exercised. Although several types of neoplasm, apart from multiple myeloma, have been shown to be monoclonal, there is equally a number of genuine neoplasms which are not demonstrably monoclonal. Even plasma cell tumours may occasionally be apparently biclonal.

Plastic Embedding

A prerequisite of accurate histological assessment is the provision of high-quality tissue sections. Prompt fixation is of prime importance, especially in lymphomas, and is properly emphasized by all authorities on this subject. Even with good fixation the results of conventional processing can be improved upon by the use of plastic embedding. A couple of examples are given here to demonstrate the superior morphological detail obtainable from plastic (ethylmethacrylate) embedding. In each instance tumour was fixed in identical fashion in formalin before being processed either in paraffin or plastic. The sections were stained identically with haematoxylin and eosin and photographed at the same magnification under the same conditions (Figures 16 to 19).

Chloroacetate Esterase

Mast cells and granulated cells of the myeloid series, excepting eosinophils, contain an enzyme called chloroacetate esterase (Moloney, McPherson and Fliegelman, 1960), which can be demonstrated after fixation in formalin and

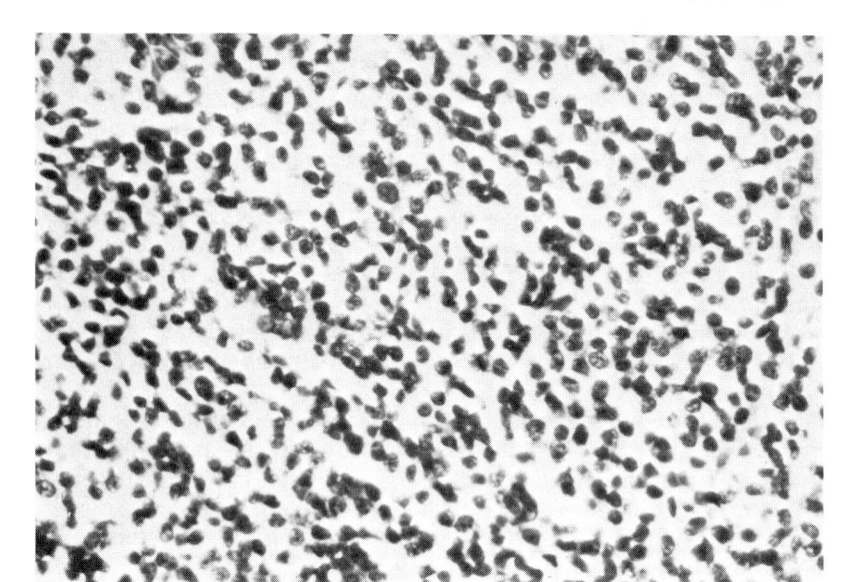

Figure 16. Centrocytic lymphoma: paraffin embedding. Haematoxylin and eosin, × 500.

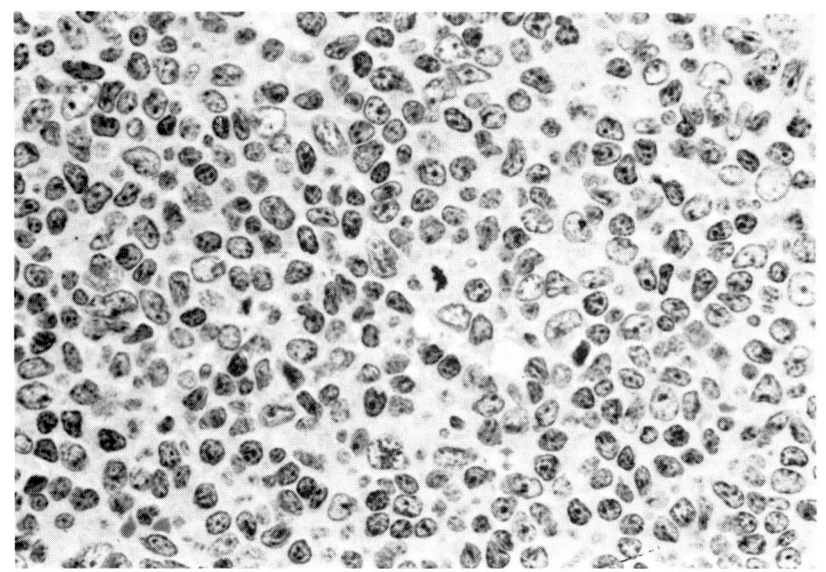

Figure 17. Same tumour as in Figure 16: methacrylate embedding. Haematoxylin and eosin, × 500.

embedding either in paraffin or ethylmethacrylate. This esterase is useful in the histological diagnosis of myeloid sarcoma. At first sight it might appear that myeloid sarcoma is unlikely to present a problem of differential diagnosis from gut lymphomas. However, the fact that myeloid sarcoma may

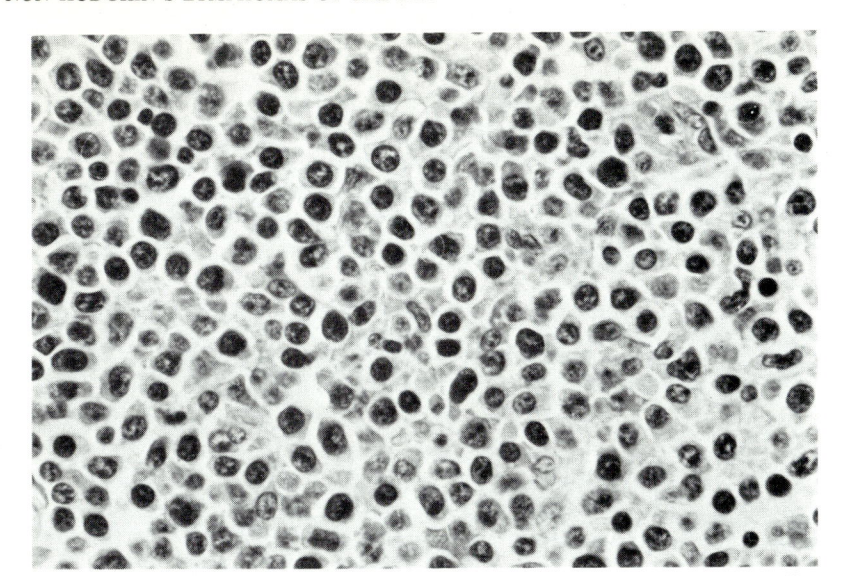

Figure 18. High-grade lymphoma: paraffin embedding. There is a hint of plasmacytoid differentiation. Haematoxylin and eosin, × 500.

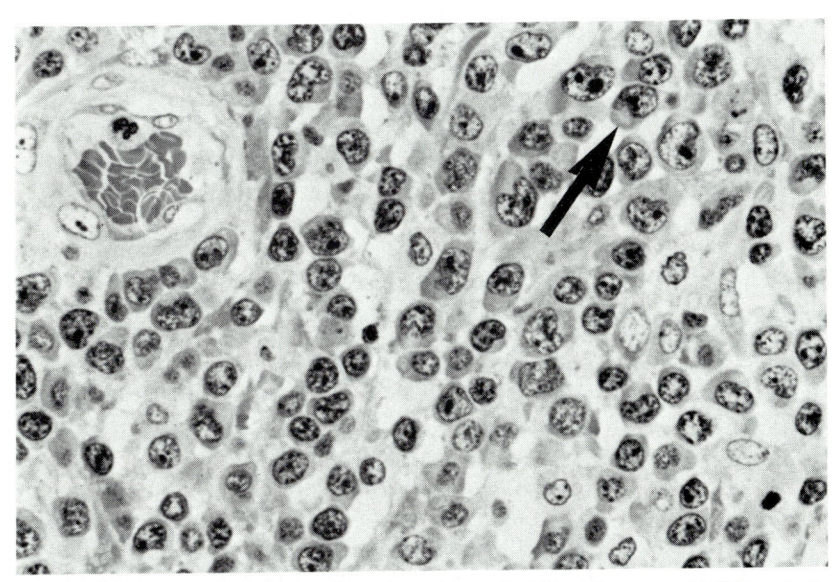

Figure 19. Same tumour as in Figure 18: methacrylate embedding. Plasmacytoid differentiation is more readily appreciated. Arrow indicates primitive plasma cell with paranuclear 'Hof'. Haematoxylin and eosin, × 500.

occasionally occur some considerable time before the demonstration of overt myeloid leukaemia is well documented (Mason, Demaree and Margolis, 1973). There are several reported instances where an initial erroneous diagnosis of malignant lymphoma had been made. The various sites at which preleukaemic myeloid sarcomas have been noted include the gut (Brugo et al, 1977). Cytologically the mimicry of malignant lymphoma can be very close (Figures 5 and 20). In the single example of preleukaemic intestinal myeloid sarcoma seen by the author even the fissuring ulceration so characteristic of many high-grade lymphomas mentioned above was present. The presence of chloroacetate esterase activity in primitive cells of a tumour will readily distinguish myeloid sarcomas from lymphoma — a differential diagnosis which might otherwise be extremely difficult.

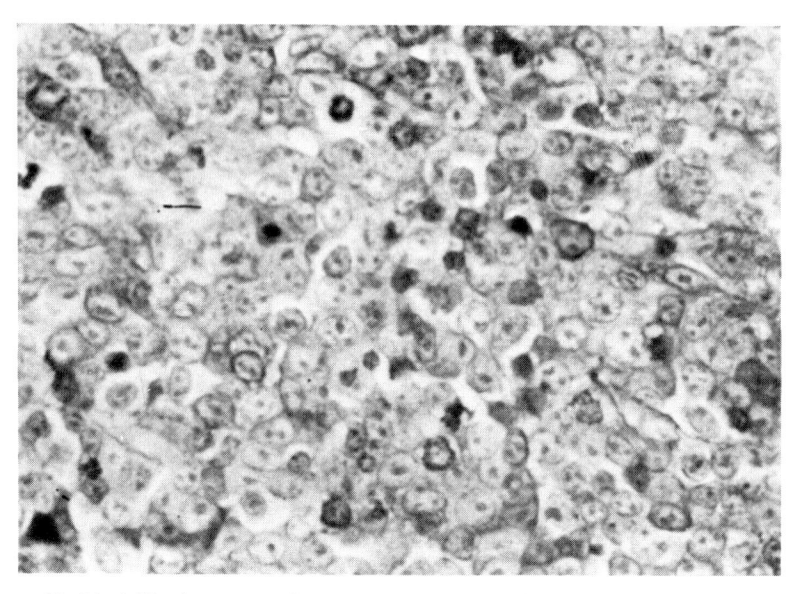

Figure 20. Myeloblastic sarcoma for comparison with Figure 5. Haematoxylin and eosin, × 550.

HODGKIN'S DISEASE

Although Hodgkin's disease of the gut is specifically excluded from consideration in this paper, it is proper to consider it in the differential diagnosis of the non-Hodgkin's lymphomas. A study of the literature would indicate that the incidence of primary Hodgkin's disease of the gut has declined markedly over the past few decades. The generally accepted view now is that Hodgkin's disease is a rare primary lesion of the gut, and indeed it is absent from several recent series of primary lymphomas (Fu and Perzin, 1972; Henry and Farrer-Brown, 1977). It is highly improbable that this represents a genuine fall in incidence and the supposition must be that the majority of the former diagnoses were erroneous. Now that the distinction between Hodgkin's and non-Hodgkin's lymphomas has important implications for the chemotherapy of these conditions, it is relevant to consider how such confusion might have arisen.

The presence of Reed-Sternberg cells is mandatory for the histological diagnosis of Hodgkin's disease (Figure 21). They are not, however, pathognomonic since cells which are very similar or even identical in appearance may be observed in an ever-growing list of other malignancies and benign reactive conditions. The background in which 'Reed-Sternberg' cells are seen is of crucial importance for the distinction of these various lesions which mimic Hodgkin's disease. Hodgkin's disease is destructive of normal architecture but the background is one of a banal inflammatory population

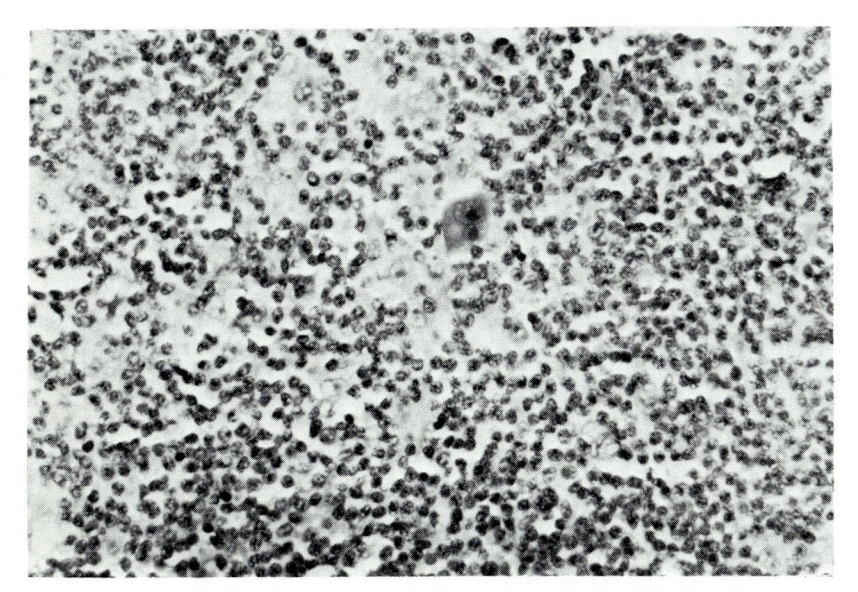

Figure 21. Hodgkin's disease showing Reed-Sternberg cell. Haematoxylin and eosin, × 250.

of cells. In some instances lymphocytes predominate in the background and in other instances eosinophil leucocytes are numerous. In the gut many examples of non-Hodgkin's lymphoma can be found in which cells resembling Reed-Sternberg cells are present, as in Figure 22. Experienced pathologists are unlikely to be seduced by appearances such as these since the rest of the infiltrate is clearly inconsistent with Hodgkin's disease. There are two particular types of non-Hodgkin's lymphoma in the gut, however, where mimicry of Hodgkin's disease can be very close, and these merit further discussion.

Centrocytic Lymphoma (Multiple Lymphomatous Polyposis)

The high degree of correlation between centrocytic lymphoma (the neoplasm composed purely of small cleaved follicular centre cells) and multiple lymphomatous polyposis (MLP) has already been mentioned. Several previously reported examples of MLP have been stated to have Hodgkin's

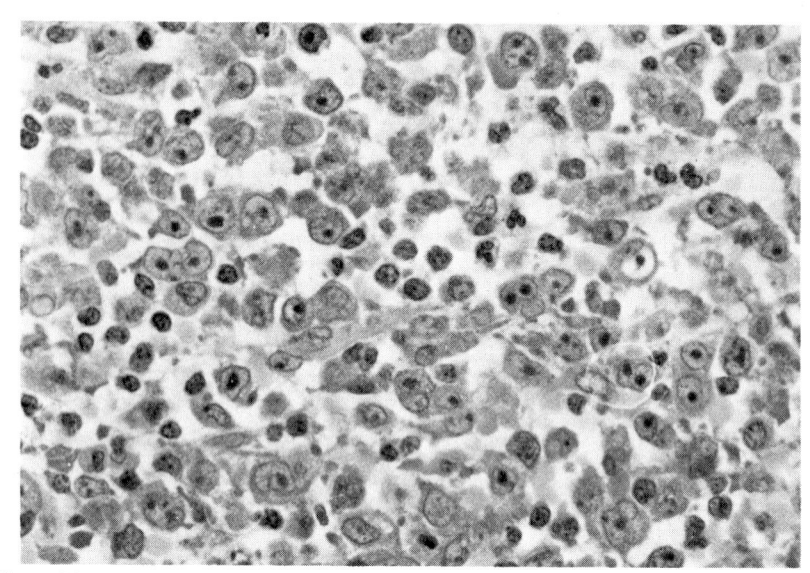

Figure 22. Non-Hodgkin's lymphoma with binucleate cells resembling Reed-Sternberg cells. Haematoxylin and eosin, × 500.

disease as their histological basis. The presence within centrocytic lymphoma of reactive histiocytes which may be numerous and are often binucleate gives a close resemblance of this lesion to lymphocytic predominant Hodgkin's disease (Figure 23). Critical inspection reveals that the

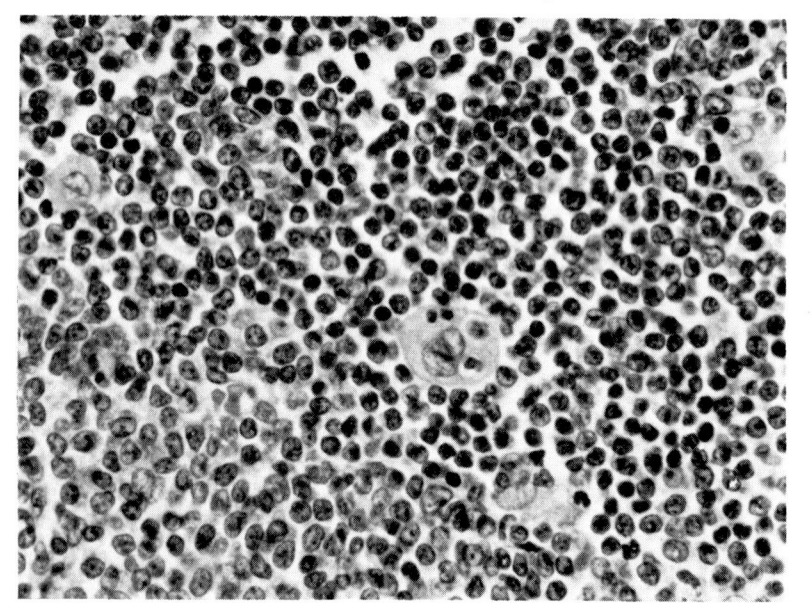

Figure 23. Binucleate histiocyte in centrocytic lymphoma. Phagocytosed material is present in the cytoplasm of the histiocyte. Haematoxylin and eosin, × 300.

binucleate cells lack the nuclear characteristics of classical Reed-Sternberg cells, and the presence of phagocytosed debris within many of them indicates their histiocytic nature. Moreover, the cells in the background are not lymphocytes as in Hodgkin's disease but centrocytes with characteristic angulated and irregular nuclear outline and finely dispersed chromatin (see Figure 17). All the mitotic activity is seen in this centrocytic population and not in the larger histiocytic cells. Distinction between lymphocytes and centrocytes may be extremely difficult in poorly preserved material. This serves to underline again the necessity for sections of high technical quality in the study of lymphoma.

Malignant Lymphoma with Eosinophilia

There is a particular variety of gut lymphoma, found predominantly in small bowel, whose major distinctive property is intense infiltration of the affected tissue by eosinophil leucocytes. The eosinophilia may be so marked that the presence of underlying malignancy is completely overlooked. If the neoplastic nature of the lesion is recognized then the finding of binucleate large lymphoma cells with a background of eosinophilic leucocytes leads often to a diagnosis of Hodgkin's disease. When a careful search is made, however, it is usually possible to discover areas where the eosinophilia is diminished and a uniform population of the blast cells of a non-Hodgkin lymphoma is revealed (Figure 24). This type of lymphoma has not yet received a convenient histological label. Since its exact histogenesis is at the moment undetermined, the noncommittal terminology used here seems appropriate, at least for the time being. There is little doubt that a definite, though not

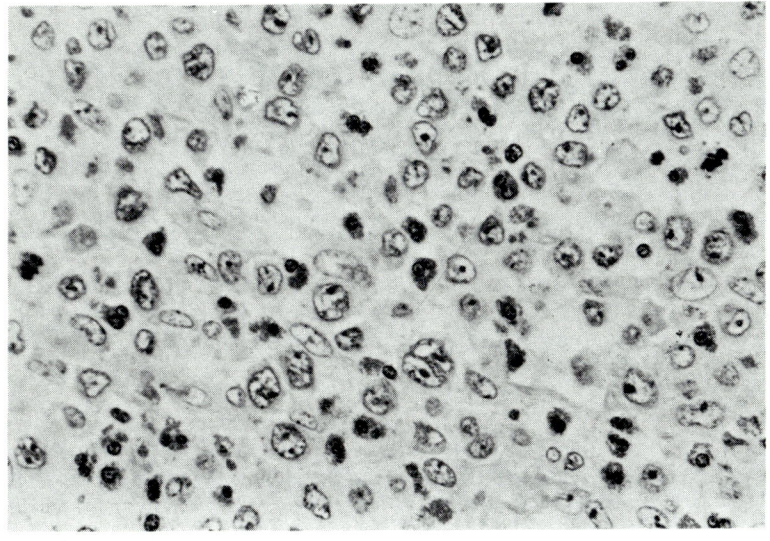

Figure 24. Malignant lymphoma with eosinophilia. In this area eosinophils are diminished in number revealing underlying malignant lymphoma. Haematoxylin and eosin, × 500.

exclusive, relationship exists between this type of lymphoma and malabsorptive syndromes with partial or total villous atrophy (Blackshaw, 1980, unpublished observations). This provides a possible explanation for the previously claimed high incidence of Hodgkin's disease of the small bowel in patients with malabsorption (Cornes, 1967). The natural behaviour and the mode of spread of malignant lymphoma with eosinophilia are unlike those of genuine Hodgkin's disease.

COOPERATION

The purpose behind all classification, grading and staging is to produce accurate prognoses as a guide to management of a disease. With regard to malignant lymphomas of the gut it is clear that tumours at different major sites must be considered separately since different surgical approaches are required for each. At each site lymphomas must be divided into the different categories since these in fact represent distinct diseases rather than grades of a single tumour. Furthermore, each type of lymphoma should be subdivided by stage. When these facts are taken into account and the number of possible permutations are considered, it is evident that only very large series of primary gut lymphomas will produce statistically valid conclusions. Even series of 200 or more cases, such as that studied by the author, are probably insufficient for this purpose. The long period of time necessary for series of this order of size to accumulate in a single institution completely abolishes their usefulness. Although combined series from several centres suffer from some obvious disadvantages this appears to be the only feasible means of obtaining the necessary answers in a reasonably short period of time.

Cooperation between individual pathologists and between institutions can therefore be considered as the advance of greatest potential importance for the future. It must be acknowledged that such cooperation is already in existence but there is a need for it to be consolidated and extended. Only in this fashion will there be an early end to the uncertainties in the pathology of gut lymphomas.

If the incidence quoted above of 1.6/100 000 persons per year is representative of the United Kingdom as a whole, then the greater London area alone will produce about 110 new cases of primary gut lymphoma every year. In England and Wales together nearly 800 new cases per year can be expected. It therefore appears that there would be sufficient material available for a cooperative effort to yield an accurate statistical analysis of the factors bearing on the prognosis of patients with primary gastrointestinal lymphoma.

ACKNOWLEDGEMENTS

Mr Bill Brackenbury of Nottingham University, Mr Norman Mackie of St Mark's Hospital, and the Department of Medical Illustration, St Bartholomew's Hospital, all contributed some of the photographs used here. Mr Stephen Jones, FIMLS, provided the ethylmethacrylate sections and Ms Jill Latham, FIMLS, and Ms Alison Field, FIMLS, performed the esterase and immunoperoxidase stains. Mrs Geraldine Northey typed the manuscript.

REFERENCES

Al-Saleem, T. & Zardawi, I.M. (1979) Primary lymphomas of the small intestine in Iraq: a pathological study of 145 cases. *Histopathology*, **3**, 89-106.

Blackledge, G., Bush, H., Dodge, O.G. & Crowther, D. (1979) A study of gastrointestinal lymphoma. *Clinical Oncology*, **5**, 209-219.

Brugo, E.A., Marshall, R.B., Riberi, A.M. & Pautasso, O.E. (1977) Preleukaemic granulocytic sarcomas of the gastrointestinal tract. *American Journal of Clinical Pathology*, **68**, 616-621.

Cornes, J.S. (1961) Multiple lymphomatous polyposis of the gastrointestinal tract. *Cancer*, **14**, 249-257.

Cornes, J.S. (1967) Hodgkin's disease of the gastrointestinal tract. *Proceedings of the Royal Society of Medicine*, **60**, 732-733.

Dawson, I.M.P., Cornes, J.S. & Morson, B.C. (1961) Primary malignant lymphoid tumours of the gastrointestinal tract. *British Journal of Surgery*, **49**, 80-89.

Friedman, A.I. (1959) Primary lymphosarcoma of the stomach: a clinical study of seventy-five cases. *American Journal of Medicine*, **26**, 783-796.

Fromke, V.L. & Weber, L.W. (1974) Extensive leukaemic infiltration of the gastrointestinal tract in chronic lymphosarcoma cell leukaemia. *American Journal of Medicine*, **56**, 879-882.

Fu, Y.-S. & Perzin, K.H. (1972) Lymphosarcoma of the small intestine: a clinicopathologic study. *Cancer*, **29**, 645-659.

Galian, A., Lecestre, M.-J., Scotto, J., Bognel, C., Matuchansky, C. & Rambaud, J.-C. (1977) Pathological study of alpha-chain disease, with special emphasis on evolution. *Cancer*, **39**, 2081-2101.

Green, J.A., Dawson, A.A., Jones, P.F. & Brunt, P.W. (1979) The presentation of gastrointestinal lymphoma: a study of a population. *British Journal of Surgery*, **66**, 798-801.

Halkin, H., Meytes, D., Militeanu, J. & Ramot, B. (1973) Multiple lymphomatous polyposis of the gastrointestinal tract. *Israel Journal of Medical Sciences*, **9**, 648-654.

Henry, K. & Farrer-Brown, G. (1977) Primary lymphomas of the gastrointestinal tract: I. Plasma cell tumours. *Histopathology*, **1**, 53-76.

Heyderman, E. (1979) Immunoperoxidase technique in histopathology: applications, methods and controls. *Journal of Clinical Pathology*, **32**, 971-978.

Jaffe, N., Buell, D., Cassady, J.R., Traggis, D. & Weinstein, H. (1977) Role of staging in childhood non-Hodgkin's lymphoma. *Cancer Treatment Reports*, **61**, 1001-1007.

Kahn, L.B. & Novis, B.H. (1974) Nodular lymphoid hyperplasia of the small bowel associated with primary small bowel reticulum cell sarcoma. *Cancer*, **33**, 837-844.

Lewin, K.J., Kahn, L.B. & Novis, B.H. (1976) Primary intestinal lymphoma of 'Western' and 'Mediterranean' type, alpha chain disease and massive plasma cell infiltration: a comparative study of 37 cases. *Cancer*, **38**, 2511-2528.

Lim, F.E., Hartman, A.S., Tan, E.G.C., Cady, B. & Meissner, W.A. (1977) Factors in the prognosis of gastric lymphoma. *Cancer*, **39**, 1715-1720.

Mason, T.E., Demaree, R.S. & Margolis, C.I. (1973) Granulocytic sarcoma (chloroma), two years preceding myelogenous leukaemia. *Cancer*, **31**, 423-432.

McGovern, V.J. (1977) Lymphomas of the gastrointestinal tract. In *The Gastrointestinal Tract* (International Academy of Pathology Monograph No. 18) (Ed.) Yardley, J.H., Morson, B.C. & Abell, M.R. Baltimore: Williams and Wilkins Co.

Moloney, W.C., McPherson, K. & Fliegelman, L. (1960) 1. Esterase activity in leukocytes demonstrated by the use of naphthol As-D chloroacetate substrate. *Journal of Histochemistry and Cytochemistry*, **8**, 200-207.

Ramot, B., Levanon, M., Hahn, Y., Lahat, N. & Moroz, C. (1977) The mutual clonal origin of the lymphoplasmacytic and lymphoma cell in alpha-heavy chain disease. *Clinical and Experimental Immunology*, **27**, 440-445.

Renton, P. & Blackshaw, A.J. (1976) Colonic lymphoma complicating ulcerative colitis. *British Journal of Surgery*, **63**, 542-545.

Rosenberg, S.A. (1977) Validity of the Ann Arbor Staging Classification for the non-Hodgkin's lymphomas. *Cancer Treatment Reports*, **61**, 1023-1027.

Scott, F.E.T., Dupont, P.A. & Webb, J. (1978) Plasmacytoma of the stomach: diagnosis with the aid of the immunoperoxidase technique. *Cancer*, **41**, 675-681.

Sheahan, D.G., Martin, F., Baginsky, S., Mallory, G.K. & Zamchek, N. (1971) Multiple lymphomatous polyposis of the gastrointestinal tract. *Cancer*, **28**, 408-425.

Skinner, J.M., Manousos, O.N., Economidou, J., Nicolau, A. & Merikas, G. (1976) Alpha-chain disease with localised plasmacytoma of the intestine. *Clinical and Experimental Immunology*, **25**, 112-116.

Taylor, C.R. (1978) Immunoperoxidase techniques: practical and theoretical aspects. *Archives of Pathology and Laboratory Medicine*, **102**, 113-121.

Whitehead, R. (1968) Primary lymphadenopathy complicating idiopathic steatorrhoea. *Gut*, **9**, 569-575.

14

Cytodiagnosis of Gastric Cancer

O.A.N. HUSAIN
R. ZEEGEN
R.A. PARKINS
K.S. IBRAHIM
J. GRAINGER
R. BASU

In discussing recent advances in the cytodiagnosis of gastric neoplasia one needs to consider not only the current potential of standard techniques but also those more specific tests, cytochemical and enzymic, which are designed to achieve a more functional assessment of the lesion. As these latter tests will be dealt with fully by Professor Munro Neville (see Chapter 15) we shall concentrate on the more traditional techniques which have improved considerably over the past 10 years, due mainly to the development of endoscopic fibreoscopy. Moreover, cytology, both by the conventional and specific techniques for the screening for gastric cancer in its earliest stages, should be evaluated as this has produced a significant contribution from Japan.

The cytodiagnosis of gastric cancer depended on simple gastric aspirates or washings until the 1940s when instruments in the form of sponges, brushes and abrasive balloons were devised, and the continuous-irrigation Faucher tube and the Woods gastroscope were introduced. None of these techniques was successful in effecting a persistently reliable sample or acceptable to the patient, and it was not until Hirschowitz introduced the gastrofibrescope in 1958 that real progress was made (Table 1). Its subsequent development permitted sampling by biopsy, brush, suction and directional lavage of anatomical sites which had previously been inaccessible (Kasugai, 1976; Winawer et al, 1976) and has had an important impact on diagnostic accuracy over the past 16 years (Kameya et al, 1964; Kasugai, 1964; Kidokoro et al, 1966; Liavag, Marcussen and Serck-Hanssen, 1971; Kasugai and Kobayashi, 1974; Winawer et al, 1975; Shida, 1976; Witzell et al, 1976; Table 2). In fact, in Japan in the decade from 1956 to 1966 the percentage of early cancers diagnosed rose from 3.8 to 34.5 per cent (Prolla, Kobayashi and Kirsner, 1969).

Several studies from the United Kingdom (Roca, Whitehead and Boddington, 1974; Smithies et al, 1975; MacKenzie et al, 1977; Boddington,

© 1980 W.B. Saunders Company Ltd.

Table 1. *Gastric washing techniques*

A. Abrasive		
	(i)	Zelltopfsonde
	(ii)	Abrasive balloon
	(iii)	Antral abrasive balloon
	(iv)	Gastric brush
B. Lavage		
	(i)	Papain
	(ii)	α-Chymotrypsin
	(iii)	Simple washout: saline, Ringer's or Hartmann's solution
	(iv)	Martinez' continuous irrigation (Faucher tube)
C. Gastrofibrescopes		

1978; Evans et al, 1978; Hughes, Lee and MacKenzie, 1978) have shown accuracies of up to 90 per cent. On the other hand, accuracy of blind tube washes has varied from 30 per cent (Segal et al, 1975) to over 90 per cent (Schade, 1960; MacDonald et al, 1963; Cantrell, 1971).

It is of interest that the early reports from Japan indicated a high level of sensitivity of 97 per cent (Kasugai, 1968) using a jet-wash technique, though Halter et al (1977) could achieve only a 50 per cent accuracy. Moreover, it was claimed that this technique was superior to direct biopsy (Fakuda et al, 1967; Kasugai, 1968). In summary, the Japanese have preferred the jet-wash technique to the nylon-brush technique though there have been some (Kasugai and Kobayashi, 1974) who now believe washing need be used only

Table 2. *Gastric cytology: efficiency of various techniques*

Series	No. with cancer	% Accuracy	Method
Papanicolaou and Cooper (1947)	27	37	Fasting aspirate
Graham, Ulfelder and Green (1948)	24	62	Fasting aspirate
Traut et al (1952)	42	71	Papain lavage
Crozier, Middleton and Ross (1956)	29	69	Lavage and brush abrasion
Seybolt and Papanicolaou (1957)	114	66	Abrasive balloon
Fukuda (quoted by Tazaki, 1959)	76	85	Modified balloon
Cabre-Fiol, Olo-Garcia and Vilardell (1959)	94	90	Mandril-sound
Raskin, Kirsner and Palmer (1959)	131	95	Gastric washings
Schade (1960)	258	97	Gastric washings
Witte (1959)	184	65	Zelltopfsonde
MacDonald et al (1963)	89	93	Chymotrypsin wash
Taebel, Prolla and Kirsner (1965)	282	81	Gastric washings
Blendis et al (1967)	100	81	Gastric washings
Kasugai (1968)	375	97	Fibregastroscopic lavage
Shida (1971)	60	90	Fibregastroscopic brush
Witzell et al (1976)	73	84	Fibrescopic brush
Thompson et al (1977)	59	90	Fibrescopic brush
Young and Hughes (1977)	61	92	Fibrescopic brush
MacKenzie et al (1977)		94	Fibrescopic brush
Boddington (1978)	84	79	Fibrescopic brush

if biopsy fails. It seems that the nylon brush has become the method of choice of Western workers on the grounds that it gives a better and more reliable sample than the jet-wash technique. Some have used the imprint smear in order to achieve cytological sampling of deeper tissue than is given by surface brushing (Yoshii et al, 1970), with better results than directional washes show (Tamura et al, 1977), but most pathologists believe that it is of little value and we ourselves no longer use this.

Biopsy has rightly achieved a pre-eminent position with an acknowledged high sensitivity and specificity rate. On the other hand, some authors often present their histological results on the basis of biopsy and excised organ diagnosis. When the biopsy is considered separately the sensitivity, if not the specificity, resembles that of the brush sample. Here, the histologists do not always do themselves justice when they examine one or two sections from a minute biopsy. The cytopathologist is accustomed to having his whole cell sample laid out on slides, but the biopsy needs step or serial sections to effect a full review of the material biopsied.

COLLECTION AND PREPARATION TECHNIQUES

Details of our own technical procedures for collecting and processing the blind-tube wash and gastroscopic-brush sample are worth relating here, both because they achieve a high accuracy rate and also because they provide useful information for the gastroscopist as well as the laboratory personnel.

Blind tube wash

This is still used on those patients unable or unwilling to undergo gastroscopy (e.g., with oesophageal stenosis), or for screening purposes, as it is still the cheapest technique for the collection of those cell samples, using cytochemical techniques for more functional cellular assessment. Here, the procedure is to have the patient fast overnight though kept adequately hydrated by a plentiful allowance of water by mouth to maintain good cell exfoliation. A Levin tube is passed through the nose or mouth to the mid-gastric position and the resting juice aspirated. This is followed by the introduction down the tube of 250 to 300 ml of buffered saline, after which the abdomen is massaged and the patient made to flex the body so as to agitate the cells from the mucosal surface. This washing is then aspirated and the procedure repeated if desired. Each resting juice and gastric wash is immediately neutralized, if necessary to pH 6, and rapidly centrifuged, preferably in ice-cold siliconized tubes, and about six smears made from each sample. Most of these smears are rapidly wet-fixed in absolute alcohol for staining by the Papanicolaou technique, and one or two thin smears rapidly air-dried for staining by one of the Romanovsky stains (May Gruenwald Giemsa). Should there be much mucus present we give the patient 7 mg of α-chymotrypsin in a glass of water half an hour before washing, which is then carried out using a further 7 mg of α-chymotrypsin in a sodium acetate buffer at pH 5.6. At this pH the enzyme digests the mucus but not the mucosa.

The screening of such smears calls for much patience and skill in interpretation as the criteria of malignancy are often less well displayed than in brush preparations.

The fibrescopic brush sample

We have used the Olympic instruments, either the GFD end-viewing for the oesophagus, or the GFK (oblique viewing) which has become more popular for both stomach and oesophagus, one of us preferring the paediatric model. Patients are asked to attend after fasting overnight and are sedated with diazepam intravenously and the larynx is anaesthetized with lignocaine 1 per cent. The saline or glycerol-lubricated fibrescope is passed with the patient lying in the supine or left-lateral position, with or without an airway. After inspection of the stomach, any lesion is photographed and the brush and biopsy samples are collected. It is preferable to obtain the brush samples first to avoid obscuring the lesion following the bleeding that invariably results from the biopsy. That it is not detrimental to the biopsy to do so was shown in a prospective randomized trial (Thompson et al, 1977), where biopsy and brush samples alternated as the first sample to be taken. In the study by Thompson and his colleagues of 211 patients (which included 59 cancers, 109 benign gastric ulcers and 33 cases with polyps or atrophic gastritis), the diagnosis of the cancers was made by histology alone in 76 per cent of cases; by cytology alone in 90 per cent and by both in 98 per cent, with only one case being negative by both techniques.

Collection of Brush Samples

The collection of a satisfactory brush sample requires an assistant, as the gastroscopist may well be manoeuvring the end of the scope and holding the lesion in focus whilst the brush is manipulated by the associate. To obtain a good cellular sample the brush must be thrust vigorously 10 to 15 times into the mucosal lesion so that the lamina propria is penetrated and a small amount of blood produced. This manoeuvre is not always carried out with sufficient vigour or enough sweeps of the brush, and may then result in a false negative result. At one time a large uncovered brush, which served only to clean both the gastroscope and the brush, was marketed and used. As a result the manufacturers have produced a range of smaller brushes encased in transparent Teflon sheaths which permit the removal of a brush sample intact by just withdrawing it into the end of the sheath before removal from the scope, and in this way multiple brush samples can be obtained. We in the United Kingdom do not collect nearly enough brush or biopsy samples. In America, Europe and Japan anything from five to ten brush and biopsy samples are obtained per gastroscopy, whereas in this country we are lucky to be given more than one of each.

Preparation of Brush Smears

The brush is protruded from the Teflon sheath over a small one-ounce plastic vial or 'universal container' containing about 5 to 10 ml of saline. Any drop of fluid-containing cells is thus not lost. The brush is then rolled rather than rubbed on to the slide surface. About six to eight smears can be made from each brush sample, most of which are wet-fixed in alcohol for Papanicolaou staining, whilst one or two thinner smears are rapidly air-dried for staining by the May Gruenwald Giemsa technique. Even after this the brush still contains a considerable amount of cells and these are vortexed off in the vial containing saline. This cell suspension is then aspirated on to a Millipore membrane which is stained by the Papanicolaou technique. This often salvages a remarkable amount of cells and on more than one occasion has been the best or only evidence of neoplasia in a brush sample. The brushes, which are sold as disposable, can with care be thoroughly and safely cleaned by a needle or another firm nylon brush, by brushing towards the tip of the wire under running water, then sterilized by formalin steam at 70 to 80°C for four to six hours. In this way, and with microscopic inspection of the bristle ends, these tiny fragile brushes can be re-used up to 12 to 15 times. We have made the cleansing, processing and repacking of these brushes the responsibility of the cytology department in order to ensure the removal of any residual cell material and to preserve the tiny brush heads as long as possible, which is well worth doing.

THE CYTOLOGY OF GASTRIC SMEARS

The cytology of gastric brush and wash samples can be easy or difficult. Our practice has been to make an immediate diagnosis if possible, and if neoplasia is present in the first set of slides stained a telephoned report is given within half to one hour. If, on the other hand, there is no evidence of malignancy, or there are changes of atrophic gastritis with marked metaplasia, all slides have to be stained and fully scanned before a negative report can be issued.

There is no doubt that prompt reporting of malignancy reduces delay in operating, and anxiety and concern on the part of both patient and clinicians, but it may be demanding in terms of technicians' and pathologists' time. It is the gastric mucosal hyperplasias, the atrophic gastritis atypias and the extreme epithelial activity found on the edge of otherwise benign ulcers due to regenerative changes that need most skilled attention. As over 70 per cent of cancers develop in stomachs displaying atrophic gastritis with marked intestinal metaplasia (Mason, 1965) there is need to analyse these changes meticulously. This does consume skilled cytologist time, and an efficient team has to be built up to tackle such a substantial gastroenterological service.

Reporting of cytology results

The problem of presenting results is bedevilled by the traditional restraints on reporting both histology and cytology and it is here that close liaison between pathologist and clinician is necessary. The standard practice of presenting a simple black and white report relating to cancer is outmoded, if not unacceptable, for two main reasons. The first is the possible inadequacy or incorrect sampling of the lesion which will mislead, and the second is the fact that there are well-recognized precancerous states ranging from marked atrophic gastritis with atypical metaplastic changes to true surface cancer, and it would be unintelligent not to report such cellular changes as being worthy of follow-up, if not an immediate repeat examination. We therefore utilize a modified Papanicolaou grading of samples, namely: I for normal (Figure 1); II for inflammatory change; IIR for marked atypia that necessitates continued follow-up (and these include the more atypical pictures of

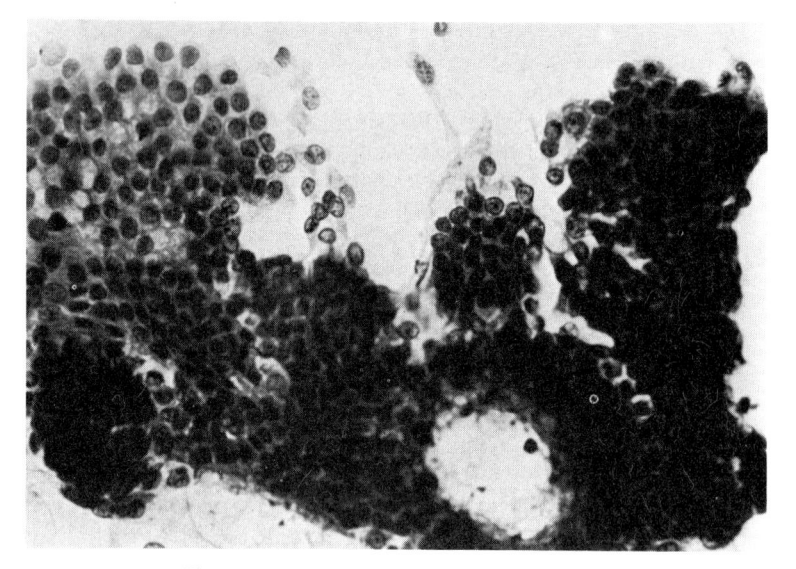

Figure 1. Normal gastric mucosal cells. × 30.

atrophic gastritis, often with considerable pleomorphism and nucleolation but not obvious neoplasia (Figure 2); Grade III is used to denote a picture suspicious of malignancy, usually inconclusive because the evidence is scanty; and finally, Grade IV, which presents a picture characteristic of malignancy (Figure 3). In this context we do not provide different grades for preinvasive and invasive stages, as in glandular cancers generally it is often difficult if not impossible to distinguish between them.

The clinicians using the service are thus given a fairly refined grading of a report as well as a proper description conveying the nature of the cell picture and the histological lesion it reflects. We believe that this method of reporting presents a significant advance in the use of a cytological service and does not lead to confusion.

The natural outcome to this should be a clearer method of analysis of reports, both of histological and cytological biopsies. This is given in Tables 3 and 4, which show our results over the past two years presented in this way.

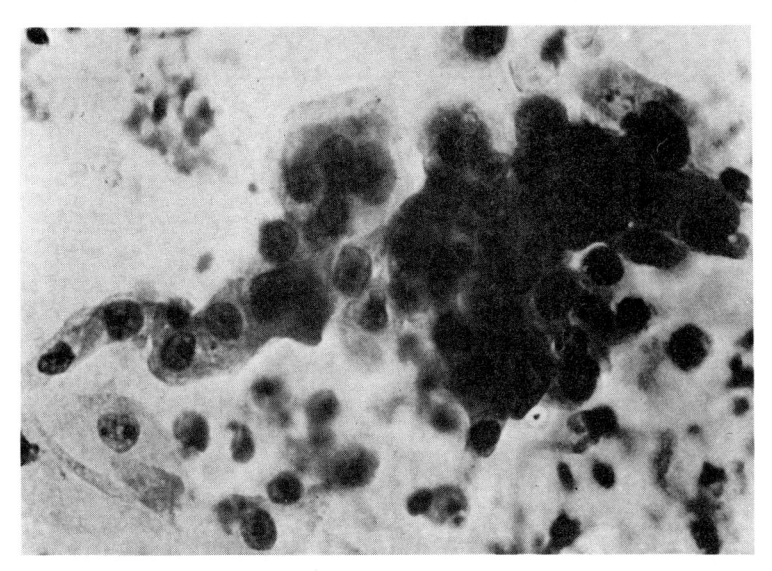

Figure 2. Atypical cell changes worthy of continued surveillance. × 120.

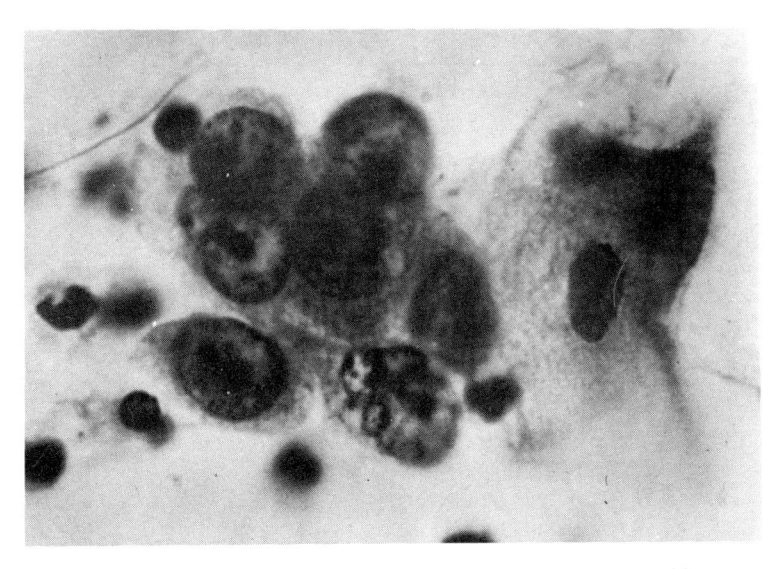

Figure 3. Malignant cells from adenocarcinoma of stomach. × 120.

These include both gastric and oesophageal brush cytology and demonstrate an accuracy for cytology of between 80 and 90 per cent, depending on whether unsatisfactory samples are included, compared with an almost equivalent figure for biopsy, but the sensitivity of both tests combined gives a figure of 98 per cent, which is presumably the result of continued practice and experience over the past 10 to 15 years.

Table 3. *Gastric and oesophageal brush cytology examination, Charing Cross and St Stephen's Hospital, 1978/79*

Normal (I)	Inflammatory (II)	Atypical (to follow) (IIR)	Suspect (III)	Positive (IV)	Total
60(10)	132(4)	8(1)	16(3)	36	252

Unsatisfactory samples in parenthesis.

Table 4. *Accuracy of biopsy and cytology diagnosis in gastric cancer, Charing Cross and St Stephen's Hospital, 1978/79*

Total cases	Pos. cytol. Pos. hist.	Pos. cytol. Neg. hist.	Neg. cytol. Pos. hist.	Pos. cytol. No biopsy	Pos. hist. Inadequate cytol	False neg. Both
61	34	9	5	7	5	1

Cytology sensitivity (overall)	50/61 = 83.3%
Cytology sensitivity (− unsatis.)	50/56 = 89.2%
Histology sensitivity	44/54 = 81.4%
No false positive cytology	
Total sensitivity	60/61 = 98%

(− unsatis.) = minus the five cytologically inadequate cases recorded above.

It so happens that we have not produced a false positive result in the past two years though we do have a category of IIR to denote the atypical and overactive cell picture which we believe may one day develop into neoplasia and warrants regular follow-up.

We will not know fully what false negative results we have in either cytology or histology until cases have been followed for some years, and some of our early series will be worth analysing soon.

A review of the cytology-negative/histology-positive cases has not disclosed any atypical or malignant cells in the smears and one can only presume that here sampling was at fault. Again, multiple biopsies and brushes would help to reduce such an error.

False positives have been reported by most skilled workers (Richards and Spriggs, 1961; Prolla et al, 1977), including ourselves, but in any event it is a moot point whether an adequate search for a focus of surface cancer on the excised organ has been made before a cytology result is established as being a false positive.

Table 5 gives our results in perspective against others and demonstrates the advantages of carrying out both biopsy and brush cytology and in many instances the greater success rate in detection by brush cytology. Again, this may well be due to the fact that not all the biopsy fragment is sectioned and if the paediatric gastroscope is used, the biopsy may be too superficial to evaluate fully.

Table 5. *Percentage accuracy of endoscopic cytology and biopsy in the diagnosis of gastric tumours*

Author	Date	Total sample	Correct cytol.	Correct histol.	Correct combined
Kobayashi, Prolla and Kirsner	1970	26	97.0	66.7	100.0
Serck-Hanssen, Marcussen and Liavåg	1973	68	94.1	52.9	94.1
Bemvenuti et al	1975	58	77.8	82.2	?
Smithies et al	1975	34	82.4	61.8	97.1
Witzel et al	1976	73	83.6	79.5	95.9
Young and Hughes	1977	61	91.8	68.9	91.8
Boddington (incl. 1969/73 series)	1978	84	78.5	72.6	92.8
Present series	1980	61	83.3	81.4	98.4

THE EARLY SURFACE CANCERS

The aim of our efforts is to achieve detection of a greater proportion of neoplasia at the early surface cancer stage which occurs on average about 10 years earlier than invasive cancer (Friesen, Docherty and Remine, 1962). Surface cancers are known to accompany so-called benign ulcers in up to 10 per cent of cases in the surrounding mucosa, usually distal to the ulcer. Several methods of identifying these lesions have been attempted, from making smears or small biopsies of geographic areas of the excised stomach to creating giant 'Swiss roll' sections of strips of stomach wall (Mason, 1966) in order to identify the thinned areas of mucosa that betray the existence of surface cancers. A simpler method developed by J. Grainger in our Cytology Departments has been to take strips of mucosa and submucosa only, leaving the bulky muscle behind, and to make small 'Swiss rolls' mounted on microscope slides, or even on projection slides; whichever way is adopted it is essential to attempt such an assessment as even at the surface cancer stage an occasional lymph node metastasis can occur (Konjetzney, 1953; Stout, 1953).

CYTOLOGICAL TUMOUR TYPING

Mention should be made here of endeavours to type the gastric carcinomas by the Laurens Classification (Laurens, 1965; Pilotti et al, 1977). The latter reviewed 78 patients with carcinoma and made a correct diagnosis of the intestinal type in 36 out of 45 cases, and 14 out of 15 cases of the advanced diffuse carcinoma. In only 13 out of the 78 cases (i.e., 16.7 per cent) the type could not be specified, giving an overall accuracy rate of 83.3 per cent.

SCREENING FOR CANCER OF THE STOMACH

Much has been written on this subject (Shida, 1971; Husain, 1976), but perhaps the most significant demonstration of the advantage of cytology in conjunction with double-contrast fluoroscopy in the improvement in survival lies in two methods of approach to gastric cancer diagnosis. These are demonstrated on the one hand by a European seven-country cooperative study utilizing the traditional methods of diagnosis and on the other hand by the more screening-orientated or early-warning-detection programmes currently being practised in Japan.

In their series from seven centres in Europe, Lundh and his co-authors (1974) showed that, when gastric cancers present clinically, where the predominant symptoms were weight loss, pain, vomiting, anorexia and weakness, and the diagnosis confirmed by barium studies in over 96 per cent, gastroscopy in 28 per cent and cytology in less than 6 per cent, the overall four-year survival rate was 9 per cent.

This should be compared with the figures published by Shida (1971) which demonstrate a mean five-year survival due to early diagnosis. Here, the tumour cases are divided into those cancers restricted to the mucosa or submucosa where survival was around 90 per cent, and those invading the muscle where it was 77 per cent, while in those reaching the serosa only 27 per cent survived five years.

There is no reason why such an approach cannot be adopted in Great Britain, even with its lower incidence rate. Evans et al (1978) demonstrated an increase in the proportion of surface cancers detected from 0.5 per cent to 10 per cent in a Cardiff practice following the introduction of systematic gastroendoscopy in the Welsh Region; the message is obvious.

As to whether screening could be afforded in the so-called low-rate countries such as the United Kingdom and the United States of America, the original quotation still holds (Husain, 1976), though affected by inflation.

As the cost of a gastroscopy alone is now well over £20.00 and the laboratory examination not less than £12.00 to £16.00, careful selection of risk cases must be undertaken. The logistics of the Japanese experience are based not only on their high-risk rates but also on their practice of field-surveying, as demonstrated by Takahashi (1971). The initial screening of every 1000 persons, in a caravan, is by personal interview and double-contrast fluoroscopy, which detect an abnormality in 200 to 300 of them. These then have endoscopy, biopsy and cytology applied in hospital, resulting in 50 to 100 final patients with a diagnosis of gastric cancer, ulcer, polyp or other pathology. The experience of the Massachusetts General Hospital of finding eight per 1000 extra early cancers, unidentified by any other diagnostic technique, when applying routine gastric washing technique to symptomatic patients attending their gastrointestinal clinic presents another form of case selection, presumably relating to the symptomatology of atrophic gastritis (Husain, 1976).

Such logistics have been commented on in a leader in the *Lancet* (1978) where it was pointed out that, even with screening, if the mean time of over seven months from first symptoms to operation persists in European practice, as is currently prevalent (Lundh et al, 1974; Cohn, 1978), then the chance of improving on the present poor survival rates is unlikely. The fact that there is no radiologist writing in this volume does not augur well for the pursuit of this problem via double-contrast radiology which does detect 40 per cent or more of these cases. However, it is estimated that there are about 4500 dyspeptics in every 300 000 population (Barnes et al, 1974), that is, those served by a District General Hospital; most are probably over 45 years of age, and a method of selection may well have to be much more searching.

SPECIAL CYTOLOGICAL DETECTION TECHNIQUES

All the above test systems for early gastric cancer detection are probably too expensive to screen for low-risk populations as they are skilled-labour-intensive and involve expensive apparatus. Attempts at screening only known high-risk categories of the population will produce a patchy sample.

It has therefore been necessary to explore other screening approaches which would more cheaply, and with less-invasive techniques, identify the high-risk cases for more purposive investigation by gastroscopy, biopsy and brush cytology. Leaving the pure biochemical, enzymic and immunological tests to Professor Munro Neville, we shall merely present a short list of those techniques that show some likelihood of being successful in this regard (Table 6).

Table 6. *Cytochemical and DNA tests for gastric cancer*

1. Naphthylamidase
2. Cathepsins
3. 6-Phosphogluconate dehydrogenase
4. Sulphomucins
5. DNA lability
6. Aminopeptidase

Most of these cytochemically-detectable enzymes are raised specifically or excessively in neoplasia, though they show some increase in the cells of the accompanying metaplasia. This was shown in histological sections by Wattenberg (1959) in relation to aminopeptidase, and more recently Jass and Filipe (1979) have studied the sialo- and sulpho-mucins which show raised activity in neoplasia and surrounding intestinal metaplasia, but as the latter accompanies gastric lesions other than carcinoma it is admitted by these authors that this approach may be too non-specific to be of value.

We, however, have investigated the lysosomal hydrolytic enzyme, naphthylamidase, a peptidase known to be secreted by invading cancer cells. We have demonstrated progressively increasing naphthylamidase activity in cells from dysplasias, through carcinoma in-situ, to invasive cancer of the cervix (Husain and Millett, 1979), and we are now attempting to apply this technique to aspirated gastric cells. The problem is going to be one of enzymically-intact cell salvage by aspiration or wash. Brush material certainly provides better-preserved cell material but this would not be of great advantage as a prescreening technique though it would certainly help to identify the potential aggressiveness of the tumour.

Another unique approach has been along the lines of work carried out by our colleague, Dr Jacqueline Millett, in studying the nature of DNA in the neoplastic cell. Again, working with cells from precancer and cancer of the cervix, she has developed a technique of slowing down the Feulgen hydrolysis by conducting it at room temperature and using 5 N HCl. By stopping the hydrolysis at stated intervals and assessing the amount of freed aldehyde-form dioxyribose sugar which has reacted with the leuco-basic fuchsin of the Schiff reagent, and by the use of a Vickers M85 integrating microdensitometer, she has shown that there are two main moieties of DNA in non-malignant cell samples, with peaks or humps at 20 and 60 minutes. In the cell nuclei of carcinoma in-situ and invasive cancer there appears to be a more labile or derepressed fraction of DNA with a hydrolysis peak at five minutes. Not only was this fraction present in the identifiable malignant cells but it appeared to be present in the normal cells in the surrounding epithelium, suggesting a field effect which might obviate the need always to seek for malignant cells in order to carry out assessment.

We are attempting to apply such a technique to gastric aspirates in the hope of automating such a DNA assessment, or of providing a more functional test of the cell potential towards neoplasia.

As yet, none of these approaches is worthy of serious consideration and the standard wash and brush cytology with biopsy will have to provide our main armamentarium against this disease.

REFERENCES

Barnes, R.J., Gear, M.W.L., Nicol, A. & Dew, A.B. (1974) Study of dyspepsia in general practice as assessed by endoscopy and radiology. *British Medical Journal*, iv, 214-216.

Bemvenuti, G.A., Hattori, K., Levin, B., Kirsner, J.B. & Reilly, R.W. (1975) Endoscopic sampling for tissue diagnosis in gastrointestinal malignancy. *Gastrointestinal Endoscopy*, 21, 159.

Blendis, L.M., Beilby, J.O.W., Wilson, J.P., Cole, M.J. & Hadley, G.D. (1967) Carcinoma of the stomach: evaluation of individual and combined diagnostic accuracy of radiology, cytology and gastro-photography. *British Medical Journal*, i, 656-659.

Boddington, M.M. (1978) Cytological aspects. In *Topics in Gastroenterology* (Ed.) Truelove, S.C. & Heyworth, M.F. pp. 165-178, Oxford: Blackwell.

Cabre-Fiol, V., Olo-Garcia, R. & Vilardell, F. (1959) Five years of cytological diagnosis of gastric cancer by 'exfoliative biopsy'. *Proceedings of World Congress of Gastroenterology (1958), Washington.* p. 1006. Baltimore, MD: Williams and Wilkins.

Cantrell, E.G. (1971) The benefits of using cytology in addition to gastric radiology. *Quarterly Journal of Medicine*, 40, 239-248.

Cohn, I. (1978) Gastrointestinal cancer. Surgical survey of abdominal tragedy. *American Journal of Surgery*, 135, 3-11.

Cowan, W.K. & Schade, R.O.K. (1974) Gastric cytology: experience in a district general hospital. *Acta Cytologica*, 18, 122-124.

Crozier, R.E., Middleton, M. & Ross, J.R. (1956) Clinical application of gastric cytology. *New England Journal of Medicine*, 255, 1128.

Evans, D.M.D., Craven, J.L., Murphy, F. & Cleary, B.K. (1978) Comparison of 'early gastric cancer' in Britain and Japan. *Gut*, 19, 1-9.

Fakuda, T., Shida, S., Takita, T. & Sawada, Y. (1967) Cytologic diagnosis of early gastric cancer by the endoscopic method with gastrofibrescope. *Acta Cytologica*, 11, 456.

Friesen, G., Docherty, M.B. & Remine, W.H. (1962) Superficial carcinoma of the stomach. *Surgery*, 51, 300.

Graham, R.M., Ulfelder, H. & Green, T.H. (1948) Cytologic method as aid in diagnosis of gastric carcinoma. *Journal of Surgery, Gynecology and Obstetrics*, 86, 257.

Halter, F., Witzel, L., Gretillat, P.A., Scheurer, U. & Keller, M. (1977) Diagnostic value of biopsy, guided lavage and brush cytology in oesophagogastroscopy. *American Journal of Digestive Diseases*, **22**, 129-131.

Hirschowitz, B.I. Curtiss, L.E., Peters, C.W. & Pollard, M.M. (1958) Demonstration of a new gastroscope. *Gastroenterology*, **35**, 50-53.

Hughes, H.E., Lee, F.D. & MacKenzie, J.F. (1978) Endoscopic cytology and biopsy in the upper gastrointestinal tract. *Clinics in Gastric Enterology*, **7** (2), 375-396.

Husain, O.A.N. (1976) Cytological screening for cancer of the stomach. *Proceedings of the Royal Society of Medicine*, **69**, 489-494.

Husain, O.A.N. & Millett, J. (1979) The detection of malignancy in the cervix. In *Quantitative Cytochemistry and its Applications* (Ed.) Patterson, J.R., Bitensky, L. & Chayen, J. pp. 231-239. London: Academic Press.

Jass, J.R. & Filipe, M.I. (1979) A variant of intestinal metaplasia associated with gastric carcinoma: a histochemical study. *Histopathology*, **3**, 191-199.

Kameya, S., Nakamura, S., Mizutani, K, Hayakawa, H., Higashiyama, S. & Kutsuna, K. (1964) Gastrofibrescope for biopsy. *Gastroenterological Endoscopy* (Japanese), **6**, 36-40.

Kasugai, T. (1964) Gastric biopsy and cytology by the fibregastroscope. *Gastroenterological Endoscopy* (Japanese), **6**, 187-190.

Kasugai, T. (1968) Gastric lavage under direct vision by the fibregastroscope employing Hanks's solution as a working solution. *Acta Cytologica*, **12**, 345-351.

Kasugai, T. (1976) Gastrofibrescopic techniques for all collections. *Compendium on Diagnostic Cytology: Tutorials in Cytology* (Ed.) Wied, G.L., Koss, L.G. & Reagan, J.W. Vol. IV, No. 1, pp. 492-496. Illinois: Chicago University Press.

Kasugai, T. & Kobayashi, S. (1974) Evaluation of biopsy and cytology in the diagnosis of gastric cancer. *American Journal of Gastroenterology*, **62**, 199-203.

Kidokoro, T., Soma, S., Seta, R., Goto, K., Yamakara, T., Tania, L. & Katayanagi, T. (1966) Gastric cytology under direct vision with special reference to the suction method. *Japanese Society for Clinical Cytology* (Japanese), **5**, 31.

Kobayashi, S., Prolla, J.C. & Kirsner, J.B. (1970) Brushing cytology of the oesophagus and stomach under direct vision by fibrescopes. *Acta Cytologica*, **14**, 219-223.

Konjetzney, G.E. (1953) The superficial cancer of the gastric mucosa. *American Journal of Digestive Diseases*, **20**, 91.

Lancet Leader (1978), **i**, 1023-1024.

Laurens, P. (1965) The two histological main types of gastric carcinomas: diffuse and so-called intestinal type carcinoma. An attempt at histo-clinical classification. *Acta Pathologica et Microbiologica Scandinavica*, **64**, 31-49.

Liavig, I., Marcussen, J. & Serck-Hanssen, A. (1971) Direct vision brush cytology in the diagnosis of gastric disease. *Acta Chirurgica Scandinavica*, **137**, 682-688.

Lundh, G., Burn, J.I., Kolig, G., Richard, C.A., Thomson, J.W.W., van Elk, P.J. & Oszacki, J. (1974) A co-operative international study of gastric cancer. *Annals of Royal College of Surgeons of England*, **54**, 3-12.

MacDonald, W.C., Brandenborg, L.L., Taniguchi, I., Beh, J.E. & Rubn, C.E. (1963) Exfoliated cytological screening for gastric cancer. *Cancer*, **27**, 163-169.

MacKenzie, J.F., Rogers, I.M., Moule, B., Young, J.A., Hughes, H.E., Lee, F.D., Russell, R.I. & Blumgart, L.H. (1977) Comparison of double contrast radiology, standard radiology, endoscopy, also histology and cytology in the diagnosis of gastric cancer. *Gut*, **18**, A416.

Mason, M.K. (1965) Surface carcinoma of the stomach. *Gut*, **6**, 185-193.

Mason, M.K. (1966) Surface carcinomas of the stomach. Pathological features and clinical significance. *Overdruck mit Tydschrift voor Gastro-Enterologic Deel*, **9**, No. 6.

Millett, J.A. & Husain, O.A.N. (1979) Analysis of chromatin in carcinoma in-situ. In *Quantitative Cytochemistry and its Applications*. (Ed.) Patterson, J.R., Bitensky, L. & Chayen, J. pp. 37-42. London: Academic Press.

Morson, B.C. (1955) Intestinal metaplasia of the gastric mucosa. *British Journal of Cancer*, **9**, 365-376.

Papanicolaou, G.N. & Cooper, W.A. (1947) The cytology of the gastric fluid in the diagnosis of cancer of the stomach. *Journal of the National Cancer Institute*, **7**, 357.

Pilotti, S., Rilke, F., Clemente, C., Alasia, L. & Grigioni, M. (1977) The cytologic diagnosis of gastric carcinoma related to the histologic type. *Acta Cytologica*, **21**, 48-59.

Prolla, J.C., Kobayashi, S. & Kirsner, J.B. (1969) Gastric cancer: some recent improvements in diagnosis based upon the Japanese experience. *Archives of Internal Medicine*, **24**, 238-246.

Prolla, J.C., Reilly, R.W., Kirsner, J.B. & Cockerham, L. (1977) Direct vision endoscopic cytology and biopsy in the diagnosis of oesophageal and gastric tumours. Current experience. *Acta Cytologica*, **21**, 399-402.

Raskin, H.F., Kirsner, J.B. & Palmer, W.L. (1959) Role of exfoliative cytology in the diagnosis of cancer of the digestive tract. *Journal of the American Medical Association*, **169**, 789.

Richards, W.C.D. & Spriggs, A.I. (1961) Cytology of gastric mucosa. *Journal of Clinical Pathology*, **14**, 132-139.

Roca, M., Whitehead, R. & Boddington, M.M. (1974) Upper gastrointestinal endoscopy. 3. Tissue diagnosis. In *Topics in Gastroenterology* (Ed.) Truelove, S.C. & Trowell, J. Vol. 2, pp. 29-51. Oxford: Blackwell.

Schade, R.O.K. (1960) *Gastric Cytology*. London: Edward Arnold.

Segal, A.W., Healy, M.J.R., Cox, A.G., Williams, I., Slavin, G., Smithies, A. & Levi, A.J. (1975) Diagnosis of gastric cancer. *British Medical Journal*, **ii**, 669-672.

Serck-Hanssen, A., Marcussen, J. & Liavig, I. (1973) In cancer detection and prevention. *Proceedings of the Second International Symposium on Cancer Detection and Prevention, Bologna* (Ed.) Maltoni, C. Amsterdam: Excerpta Medica.

Seybolt, F.F. & Papanicolaou, G.N. (1957) The value of cytology in the diagnosis of gastric cancer. *Gastroenterology*, **33**, 369.

Shida, S. (1971) Biopsy smear cytology with the fibregastroscope for direct observation. *Early Gastric Cancer* (Gann Monograph on Cancer Research 11). pp. 207-222, 223-232. Tokyo: University of Tokyo Press.

Shida, S. (1976) Gastric cytology. Its evaluation for the diagnosis of early gastric cancer. *Compendium on Diagnostic Cytology, Tutorial in Cytology* (Ed.) Wied, G.L., Koss, L.G. & Reagan, J.W. 4th edn, pp. 457-467. Illinois: Chicago University Press.

Smithies, A., Lovell, D., Hishon, S., Pounder, R.E., Newton, C., Kellock, J.D., Misiewicz, J.J. & Blendis, L.M. (1975) Value of brush cytology in diagnosis of gastric cancer. *British Medical Journal*, **iv**, 326.

Stout, A.P. (1953) *Atlas of Tumour Pathology in Tumours of the Stomach*. Section VI, Fascicle 21. Washington, DC: Armed Forces Institute of Pathology.

Taebel, D.W., Prolla, J.C. & Kirsner, J.B. (1965) Exfoliative cytology in the diagnosis of stomach cancer. *Annals of Internal Medicine*, **63**, 1018-1026.

Takahashi, K. (1971) Outline of gastric mass survey by x-ray. *Early Gastric Cancer* (Gann Monograph on Cancer Research 11). pp. 207-222. Tokyo: University of Tokyo Press.

Tamura, K., Masuzawa, M., Akiyama, T. & Rukui, O. (1977) Touch smear cytology for endoscopic diagnosis of gastric carcinoma. *American Journal of Gastroenterology*, **67**, 463-467.

Tazaki, Y. (1959) Clinical aspects of gastric carcinoma in Japan. *Proceedings of World Congress of Gastroenterology (1958), Washington*. p. 1148. Baltimore, MD: Williams and Wilkins.

Thompson, H., Hoare, A.M., Dykes, P.W., Allan, R.N. & Keighley, M.R.R. (1977) A prospective randomised trial to compare brush cytology before and after punch biopsy for endoscopic diagnosis of gastric cancer. *Gut*, **18**, A398.

Traut, H.F., Rosenthal, M., Harrison, J.T., Farber, S.M. & Grimes, O.F. (1952) Evaluation of cytological diagnosis of gastric cancer. *Journal of Surgery, Gynecology and Obstetrics*, **95**, 709.

Wattenberg, W. (1959) Histochemical study of amino-peptidase in metaplasia and carcinoma of the stomach. *American Medical Association Archives of Pathology*, **67**, 281-286.

Winawer, S.J., Posner, G., Lightdale, C.J., Sherlock, P., Melamed, M. & Fortner, J.G. (1976) Endoscopic diagnosis of advanced gastric cancer. Factors influencing yield. *Gastroenterology*, **69**, 1183-1187.

Witte, S. (1959) Die Zytodiagnostik des magen Karzinomas. *Krebsarzt*, **14**, 408-411.

Witzel, L., Halter, F., Gretillat, P.A., Scheurer, U. & Keller, M. (1976) Evaluation of specific value of endoscopic biopsies and brush cytology for malignancies of the oesophagus and stomach. *Gut*, **17**, 375-377.

Yoshii, Y., Takanashi, J., Yamaoka, Y. & Kasugai, T. (1970) Significance of imprint smears in cytologic diagnosis of malignant tumours of stomach. *Acta Cytologica*, **14**, 249-253.

Young, J.A. & Hughes, H.E. (1977) Report on a three-year trial of endoscopic cytology of stomach and duodenum. *Seventh European Congress of Cytology, Liege*.

15
Tumour Markers and the Gastrointestinal Tract

A. MUNRO NEVILLE
DONALD J.R. LAURENCE

The last decade has witnessed an increasing appreciation that many, and possibly all, human tumours synthesize, and may release a wide variety of characteristic substances. Although they are collectively referred to as 'tumour markers' none can be regarded as tumour specific. Some markers are appropriate (eutopic) to the tissue from which the tumour develops. Examples are calcitonin and medullary thyroid carcinoma, human chorionic gonadotrophin (HCG), and choriocarcinoma, α-fetoprotein (AFP) and yolk sac carcinoma, carcinoembryonic antigen (CEA) and colorectal carcinoma, steroid hormones and adrenocortical tumours (Neville and Cooper, 1976). Other markers are regarded as 'ectopic' or inappropriate in time, place and amount, the classical examples being ACTH, ADH and calcitonin production by bronchial carcinomas.

Table 1 lists representative examples of some tumour markers. They can be divided into a series of categories based in part on their functional properties and the methods used in their detection. While many markers are released by the tumour cells and may be measured in the blood or other body fluids, others appear to be integral components of the cell structure. Both categories of marker can be demonstrated at a tumour cell level through the use of immunocytochemical methods.

Many uses have been proposed for tumour markers. In addition to furthering our understanding of the biology of cancer, it has been suggested that they may have a role to play in assisting with the diagnosis and monitoring of neoplasia. For the histopathologist, markers can be used to improve tumour classification and appreciation of tumour histogenesis.

The present resumé of tumour markers and gastrointestinal tract neoplasms will attempt to demonstrate the clinical and pathological significance of markers at the cellular level and by their measurement in body fluids. Some recent studies of new markers, and the uses which they may have, will be highlighted while placing in perspective those tumour products with proved significance in the laboratory and in relation to patient care.

© 1980 W.B. Saunders Company Ltd.

Table 1. *Some examples of tumour-derived and tumour associated products ('tumour markers') and some of the characteristic tumours by which they are produced*

Product	Typical tumours
Hormones and their subunits	
ACTH and related MSH, LPH	Pituitary, bronchus
ADH	Bronchus
Hypothalamic releasing factors	Bronchus
Calcitonin	Thyroid, bronchus, breast
HCG and subunits	Choriocarcinoma, bronchus, teratoma
'PTH-like'	Parathyroid, bronchus
Prostaglandins	Breast, colon
Enzymes	
Prolylhydroxylase	Hepatoma, breast
Sialyltransferase	Many
Phosphatases	Prostate, hepatoma
γ-glutamyltranspeptidase	Many
Galactosyltransferase	Many
Oncofetoplacental products and other 'antigens'	
CEA and related materials	Gastrointestinal
AFP	Hepatoma, teratoma
FSA	Gastric
BOFA	Many
Pregnancy-associated proteins	Choriocarcinoma, breast, teratoma
Placental-type enzymes	Many
Other macromolecules	
Milk proteins	Breast
β-2-microglobulin	Many
Polyamines	Many
Nucleosides	Many
Monoclonal immunoglobulins	Myeloma
Ferritin	Many

CATEGORIES OF MARKERS

Hormones

The ectopic production of hormones by tumours with APUD features, such as those of the bronchus, and pancreatic islets is not uncommon. In addition, a series of previously unrecognized gastrointestinal hormones has been found and the tumours which manufacture these identified (see Polak, Chapter 2). The present consensus is that the common gastrointestinal tumours such as those of the exocrine pancreas, colon and rectum are seldom associated with the full spectrum of ectopic hormonal release. Not all workers, however, would agree (Odell et al, 1977).

Estimates of the frequency of raised blood levels of human chorionic gonadotrophin (HCG) and/or βHCG in patients with gastrointestinal tumours vary greatly from one series to another (Braunstein et al, 1973; Franchimont et al, 1976; Hattori et al, 1978). However, elevated blood HCG or βHCG levels are infrequent, occurring in association with about 10 per cent of tumours and such elevations are seldom much above normal. It is questionable whether their measurement, in general, is of value in clinical management (Franchimont et al, 1976). In contrast, biochemical extraction and immunocytochemical procedures have shown that almost half of all colorectal carcinomas contain HCG (Hattori et al, 1978; Buckley and Fox, 1979). Immunoperoxidase methods have localized HCG to the tumour cells themselves, often in single cells isolated among other tumour cells in which HCG is not demonstrable. Colorectal carcinomas containing HCG have been noted to be situated more frequently in the left than in the right colon and appear to be more locally invasive (Buckley and Fox, 1979). The presence of HCG cells did not, however, appear to correlate with a higher incidence of distant metastases. Very infrequently, such tumours may also be associated with the production of other placental proteins and hormones (Muggia et al, 1975). Primary choriocarcinomas of the gastrointestinal tract, and in particular of the stomach, may occur occasionally when the assay of HCG and other placental products would be of biological and clinical relevance in these cases (Kameya et al, 1975).

There are interesting papers reporting the presence of steroid hormone receptors for oestrogens, androgens and progesterone in some colorectal carcinomas (McClendon et al, 1977; Alford et al, 1979). Kiang and Kennedy (1977), on the contrary, failed to detect oestrogen receptor activity in colorectal carcinomas. This functional aspect of colorectal neoplasia requires further study but it is possible that receptor proteins for steroid hormones may occur more widely than was previously thought. To date, no hormonal therapy has been suggested or tried in patients harbouring such tumours. It is interesting to note that common aetiologies have been proposed for breast and colorectal carcinomas (Berg, 1975).

Enzymes

Several studies have examined the role of plasma enzyme assays in the diagnosis of primary and metastatic colorectal carcinomas (Steele et al, 1974; Munjal et al, 1976; Beck et al, 1979). The enzymes assayed have been both tumour-derived and tumour associated (Neville and Cooper, 1976). They appear to offer little or no advantage in clinical management over the assay of other products such as the carcinoembryonic antigen (CEA) (Gold and Freedman, 1965).

The demonstration of enzyme changes at a cellular level may have interesting biological and pathological relevance. Gamma-glutamyltranspeptidase levels have been shown to be raised in the rodent colon following 1,2-dimethylhydrazine administration and before overt neoplasms develop. In man, γ-glutamyltranspeptidase levels are higher in colorectal carcinomas than normal colon (Fiala et al, 1979). These changes may be regarded as field effects analogous to the glycoprotein alterations in the uninvolved colon from patients with colorectal carcinomas (Filipe, Mughal and Bussey,

1980). If the rat model is applicable to man, it may be of value to attempt to demonstrate prospectively γ-glutamyltranspeptidase levels in colorectal biopsies or cells shed from the intestinal tract as elevated amounts might be of assistance in the diagnostic assessment of dysplastic, premalignant and malignant lesions.

Antigens

Colorectal carcinoma

In contrast to the apparent paucity of hormone and/or enzyme production by gastrointestinal tumours, many groups of workers have identified 'antigenic' changes in human colorectal carcinomas (Table 2). This has been the subject of a recent comprehensive review (Kahan et al, 1979). While the continuing use of the term 'antigens' may be strictly incorrect, it serves to embrace a group of macromolecules detected by immunological techniques and without known biological function at present. Some, however, such as the neo-antigens described by Thomsom, Tataryn and Schwartz (1980) may also be antigenic in the tumour-bearing patient.

'Normal tissue common antigens' are expressed by a wide variety of normal tissues and often by their tumours. Two, namely the zinc glycinate marker (ZGM) and the epithelial membrane antigen (EMA) have been described recently. ZGM is a glycoprotein (molecular weight $\sim 2 \times 10^6$) with more than 50 per cent carbohydrate which is detectable in many organs. ZGM occurs in the cytoplasm and on the luminal membrane of the cells of the lower part of the colonic glands; this distribution being quite different from that of CEA (Doos et al, 1978; O'Brien et al, 1980). Most colorectal carcinomas express ZGM (Pusztaszeri, Saravis and Zamcheck, 1976; Doos et al, 1978) and preliminary results indicate that raised levels may occur in the blood of patients with benign and malignant colonic tumours.

EMA is also a glycoprotein, unrelated to ZGM or the carcinoembryonic antigen (CEA), with a molecular weight of $\sim 1 \times 10^6$ (Heyderman, Steele and Ormerod, 1979). It is present in small amounts in many parts of the gastrointestinal tract and is present in large amounts in the cytoplasm and on the luminal borders of the cells of most adenocarcinomas, including those of the colon and breast (Sloane and Ormerod, 1980). Antisera to EMA have a valuable immunocytochemical role to play in diagnostic histopathology as a marker of epithelial differentiation.

A series of organ-specific antigens has been described (see Table 2), two of which have been the subject of detailed immunochemical study. Thomson and his colleagues (1980), using the leucocyte adherence inhibition (LAI) test, have identified in a preliminary report the existence and nature of organ-specific colonic neo-antigens (TA) which may be immunogenic in the tumour bearing host. These antigens are not considered to be malignancy specific as they can be detected in epithelial dysplasias and benign neoplastic conditions of the colon (Thomson, Tataryn and Schwartz, 1980). None the less, their presence as determined by the LAI test may be valuable in assisting with the diagnosis of gastrointestinal carcinomas (Tataryn et al, 1979).

Table 2. *Human colon tumour antigens*[a]

Type	Nomenclature
Normal tissue common antigens	NCA (NGP, CEX) ZGM[b] EMA[c] BOFA
Antigens restricted to normal tissue	CMA-B Cytoplasmic Ag Blood group antigens
Organ-specific antigens	MTA Mucus Ag MRA CMA-BP CMA-CM CSA Colonic neo-antigens (TA)[d]
Oncofetal antigens	T antigen CEA
Tumour-specific antigens	Tennagen

From data assembled by [a]Kahan et al, 1979, and [b]Doos et al, 1978; [c]Heyderman, Steele and Ormerod, 1979 and [d]Thomson, Tataryn and Schwartz, 1980.

Goldenberg, Pegram and Vasquez (1975) prepared a glycoprotein colon-specific antigen (CSAp) from colon tumours. It has a molecular weight ~ 70 to 100KD and can be detected in small amounts in the fetal and normal gut. It is known to be a colonic tumour product but is also synthesized by ovarian mucinous cystadenocarcinomas. Antisera to this substance may be of value in identifying, at a histological level, gastrointestinal and ovarian tumours presenting as metastases of unknown origin.

To date, only one antigen expressed by colorectal tumours is thought to be tumour specific (see Table 2). This macromolecule and its role in clinicopathological studies are now under active consideration by several groups.

The carcinoembryonic antigen (CEA), first described by Gold and Freedman (1965), is one of the better-known examples of an oncofetal antigen. However, with the use of more sensitive techniques CEA has been shown to be also present in the normal adult colon. This glycoprotein has been the subject of many chemical, immunological and clinicopathological studies. The role of CEA as a tumour marker to assist with the clinical management of patients with gastrointestinal tumours continues to be the subject of numerous reports. Several studies have reaffirmed the earlier conclusions that its assay in blood has no value in screening or for the detection of localized primary colorectal neoplasms (Laurence et al, 1972; Gold, 1978; Meeker, 1978) even in at-risk populations (Anderson et al, 1978).

The follow-up of patients with colorectal cancer after surgery and the sequential assay of blood CEA levels are its major applications. Our own series, although published some time ago, serves to illustrate this point (Neville and Cooper, 1976; Table 3). While some patients will develop recurrent and/or metastatic disease in the presence of a normal CEA titre, most will show rising plasma CEA levels, many of which will predate the overt clinical detection of metastases (Table 3; Wood et al, 1978). This lead time is usually of the order of nine to 12 months, although periods in excess of 24 months have been found in some patients.

Table 3. *The role of plasma CEA in the monitoring of 771 patients with colorectal carcinomas after clinically curative operations*[a]

Clinical condition	Plasma CEA	Number of patients
NER[b]	Normal	525
	Rising[c]	54
Recurrence	Normal	66
	Synchronous rise[c]	89
	Antecedent rise[c]	37

[a]From data of Neville and Cooper (1976).
[b]NER = no evidence of recurrence.
[c]Rising to >40 ng/ml with a sustained upward trend in the plasma levels.

Failure to develop rising CEA levels with recurrent disease is more likely to occur if the preoperative CEA level was normal (Reynoso, 1978) or if immunocytochemical studies of the primary tumour histology show an absence of CEA (Goldenberg et al, 1978). Even if the preoperative level of CEA is raised, a subsequent recurrence many not be accompanied by a rise in plasma CEA (Table 3; Moertel, Schutt and Go, 1978; Neville et al, 1978; Lawton, Giles and Cooper, 1980).

It has been claimed that by estimating the postoperative levels of CEA more frequently, and submitting them to analysis by nomograms or computer, a more accurate assessment of the CEA time curves and the readier and earlier detection of metastases can be achieved (Martin et al, 1977). This has formed the basis for 'second-look' surgical intervention. The presence of recurrent or metastatic tumour has been confirmed in most but not all cases at second-look surgery (Martin et al, 1979). In a certain number (72 per cent in one series) of patients with rising CEA titres, single localized and surgically resectable recurrences were detected (Cooper et al, 1979; Martin et al, 1979).

Such operative intervention has been claimed to result in a longer period of subsequent survival, but not all groups agree that this procedure results in the detection of resectable disease (Moertel, Schutt and Go, 1978; Cohen and Wood, 1979). More time will be required to establish the clinical value of operative intervention in the presence of rising CEA titres. Certainly, our own experience and that of others, while not denying that it is possible to detect metastases earlier through the sequential assay of CEA, would tend to support the view that when rising levels of CEA are detected, such patients generally have a significant and widespread tumour load.

Study of the rate of plasma CEA levels in patients with known residual or metastatic disease may correlate with prognosis, those with the more rapid rises fairing worst (Lawton, Giles and Cooper, 1980). When patients are receiving therapy, but rising CEA levels still are noted, it would tend to point to the futility of continuing therapy (Lawton, Giles and Cooper, 1980).

Pancreas

Two antigens, CEA and, more recently, pancreatic oncofetal antigen (POA), have been proposed as being of value in the diagnosis and management of carcinomas of the exocrine pancreas.

A carefully controlled study of the role of CEA in the diagnosis of pancreatic carcinoma has been conducted by the Medical Research Council (1980). It was found that elevated CEA levels occur not infrequently with pancreatic carcinoma and are stage dependent, but that such information is of little if any help in making the initial diagnosis of neoplasia.

Until two years ago, there was some dispute as to whether the pancreas and its tumour express an oncofetal antigen other than CEA. This has been resolved by the isolation of a macromolecule of molecular weight 40 kilo Dalton (KD) from pancreatic carcinomas (Hobbs, Knapp and Branfoot, 1980). Immunocytochemical studies locate the antigen in the cytoplasm of the cells of pancreatic carcinomas and the fetal pancreas, but not, apparently, in the adult normal pancreas. A similar and probably identical antigen has been isolated by Mihas (1978) and Arndt et al (1978).

POA has been measured in the plasma by radioimmunoassay; elevated levels occurred in 97 per cent of patients with pancreatic carcinoma, but also in some patients with chronic pancreatitis (Hobbs, Knapp and Branfoot, 1980). A further glycoprotein of molecular weight 800 000 to 900 000, also called POA, has been purified from pancreatic carcinomas by Gelder et al (1978). It may share antigenic determinants with the material isolated by Hobbs, Knapp and Branfoot (1980). Enzyme immunoassay of this high molecular weight POA has shown raised plasma levels in pancreatic carcinoma and in pancreatitis (Nishida et al, 1980). Thus, the role of either of these POAs in assisting with initial diagnosis requires further study. Preliminary work suggests that they may serve a useful role in longitudinal monitoring.

THE DETECTION OF METASTASES

Metastases remain the dominant cause of death in tumour-bearing patients. It is not unreasonable, therefore, to attempt to describe methods which will facilitate their earlier detection when, hopefully, the initiation of therapy may improve the present dismal results.

While the assay of plasma tumour marker levels may have a part to play in this context in gastrointestinal tumours, current evidence tends to suggest that they enable the detection in most patients of metastases only late in the evolution of the disease. Other approaches thus seem worthy of consideration.

More than two decades have passed since Pressman (1957) showed the selective uptake of tumour-specific antibodies by animal tumours and suggested that such an approach might be valuable in human cancer detection and/or therapy. Since then, several groups of workers have reported the apparently specific uptake of radiolabelled antibodies by experimental tumours and by human tumours growing in immune-deprived animals (Izzo, Buchsbaum and Baie, 1972; Primus et al, 1973; Mach et al, 1974). Success using this approach at a clinical level has been difficult to achieve but was recently recorded by some (Belitsky et al, 1978; Goldenberg et al, 1978; Dykes et al, 1980) but not all workers (Reif et al, 1974).

In the absence of a known human tumour-specific property or antigen, attention has once more turned to the cell surface glycoprotein expressed by many human tumour cells, namely CEA. Using xenogeneic anti-CEA labelled with radioactive iodine, Goldenberg and his associates have demonstrated by scanning techniques that this approach can result in the successful localization of both primary and metastatic tumours of colon, rectum, uterus, ovary and breast (Goldenberg et al, 1978). Moreover, radioimmunodetection was successful when other physical diagnostic techniques did not locate the various lesions. These results have recently been corroborated by Dykes and his colleagues (1980) who, using labelled anti-CEA, successfully detected four of five primary gastrointestinal tumours and eight of 11 metastatic deposits.

The success achieved by these workers may reside partly in the quality of reagent employed but probably more in the efficient computer programme which helped them to distinguish specific ^{131}I-radioactive binding from the background non-specific activity that was assessed by the distribution of ^{99}Tc^{m}-labelled human serum albumin and ^{99}Tc^{m}-pertechnetate. Uptake by the tumours was small but occurred even when there was a raised plasma CEA level. Whether this uptake is specific remains to be proved definitely. In addition, the site of anti-CEA binding remains unknown so that a considerable number of fundamental studies is still required. None the less, these initial results are promising, and with improvements in emission tomographic techniques and using ^{123}I instead of ^{131}I further success at a clinical level may be anticipated.

If organ- or even tumour-specific antibodies can be found, this could also improve the results obtained. In this context the mouse myeloma hybridoma system for the preparation of monoclonal antibodies (Kohler and Milstein, 1975) will have much to offer and has already yielded an immunological reagent with apparent human colorectal carcinoma specificity (Herlyn et al, 1979).

From the current results and those presented at a recent workshop (Goldenberg, 1980), the limit of radioimmunodetection would appear to be a tumour of approximately 2 cm diameter. This would suggest that methods of detecting metastases, not dependent on physical diagnostic techniques, are worthy of examination. With the demonstration, as described above, of the relative insensitivity of assays for marker substances in blood, how is this to be achieved?

The introduction of immunocytochemical and, more particularly, immunoperoxidase methods capable of detecting tumour products and antigens at a cellular level in formalin-fixed paraffin-embedded sections may offer an alternative approach to the detection of metastatic foci. Mention has been made of the epithelial membrane antigen (EMA) (Heyderman, Steele and Ormerod, 1979) and its value as a marker of both normal and malignant epithelial cells (Sloane and Ormerod, 1980). By immunoperoxidase methods, these workers have shown that they can detect in needle biopsy and aspiration specimens small foci of microscopic metastases, even those occurring as single cells in the liver and bone marrow from patients with breast carcinomas. Many other antigens of relevance to gastrointestinal tumours, such as CEA, NCA, ZGM and POA, can be detected immunocytochemically and this method can be extended to antigens detected by monoclonal antibodies (McIlhinney and Ormerod, 1980, personal communication). With a knowledge of the commonest sites to which tumours may metastasize, such technology would therefore afford an alternative approach to the detection of metastases which could complement radio-immunolocalization and the assay of markers in the body fluids.

SUMMARY

A brief review is presented of the range of products, in particular so-called 'antigens', expressed by colorectal and pancreatic carcinomas. They appear to have limited value in assisting with the detection and diagnosis of primary and metastatic lesions at these sites. Attention is drawn to the use of antibodies to such markers both in vivo and at a cellular level as a further approach to aid in tumour detection.

REFERENCES

Alford, T.C., Do, H.M., Geelhoed, G.W., Tsangaris, N.T. & Lippman, M.E. (1979) Steroid hormone receptors in human colon cancers. *Cancer*, **43**, 980-984.

Anderson, H.A., Snyder, J., Lewinson, T., Woo, C., Lilis, R. & Selikoff, I.J. (1978) Levels of CEA among vinyl chloride and polyvinyl chloride exposed workers. *Cancer*, **42**, 1560-1567.

Arndt, R., Nishida, K., Becker, W.-M. & Thiele, H.-G. (1978) Partial molecular characterisation of onco-fetal pancreas antigen and preliminary experiences concerning its diagnostic value. In *Proceedings of the Sixth Meeting of the International Society for Oncodevelopmental Biology and Medicine*, Abstract 229. Amsterdam: Elsevier.

Beck, P.R., Belfield, A., Spooner, R.J., Blumgart, L.H. & Wood, C.B. (1979) Serum enzymes in colorectal cancer. *Cancer*, **43**, 1772-1776.

Belitsky, P., Ghose, T., Aquino, J., Norvell, S.T. & Blair, H.A. (1978) Radionuclide imaging of primary renal-cell carcinoma by I-131-labeled antitumor antibody. *Journal of Nuclear Medicine*, **19**, 427-430.

Berg, J.W. (1975) Can nutrition explain the pattern of international epidemiology of hormone-dependent cancers? *Cancer Research*, **35**, 3345-3350.

Buckley, C.H. & Fox, H. (1979) An immunohistochemical study of the significance of HCG secretion by large bowel adenocarcinomata. *Journal of Clinical Pathology*, **32**, 368-372.

Cohen, A.M. & Wood, W.C. (1979) Carcinoembryonic antigen levels as an indicator for reoperation in patients with carcinoma of the colon and rectum. *Surgery, Gynecology and Obstetrics*, **149**, 22-26.

Cooper, M.J., Mackie, C.R., Skinner, D.B. & Moossa, A.R. (1979) A reappraisal of the value of carcinoembryonic antigen in the management of patients with various neoplasms. *British Journal of Surgery*, **66**, 120-123.

Doos, W.G., Saravis, C.A., Pusztaszeri, G., Burke, B., Oh, S.K., Zamcheck, N. & Gottlieb, L.S. (1978) Tissue localization of zinc glycinate marker and carcinoembryonic antigen by immunofluorescence. II. Immunofluorescence microscopy. *Journal of the National Cancer Institute*, **60**, 1375-1382.

Dykes, P.W., Hine, K.R., Bradwell, A.R., Blackburn, J.C., Reeder, T.A., Drolc, Z. & Booth, S.N. (1980) Localisation of tumour deposits by external scanning after injection of radiolabelled anti-carcinoembryonic antigen. *British Medical Journal*, **i**, 220-222.

Fiala, S., Trout, E., Pragani, B. & Fiala, E.S. (1979) Increased γ-glutamyl transferase activity in human colon cancer. *Lancet*, **i**, 1145.

Filipe, M.I., Mughal, S. & Bussey, H.J. (1980) Patterns of mucus secretion in the colonic epithelium in familiar polyposis. *Investigative and Cell Pathology*, in press.

Franchimont, P., Zangerle, P.S., Nogarede, J., Bury, J., Molter, F., Reuter, A., Hendrick, J.C. & Collette, J. (1976) Simultaneous assays of cancer-associated antigens in various neoplastic disorders. *Cancer*, **38**, 2287-2295.

Gelder, F.B., Reese, C.J., Moossa, A.R., Hall, T. & Hunter, R. (1978) Purification, partial characterisation and clinical evaluation of a pancreatic oncofoetal antigen. *Cancer Research*, **38**, 313-324.

Gold, P. (1978) Immunology and immunotherapy of colorectal cancer. *Canadian Journal of Surgery*, **21**, 212-213.

Gold, P. & Freedman, S.O. (1965) Specific carcinoembryonic antigens of the human digestive system. *Journal of Experimental Medicine*, **122**, 467-481.

Goldenberg, D. (1980) Radioimmunodetection. *Cancer Research*, in press.

Goldenberg, D.M., Pegram, C.A. & Vasquez, J.J. (1975) *Journal of Immunology*, **114**, 1008-1013.

Goldenberg, D.M., Sharkey, R.M. & Primus, F.J. (1978) Immunocytochemical detection of carcinoembryonic antigen in conventional histophathology specimens, *Cancer*, **42**, 1546-1553.

Goldenberg, D.M., DeLand, F., Kim, E., Bennett, S., Primus, F.J., Van Nagell, Jr, J.R., Estes, N., De Simone, P. & Rayburn, P. (1978) Use of radiolabeled antibodies to carcinoembryonic antigen for the detection and localization of diverse cancers by external photoscanning. *New England Journal of Medicine*, **298**, 1384-1388.

Hattori, M., Fukase, M., Yoshimi, H., Matsukura, S. & Imura, H. (1978) Ectopic production of human chorionic gonadotropin in malignant tumours. *Cancer*, **42**, 2328-2333.

Herlyn, M., Steplewski, Z., Herlyn, D. & Koprowski, H. (1979) Colorectal carcinoma-specific antigen: detection by means of monoclonal antibodies. *Proceedings of the National Academy of Sciences of the United States of America*, **76**, 1438-1442.

Heyderman, E., Steele, K. & Ormerod, M.G. (1979) A new antigen on the epithelial membrane: its immunoperoxidase localisation in normal and neoplastic tissue. *Journal of Clinical Pathology*, **32**, 35-39.

Hobbs, J.R., Knapp, M.L. & Branfoot, A.C. (1980) Pancreatic oncofoetal antigen (POA): its frequency and localisation in humans. *Journal of the International Society for Oncodevelopmental Biology and Medicine*, in press.

Izzo, M.J., Buchsbaum, D.J. & Baie, W.F. (1972) Localization of an ^{125}I-labeled rat transplantation antibody in tumours carrying the corresponding antigen. *Proceedings of the Society for Experimental Biology and Medicine*, **139**, 1185-1188.

Kahan, B.D., Rutzky, L.P., Legrue, S.J. & Tom, B.H. (1979) Molecular approaches to human colon cancer. In *Methods in Cancer Research* (Ed.) Fishman, W.H. & Busch, H. Vol. VIII, pp. 197-275. London: Academic Press.

Kameya, T., Kuramoto, H., Suzuki, K., Kenjo, T., Oshikiri, T., Hayashi, H. & Itakura, M. (1975) A human gastric choriocarcinoma cell line with human chorionic gonadotropin and placental alkaline phosphatase production. *Cancer Research*, **35**, 2025-2032.

Kiang, D.T. & Kennedy, B.J. (1977) Estrogen receptor assay in the differential diagnosis of adenocarcinomas. *Journal of the American Medical Association*, **238**, 32-34.

Kohler, G. & Milstein, C. (1975) Continuous cultures of fused cells secreting antibody of predefined specificity. *Nature*, **256**, 495-497.

Laurence, D.J.R., Stevens, U., Bettelheim, R., Darcy, D., Leese, C., Turberville, C., Alexander, P., Johns, E.W. & Neville, A.M. (1972) Role of plasma carcinoembryonic antigen in diagnosis of gastrointestinal, mammary and bronchial carcinoma. *British Medical Journal*, **iii**, 605-609.

Lawton, J.O., Giles, G.R. & Cooper, E.H. (1980) Evaluation of CEA in patients with known residual disease after resection of colonic cancer. *Journal of the Royal Society of Medicine*, **73**, 23-28.

Mach, J.-P., Carrel, S., Merenda, C., Sordat, B. & Cerottini, J.C. (1974) In vivo localisation of radiolabelled antibodies to carcinoembryonic antigen in human colon carcinoma grafted into nude mice. *Nature*, **248**, 704-706.

Martin, Jr, E.W., James, K.K., Hurtubise, P.E., Catalano, P. & Minton, J.P. (1977) The use of CEA as an early indicator for gastrointestinal tumour recurrence and second-look procedures. *Cancer*, **39**, 440-446.

Martin, Jr, E.W., Cooperman, M., King, G., Rinker, L., Carey, L.C. & Minton, J.P. (1979) A retrospective and prospective study of serial CEA determinations in the early detection of recurrent colon cancer. *American Journal of Surgery*, **137**, 167-169.

McClendon, J.E., Appleby, D., Clandon, D.B., Donegan, W.L. & DeGosse, J.J. (1977) Colonic neoplasms, tissue estrogen receptor and carcinoembryonic antigen. *Archives of Surgery*, **112**, 240-241.

Medical Research Council, Tumour Products Committee (Clinical Subgroup), Bagshawe, K.D., et al (1980) The diagnostic value of plasma carcinoembryonic antigen (CEA) in pancreatic disease. *British Journal of Cancer*, in press.

Meeker, W.R. (1978) The use and abuse of CEA test in clinical practice. *Cancer*, **41**, 854-862.

Mihas, A.A. (1978) Immunologic studies on a pancreatic oncofoetal protein. *Journal of the National Cancer Institute*, **60**, 1439-1444.

Moertel, C.G., Schutt, A.J. & Go, V.L.W. (1978) Carcinoembryonic antigen test for recurrent colorectal carcinoma. *Journal of the American Medical Association*, **239**, 1065-1066.

Muggia, F.M., Rosen, S.W., Weintraub, B.D. & Hansen, H.H. (1975) Ectopic placental proteins in nontrophoblastic tumors. *Cancer*, **36**, 1327-1337.

Munjal, D., Chawla, P.L., Lokich, J.J. & Zamcheck, N. (1976) Carcinoembryonic antigen and phosphohexose isomerase, Gamma-glutamyl transpeptidase and lactate dehydrogenase levels in patients with and without liver metastases. *Cancer*, **37**, 1800-1807.

Neville, A.M. & Cooper, E.H. (1976) Biochemical monitoring of cancer. *Annals of Clinical Biochemistry*, **13**, 283-305.

Neville, A.M., Patel, S., Capp, M., Laurence, J.D.R., Cooper, E.H., Turberville, C. & Coombes, R.C. (1978) Long-term follow-up of colorectal carcinoma patients by repeated CEA radioimmunoassay. *Cancer*, **42**, 1448-1451.

Nishida, K., Sugiura, M., Yoshikawa, T. & Kondo, M. (1980) Enzyme immunoassay of pancreatic oncofetal antigen as test for pancreatic cancer. *Lancet*, **i**, 262-263.

O'Brien, M.J., Kirkham, S.E., Burke, B., Ormerod, M.G., Saravia, C.A., Gottlieb, L.S., Neville, A.M. & Zamcheck, N. (1980) CEA, ZGM and EMA-localization in cells of pleural and peritoneal effusions. A preliminary study. *Investigative and Cell Pathology*, in press.

Odell, W., Wolfsen, A., Yoshimoto, Y., Weitzman, R., Fisher, D. & Hirose, F. (1977) Ectopic peptide synthesis: a universal concomitant of neoplasia. *Transactions of the Association of American Physicians*, **90**, 204-227.

Pressman, D. (1957) Radiolabeled antibodies. *Annals of the New York Academy of Sciences*, **69**, 644-650.

Primus, F.J., Wang, R.H., Goldenberg, D.M. & Hansen, H.J. (1973) Localisation of human GW-39 tumors in hamsters by radiolabeled heterospecific antibody to carcinoembryonic antigen. *Cancer Research*, **33**, 2977-2982.

Pusztaszeri, G., Saravis, C.A. & Zamcheck, N. (1976) The zinc glycinate marker in human colon carcinoma. *Journal of the National Cancer Institute*, **56**, 275-278.

Reif, A.E., Curtis, L.F., Duffield, R. & Shauffer, I.A. (1974) Trial of radiolabeled antibody localization in metastases of a patient with a tumor containing carcinoembryonic antigen (CEA). *Journal of Surgical Oncology*, **6**, 133-150.

Reynoso, G. (1978) The analytical reliability of the zirconyl phosphate method of plasma carcinoembryonic antigen. *Cancer*, **42**, 1406-1411.

Sloane, J.P. & Ormerod, M.G. (1980) Distribution of epithelial membrane antigen in normal and neoplastic tissues and its value in diagnostic tumor pathology. *Cancer*, submitted for publication.

Steele, L., Cooper, E.H., Mackay, A.M., Losowsky, M.S. & Goligher, J.C. (1974) Combination of carcinoembryonic antigen and gamma glutamyl transpeptidase in the study of the evolution of colorectal cancer. *British Journal of Cancer*, **30**, 319-324.

Tataryn, D.N., MacFarlane, J.K., Murray, D. & Thomson, D.M.P. (1979) Tube leukocyte adherence inhibition (LAI) assay in gastrointestinal (GIT) cancer. *Cancer*, **43**, 898-912.

Thomson, D.M.P., Tataryn, D.N. & Schwartz, R. (1980) Partial purification of organ-specific neoantigens from human colon and breast cancer by affinity chromatography with human tumour-specific γ-globulin. *British Journal of Cancer*, **41**, 86-99.

Wood, C.B., Horne, C.H.W., Towler, C.M., Burt, R.W., Ratcliffe, J.G. & Blumgart, L.H. (1978) A critical comparison of the value of pregnancy-associated alpha$_2$-glycoprotein and carcinoembryonic antigen assays in patients with colorectal cancer. *Journal of Clinical Pathology*, **31**, 1065-1067.

16

The Epidemiology and Pathology of Cancer of the Oesophagus

PAULA COOK-MOZAFFARI

Cancer of the oesophagus has a pattern of incidence which is remarkable in almost all its aspects. In the first place, the range of incidence between different regions of the world is around 500-fold (Table 1) and is greater than the range for almost any other commonly occurring type of cancer. Cancer of the lung, for example, shows only a 40-fold variation between the highest and lowest recorded incidence levels; cancer of the stomach, 20-fold; cancer of the colon, 50-fold variation (Doll, 1967). Within Britain, the tumour which shows greatest regional variation is cancer of the stomach which is around twice as common in parts of Wales as in the lowest incidence areas of England. Lung cancer is around four times as common in our most urban compared with our rural areas.

Secondly, sharp gradients of incidence (with a range greater than the total world variation for most types of cancer) occur between regions only a few hundred miles apart. Between Gurjev town in Kazakhstan and the towns of Georgia, 500 miles away, the incidence of cancer of the oesophagus drops 70-fold for men and 230-fold for women (Doll, 1969). In northern China there is a 60-fold decrease for men and a 90-fold decrease for women between the northeast of Honan Province and northern Shansi 300 miles away (Coordinating committee, Chinese, 1974a*). Similar, but slightly less extreme gradients have been reported from northern Iran (Mahboubi et al, 1973); from southern and East Africa (within the Transkei, between Natal and southern Mozambique, and between western Kenya and Uganda) (Prates and Torres, 1965; Schonland and Bradshaw, 1968; Ahmed and Cook, 1969; Rose 1973; Rose and McGlashan, 1975); and between Normandy and Brittany, in northern France, and other parts of western Europe.

Furthermore, the levels of incidence for cancer of the oesophagus which occur around the Caspian Sea, in Kazakhstan and northern Iran, are the highest observed for any type of cancer, in general populations, anywhere in the world. They are comparable with the incidence rates that have been

---

* A map is provided (Figure 1) because of the difficulty encountered in locating places mentioned in Chinese research reports in Western atlases due to changes in place names and to lack of standardization of spelling.

© 1980 W.B. Saunders Company Ltd.

Table 1. Annual truncated incidence rates and estimated incidence rates (for the age group 35 to 64 years) for cancer of the oesophagus (age standardized using the World Standard Population)

Area	Refs	Incidence/100 000 men aged 35–64	Male/female incidence	Area	Refs	Incidence/100 000 men aged 35–64	Male/female incidence
Western Europe				Nn Gorgan	8	173.7	0.9
W. Germany (Hamburg)	3	3.7	3.4	Sn Gorgan	8	104.1	0.9
Austria	4	4.9†	6.5	Central Mazandaran	8	62.8	1.4
Belgium	4	6.2†	4.9	Wn Mazandaran	8	44.5	2.0
Netherlands (3 Provinces)	1	2.5	3.2	NW Gilan	8	48.7	3.4
UK (av. of 6 registries)	3	5.6	1.4	SE Gilan	8	20.0	3.5
Ireland	4	8.0†	1.4	Azerbaidjan (Ardebil)	8	109.8	2.1
Switzerland (Geneva)	3	11.2	11.5	Asia — Central Soviet Asia (towns)			
France	4	25.5†	18.2	Kazakhstan (Gurjev)	4	547.2	1.6
France (Normandy and Brittany)	5	40.8†*	25.0	Kazakhstan	4	64.9†*	1.3
Northern Europe				Uzbekistan	4	48.6†*	2.3
Iceland	3	3.4	1.8	Turkmenistan	4	110.5†*	1.1
Sweden	3	3.5	3.2	Kirghizia	4	23.6†*	2.4
Norway (urban)	3	4.6	7.7	Tajikstan	4	32.5†*	10.5
(rural)	3	1.9	3.8	Asia — Far East			
Denmark	3	3.7	4.1	India (Bombay)	3	21.0	1.
Finland	3	8.1	1.8	Singapore (Chinese)	3	30.0	3.
Eastern Europe				(Malay)	3	(4.4)	(0.
E. Germany	3	3.8	5.4	(Indians)	3	7.9	(0.
Poland (Warsaw City)	3	9.7	4.0	Japan (Miyagi)	3	20.1	5.
(4 rural areas)	3	4.9	8.2	(Okayama)	3	4.9	(1.
Hungary (Vas)	3	2.7	(9.0)	(Osaka)	3	11.2	(3.
Czechoslovakia	4	3.3†	5.4	China			
Bulgaria	4	2.5†*	2.0	NE Honan (Yangcheng and Hehpih			
Rumania (Banat Region)	3	2.3	7.7	Counties)	6	236.6†*	1
Western Soviet Union (towns)				NE Honan (Linhsien County)	7	123.4	1
Belorussia	4	9.3†*	3.6	Nn Shansi (Hunyuan and Tatung			
Estonia	4	15.0†*	7.2	Counties)	6	3.9†*	2
Latvia	4	11.6†*	9.9	Shanghai City	7	24.3	2
Lithuania	4	5.2†*	2.4	Kwantung (Chung Shan County)	7	3.9	2
Moldavia	4	9.1†*	5.7	Canada (av. of 7 registries)	3	4.8	4
Ukraine	4	10.7†*	3.5	Eastern and Central USA			
RSFSR	4	24.1†*	9.8	Connecticut	3	9.4	
Georgia	4	7.9†*	5.1	New York State	3	6.6	
Armenia	4	9.1†*	6.3	Western USA			
Azerbaidjan	4	28.6†*	1.7	Utah	3	4.1	
Southern Europe				Nevada	3	5.0	
Portugal	4	11.5†	3.7	California (Alameda, white)	3	7.2	
Spain (Zaragoza)	3	6.5	9.2	(Alameda, black)	3	19.8	(
Italy	4	6.5†	5.7	(San Franc. Bay, white)	3	6.4	
Malta	3	3.4	(8.5)	(San Franc. Bay, black)	3	27.9	
Yugoslavia (Slovenia)	3	9.6	16.0	(San Franc. Bay, Chinese)	3	12.5	(
Asia — Middle East				Southern USA			
Israel (Jews born in Israel)	3	(1.1)	(1.2)	Texas (El Paso, Spanish)	3	(3.1)	3.
(Jews born in Africa/Asia)	3	3.2	0.9	(El Paso, other white)	3	2.7	(
(Jews born in Europe/America)	3	3.4	1.5	New Mexico (Spanish)	3	2.4	(
(non-Jews)	3	(0.9)	0.9/0.0	(other white)	3	4.0	
Iran				(Amer. Indian)	3	(4.6)	4
NE Gonbad	8	515.6	1.1				
Central Gonbad	8	217.7	0.7				
Sn Gonbad	8	151.6	1.2				

Table 1. (*continued*)

Area	Refs	Incidence/100 000 men aged 35–64	Male/female incidence	Area	Refs	Incidence/100 000 men aged 35–64	Male/female incidence
Caribbean				(Natal)	2	93.1	3.5
Puerto Rico	3	29.6	2.7	(Johannesburg)	12	54.5‡	4.2
Cuba	3	7.4	2.6	Mozambique (Lourenco Marques)	1	11.8	11.8/0.0
Jamaica	3	13.0	2.3	Rhodesia (Bulawayo)	2	94.9	3.3
Curacao	9	44.4*	18.7	Africa (other)			
South America				S. Africa (Cape Prov., white)	2	9.0	6.4
Colombia (Cali)	3	7.3	4.1	(Cape Prov., coloured)	2	21.3	21.3/0.0
Venezuela	4	4.8†	1.0	(Natal, Indian)	2	(14.7)	0.6
Brazil (Recife)	3	10.5	5.5	Oceania			
(Sao Paulo)	3	22.0	7.3	Australia	4	5.0†	2.9
Uruguay	4	23.6†	2.8	New Zealand (Maori)	3	(4.3)	(4.0)
Africa (blacks)				(non-Maori)	3	7.0	2.4
Nigeria (Ibadan)	2	(2.5)	(8.3)	Hawaii (Hawaiian)	3	(16.1)	16.1/0.0
Uganda (Kyadondo)	1	5.5	1.6	(Caucasian)	3	10.5	(3.6)
Kenya (C. Nyanza)	10	106.0‡	11.8	(Japanese)	3	6.6	(0.7)
S. Africa (Cape Province)	2	77.0	2.2	Fiji (Fijians)	13	4.2	4.2/0.0
(Transkei Sn (Butterworth))	11	180.7*	2.3	(Indians)	13	4.5	3.5
(Transkei Nn (Bizana))	11	26.2*	2.3				

( ) Incidence based on fewer than ten cases; * estimate from a different age group; † estimate from mortality data; ‡ adjusted for under-reporting.

1 Doll, Payne and Waterhouse (1966)
2 Doll, Muir and Waterhouse (1970)
3 Waterhouse et al (1976)
4 Doll (1969)
5 Estimate from Tuyns (1969, personal communication)
6 Estimate from Coordinating Group, Chinese (1974a)
7 Estimate from Miller (1978)
8 Mahboubi et al (1973)
9 Estimate from IARC Annual Report (1970)
10 Ahmed and Cook (1969)
11 Estimate from Rose and McGlashan (1975)
12 Estimate from Robertson, Harington and Bradshaw (1971)
13 Estimate from Boyd, Doll and Gurd (1973)

observed in known high-risk groups; with the lung cancer rate, for example, among lifelong heavy smokers in London.

Over most of Europe incidence is low, as it is also among the white populations of the United States, Canada, Africa, Australia and New Zealand. American blacks, however, have a risk of the disease that is two to four times higher than that in whites, and in both black and white populations in the Caribbean and South America moderate levels of incidence have been recorded. In Asia there are isolated reports of moderate incidence from India, Singapore and Japan.

All the incidence rates shown in Table 1 have been calculated for the age group 35 to 64 years. At younger ages few cases are reported while, over the age of 65, bias is introduced into the comparisons by the reluctance or inability of older people to avail themselves of medical facilities, particularly in the poorer communities of the world (Doll and Cook, 1967). Indeed a problem in epidemiological investigations of cancer of the oesophagus is

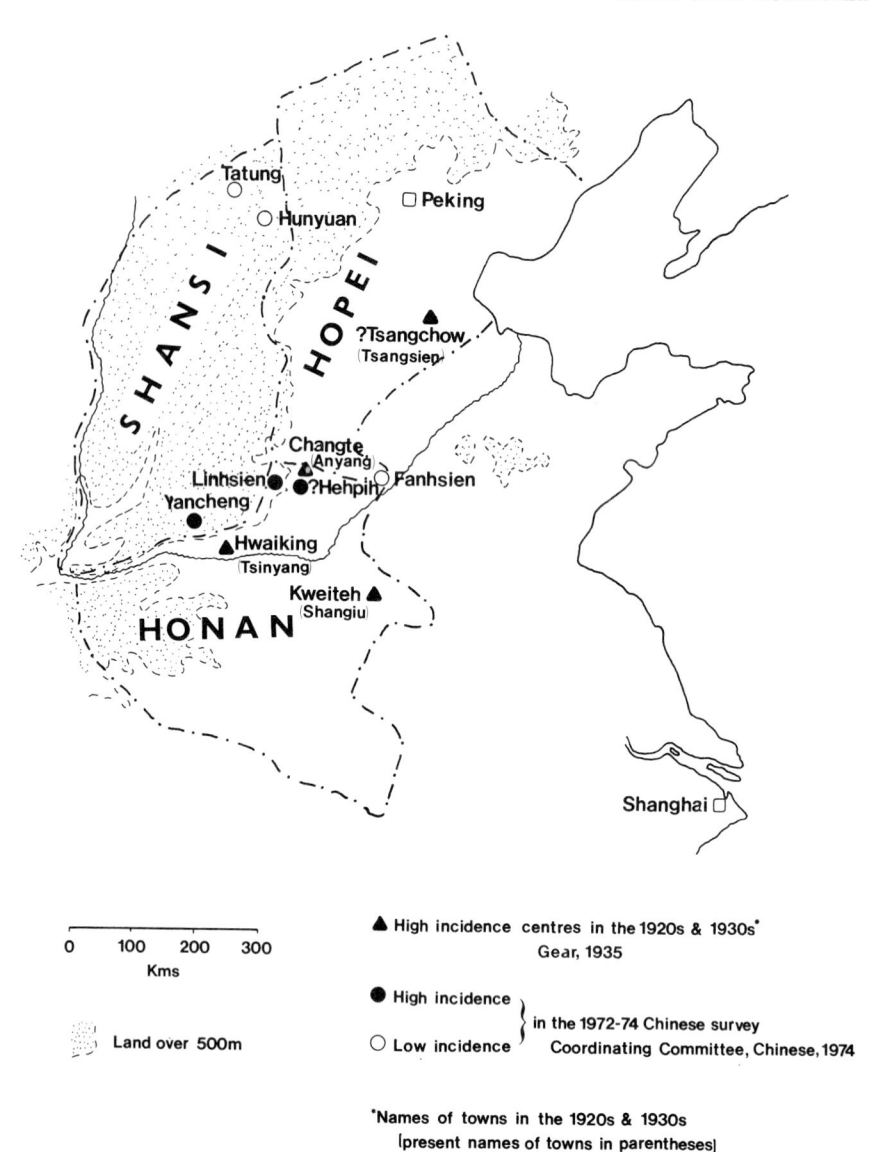

Figure 1. Cancer of the oesophagus in northern China.

that the highest recorded incidence levels occur in economically less advanced countries, where population data are often inadequate and where worthwhile cancer registration is very difficult. Pathologists working in such areas have often shown great enthusiasm for recording cancer data but their efforts have been hampered by the fact that over much of rural Africa and Asia doctors rarely attempt to take a biopsy from inaccessible tumours (Burkitt, Hutt and Slavin, 1968; Mahboubi et al, 1973). However, in the absence of other data it has been necessary to mount special surveys to establish the true incidence in areas where an exceptional situation was suspected and to stress that tumours diagnosed on radiological or even on clinical grounds alone should be included. In northern Iran, technicians were sent each month over a period of years to several hundred doctors to collect information about newly diagnosed cases (Mahboubi et al, 1973). In China and in the Transkei region of South Africa, a village-to-village search was mounted, again over a period of years, to identify all cases of cancer of the oesophagus (Burrell, 1962, 1969; Rose, 1973; Coordinating committee, Chinese, 1974a). The inclusion of the clinically diagnosed cases is admissible because the course of the disease is so distinctive, with progression through inability to swallow first solids and then liquids to death from starvation, which usually occurs within a few months of first reaching hospital. (With surgical intervention or radiotherapy the prognosis has been little better although the patient may die more comfortably.) In Iran a check was made on completeness of reporting by collecting information not just about cancer of the oesophagus but about all malignant tumours. The incidence of cancer at other sites showed a very similar level across all regions (Mahboubi et al, 1973).

Expense limits the area that can be covered in the intensive incidence investigations described above. The pattern of cancer occurrence in wide tracts of rural Africa has, however, been outlined using a less rigorous method of analysis in which, in the absence of population data, the frequency of one type of cancer is expressed proportional to the number of tumours at other sites (Cook and Burkitt, 1971) or relative to the number of hospital beds or admissions (Oettlé, 1963). In both surveys data were collected by postal questionnaire; in East Africa the forms were sent monthly over a period of years. The information of this type for cancer of the oesophagus is summarized in Figure 2. Two features are of particular interest. In the first place there are clearly several other gradients of frequency in addition to those that have been defined by the incidence surveys described above, between Johannesburg (28 per cent of cancer in men) and rural areas of the northern Transvaal, for example, and between southern Malawi and southern Tanzania and the adjacent areas of eastern Zambia. Secondly, cancer of the oesophagus is strikingly absent from West Africa.

INCIDENCE OF CANCER OF THE OESOPHAGUS IN WOMEN

All the descriptions of patterns of frequency so far have been for men. This is because the pattern of incidence for women is a partial reflection of that for men. The ratio of male to female incidence is given in the right-hand columns of Table 1 and it can be seen that whereas the rates for women sometimes show the same high frequency, often they occur at a much lower level. Furthermore, although in one or two areas of very high incidence the female risk is marginally higher than the male, there is no example of a high incidence in women unaccompanied by a high incidence in men.

The range of variation in the sex ratio and the lack of any consistent

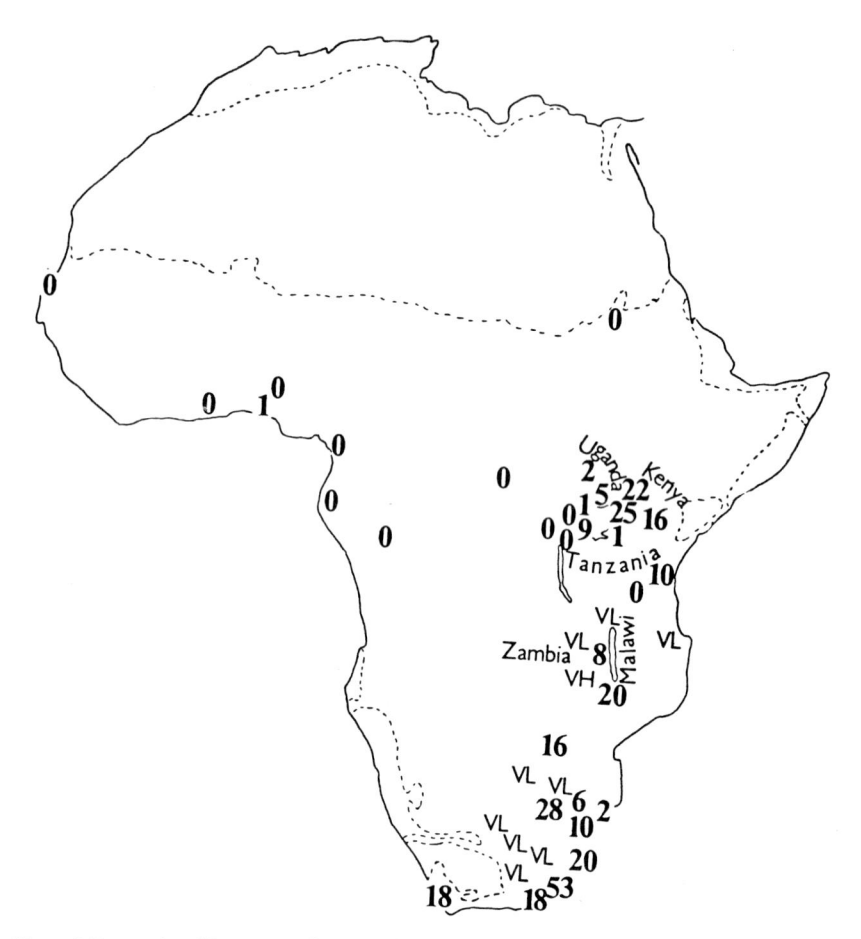

Figure 2. Proportional frequency of cancer of the oesophagus in Africa. This map is compiled from data gathered together from many sources. Detailed references are given in Cook (1971). 25 = cancer of the oesophagus in men expressed as a percentage of all male cancer. Estimated frequency by local doctors is very high (VH) or very low (VL).

relationship with the level of incidence are further distinctive features of the occurrence of cancer of the oesophagus. In the exceptionally high incidence areas of Central Soviet Asia, Iran and China, the incidence in men and women is nearly equal while, as one passes into the adjacent areas of lower incidence, there is a steeper decline of risk for women than for men. However, in Africa, although this is the pattern between the south and the north of the Transkei, in southern Malawi, Bulawayo and Kenya a high incidence in men is accompanied by a 10- to 12-fold lower risk in women while in southern Uganda there is a low but similar level of risk in both men and women. In Normandy and Brittany, cancer of the oesophagus is outstandingly a disease of men, with a sex ratio of over 25:1.

CHANGING FREQUENCIES WITH TIME

Another odd feature of the epidemiology of cancer of the oesophagus is the changing pattern of incidence with time. Well-documented but small-scale increases in incidence have been recorded for both sexes among blacks in the United States and for men in Normandy and Brittany (Schoenberg, Bailar and Fraumeni, 1971; Audigier, Tuyns and Lambert, 1975). However, in South Africa there are indications that the disease has come up like an epidemic from being very rare up to the 1930s to being one of the commonest types of cancer diagnosed at some centres by the 1960s and 1970s. The most reliable reports are from Johannesburg where, at the principal African hospital, cancer of the oesophagus represented 2 per cent of all tumours diagnosed in men in the 1930s (Berman, 1935), 10 per cent in the early 1950s, and 28 per cent in the early 1960s (Robertson, Harington and Bradshaw, 1971). The earlier figure is based on all cases diagnosed, not on histology records alone, and tumours at other internal sites occur with greater frequency in the series. Stomach cancer was six times as common and primary liver cancer 12 times as common as cancer of the oesophagus. The latter figure of 28 per cent is an overestimate in that it includes patients who have come to Johannesburg from other parts of South Africa. However, if the age-standardized incidence rate for Johannesburg residents in the early 1950s is compared with that for residents seen at the principal African hospital in the early 1960s the risk in men shows a twofold increase (Robertson, Harington and Bradshaw, 1971). The proportional frequency among 'local residents' seen at the hospital was in the order of 20 per cent (compared with the figure of 28 per cent for patients from all regions). By the early 1960s the oesophagus had become the most common individual site for cancer development in men.

In Durban the hospital admissions in the 1950s and 1960s indicate a fivefold increase in risk (Schonland and Bradshaw, 1969). Part of this may be due to changes in patterns of referral to the hospital but the majority of patients, even for a severe disease such as cancer, are likely to be local residents.

In the Transkei there are only clinical impressions that the disease was rare in the 1920s and 1930s (Burrell, 1957, 1962) but in the neighbouring Ciskei where the disease is now common (Rose, 1967) cancer of the oesophagus represented less than 1 per cent of malignancies diagnosed at Lovedale Mission hospital between 1913 and 1933 (Macvicar, 1925; Berman, 1935). In view of the regional similarity of reporting by doctors at isolated small hospitals in East Africa — all in one region saying that they never see cancer of the oesophagus; all in another region reporting it as common (Cook and Burkitt, 1971) — it seems reasonable to give credence to these early reports from small hospitals and to the clinical impressions.

The increase in southern Africa now also appears to be affecting other areas where until recently the disease was little known. There are reports of moderate frequencies from Swaziland, the Transvaal and Botswana where until the early 1960s it was not seen (Oettlé, 1963; Sutherland, 1968; Keen, 1971; Macrae and Cook, 1975).

In East Africa the picture is less clear. The pathology records at the large central hospital in Nairobi, Kenya, showed cancer of the oesophagus representing fewer than 0.1 per cent of all tumours diagnosed in the mid 1930s (Vint, 1935) compared with around 16 per cent in the late 1960s (Cook and Burkitt, 1971) and, whereas doctors at small mission hospitals may never take an oesophageal biopsy, it seems less likely that this would be the practice at a central government hospital. However, the one historical report that exists for western Kenya indicates a fairly constant frequency at around 14 per cent between 1926 and 1950, although numbers for the earlier period are very small (Cook, 1971). In Uganda, as in the lower-frequency areas of southern Africa, cancer of the oesophagus is now beginning to be seen (Templeton, 1973).

There is no evidence concerning recent change in the exceptionally high incidence areas of Iran and Soviet Central Asia. In northern China in the 1920s and 1930s several missionary doctors reported cancer of the oesophagus as one of the types of cancer most commonly diagnosed (Davies, 1924; Gear, 1935) (see Figure 1) while the Chinese epidemiologists who are now investigating the disease say that it has been known in the high-incidence areas for over 2000 years (Kaplan and Tsuchitani, 1978). In Iran a medical text from the twelfth century describes and illustrates cancer of the oesophagus, suggesting that there too it is of long-standing origin (Elgood, 1951).

THE SEARCH FOR AETIOLOGICAL HYPOTHESES

By the end of the 1960s case-control investigations in different parts of the world had repeatedly shown that the consumption of alcohol and to a lesser extent tobacco was involved in the development of cancer of the oesophagus (Higginson and Oettlé, 1960; Wynder and Bross, 1961; Burrell, 1962; Martinez, 1969). However, these higher risks had been demonstrated equally within areas of low, moderate and high incidence and the worldwide differences in the consumption of alcohol or tobacco were quite insufficient to explain the enormous variation in the incidence of cancer of the oesophagus between such areas (Doll, 1967). Furthermore, information was beginning to percolate through from Iran that in the rural areas of very high incidence the proscriptions of the Moslem religion were still widely observed — especially by the women, among whom the incidence was as high as in men — and that virtually no alcohol at all was consumed (Kmet and Mahboubi, 1972). There was an urgent need at this point for new hypotheses of causation and it seemed that the best way to generate ideas would be to exploit the geographical clues and examine in detail the environment and way of life of the regions where sharp gradients of incidence had been observed (IARC Internal Report, 1968).

Iran

Work has progressed furthest along these lines in Iran. Perusal of available environmental and sociological information showed a strong negative association with rainfall and partial correlations with the many variables dependent on rainfall, such as vegetation, soil types and crop patterns (Kmet and Mahboubi, 1972).

The highest incidence levels occurred in Turkomans who are the most western of the mongoloid peoples of Central Asia but the incidence seems to cut across ethnic boundaries with Persians, Turks and Turkomans all suffering the disease at varying levels (Mahboubi et al, 1973; Cook-Mozaffari, 1979).

The limits of what could be learned from published sources were quickly reached and a survey was mounted to collect additional information. Field teams lived during the course of a year in some 40 villages around the south of the Caspian Sea and carried out detailed dietary, sociological and physiological surveys on the general population of the area (Iran—IARC, Joint Study Group, 1977). This work confirmed the absence of alcohol as a risk factor and focused attention on the very restricted diet of the highest incidence areas. For most of the year little besides home-baked bread, tea and sugar is consumed. The flocks of sheep and goats give milk for yogurt in the spring before the pastures are scorched dry with the approach of summer. The bare steppe grasslands provide virtually no vegetables or fruit and the traditional diet of the Turkomans is almost completely lacking in either. Such a diet has very low levels of animal protein, vitamin A, riboflavin and vitamin C (Hormozdiari et al, 1975). Overt clinical signs of riboflavin deficiency are widespread (Kmet, McLaren and Siassi, 1980).

Intensive analysis of constituents of the diet for known carcinogens such as nitrosamines, aflotoxins and polycyclic hydrocarbons showed very low levels of these contaminants throughout the different incidence zones and no significant correlations with incidence (IARC Annual Report, 1975).

The few variables which did show some degree of geographical variation with incidence were followed up in a case-control study in which each patient was matched with two controls from the same village (Cook-Mozaffari et al, 1979). At this stage, factors such as the consumption of sheep's milk, the use of a special pregnancy diet made of crushed pomegranate seeds, raisins and pepper, the chewing of 'nass' (a mixture of tobacco and woodash), the use of sesame oil for cooking, the dyeing of wool for carpets, and the occasional consumption of a wild spinach high in nitrates were eliminated from further consideration as potential risk factors. However, the case-control study confirmed the risk attributable to a low intake of fruit and vegetables and demonstrated that within the generally poor rural communities of northern Iran it is those of lowest economic status who are most at risk for cancer of the oesophagus.

A result that was almost overlooked in the population investigation was the possible role of opium. Logistic problems with the collection of urine samples for the measurement of morphine metabolites meant that relatively few specimens were available. However, a broad regional analysis demonstrated that in the higher-incidence areas 50 per cent of the men and women over the age of 35 years had 'consumed' opium in the previous 24 hours and that the questionnaire responses for this largely illegal activity had greatly underestimated the extent of its use.

The use of opium could not be investigated in the case-control study because many of the patients would have been taking the drug to relieve their symptoms, but a survey is under way to investigate the use in 'case families' and 'control families' and to find out more about eating the dross scraped from the inside of the opium pipe, a habit which is said to be most common in the highest incidence areas (Hewer et al, 1978). The opium dross has been shown to be highly mutagenic (Day, 1980, personal communication), but the exact role it might play is difficult to interpret in view of its apparent lack of use in the neighbouring high-incidence areas of Soviet Central Asia where one might expect a similar aetiology for the disease but where the traditional drug used was hashish (Vambery, 1869; Schuyler, 1876; Bogovski, 1977, personal communication).

What the Iranian and the Central Asian areas of high incidence do have in common is that they are all wheat areas and much interest has centred on the possible fungal contamination of bread or its adulteration with seeds from other plants. However, analysis of bread and wheat samples from Iran have demonstrated no carcinogenic mycotoxins, and although there is widespread admixture of other seeds in the wheat the worst that can be said of these is that they are potentially abrasive (IARC Annual Report, 1978).

China

Wheat seemed to be a common factor which could embrace also the high-incidence areas of China where it is one of the main crops. However, in the county of Linhsien where most epidemiological investigation has taken place, a maize bread cooked by steaming is the staple diet and, there, fungal mould is apparently widespread, grown during weeks of storage and relished as the preferred taste of bread (Kaplan and Tsuchitani, 1978).

Poverty is also a factor which could provide a link between the aetiology of cancer of the oesophagus in China and in Central Asia and Iran. Before the completion of the Red Flag Canal in 1969 the county of Linhsien was renowned for 'extreme poverty, periodic drought and chronic water shortages'. The American delegation to China, who commented on this poverty (Kaplan and Tsuchitani, 1978), were also impressed by the limited nature of the diet which consists mainly of ground cornmeal and wheat and 'pickled'* vegetables. As in Iran, few fresh vegetables are taken and little protein of animal origin. The 'pickled' vegetables, as well as the mouldy bread, are suspect as a source of nitrosamines or nitrosamine precursors and vigorous attempts are being made to change the traditional eating habits. Strong confirmation of the carcinogenic potential of the diet was felt to come from the high incidence of oesophageal and pharangeal carcinomas in domestic chickens in Linhsien. These are fed principally on table scraps and, when some 50 000 people were moved from Linhsien to low-incidence Fanhsien, because their land was needed for building a reservoir, the new chickens which they acquired from previously cancer-free flocks also contracted cancer after a lifetime on a Linhsien-type diet.

---

*Cabbage leaves are covered in water in an earthenware container and left to rot for several months.

Singapore, Japan and Puerto Rico

Case-control studies in moderate-incidence populations in Singapore, Japan and Puerto Rico have incriminated alcohol, cigarette smoking and a preference for burning-hot drinks as risk factors. However, the disease was also found to occur more in groups of low socioeconomic status, and in Japan, the only study in which the question was asked, the patients had a lower consumption of fruit (Martinez, 1969; Hirayama, 1971; de Jong et al, 1974). A description of the diet in rural Puerto Rico commented on the low intakes of vitamin A, riboflavin, iron, calcium and calories (Fernandez, 1975).

Africa

With the poor economic situation in most African countries, a restricted diet could clearly be a necessary background factor for the development of cancer of the oesophagus there. Low intakes of vitamin A and riboflavin, for example, are characteristic of the diet in the high-incidence areas of central and western Kenya (Bohdal, Gibbs and Simmons, 1969). From the Transkei there has been a suggestion that molybdenum deficiencies in the soil cause a build-up of nitrates in plants which could be converted to nitrosamines in the stomach (Burrell, Roach and Shadwell, 1966).

The soils of Linhsien are also low in molybdenum and its addition to seeds before planting has considerably reduced the nitrate content of grains and increased the vitamin C content of vegetables (Kaplan and Tsuchitani, 1978). However, in Africa it is difficult to see how general items of diet eaten by both men and women could account for the 10- to 12-fold male excess of cancer of the oesophagus which has been observed in many regions of higher incidence. It would seem rather that some social habit such as drinking or smoking must be a predominant risk factor. There is no association with mere quantity of alcohol consumed. A Liquor Commission in low-incidence Uganda established that illicit distilling was the third industry of the country after the production of cotton and coffee (Uganda Government, 1963) while in west Africa where the disease is virtually unknown the drinking of palm wine is common. Interest centred more on the possible contamination of home-made spirits distilled through old exhaust pipes, for example, or laced with metal polish (Burrell, 1957; McGlashan, 1969). However, these were features of distilling in urban areas and could not explain the high rural frequencies of cancer of the oesophagus. A more promising lead was the report that nitrosamines had been found in maize spirit from a high-incidence region of Zambia (McGlashan, Walters and McLean, 1968). Nitrosamines appear repeatedly in epidemiological studies of cancer of the oesophagus. Not only are they strongly carcinogenic but they are also the only group of chemicals which give rise to oesophageal tumours in experimental animals (Magee and Barnes, 1967). However, at this stage the chemists were continuously revising their techniques for measuring nitrosamines and when spirit samples from high- and low-incidence areas in East Africa were measured by more rigorous methods they showed no trace of nitrosamine contamination (Collis et al, 1971). Re-analysis of the Zambia samples had led to the same conclusion (McGlashan, Patterson and Williams, 1970).

An association which could account for both the geographical variation and the continuing patchy increases of incidence with time within Africa is the current use of maize as the principal ingredient of home-made beer. In much of East and southern Africa maize has replaced the traditional millets and sorghum for beer making during the past 50 years. In Uganda, however, maize beer has only recently begun to usurp the traditional banana or millet brews (Cook, 1971).

Beer drinking is very widespread in African communities and the fact that it has not been implicated as a risk factor in case-control studies could merely reflect its ubiquity. Also, however, questioning has concentrated more on the consumption of spirits.

A factor which has stood out in case-control investigations is the smoking of pipes or the use of pipe tobacco for cigarettes (Bradshaw and Schonland, 1969, 1974; Rose, 1979). Particular interest has centred on the habit of sucking the dottle from the stem of pipes in the Transkei which parallels the use of opium dross in Iran (Hewer et al, 1978).

France

In France as well as Africa there was no clear geographical association with quantity of alcohol consumed (Tuyns, 1970) although both cancer of the oesophagus and mortality from alcoholism are very common in Normandy and Brittany. Suspicion again fell on the local drinks— on home-made ciders and apple brandies — and low levels of nitrosamines were detected (IARC Annual Report, 1975). At about the same time, however, similarly low levels were found in food samples from both the high- and the low-incidence areas in Iran (IARC Annual Report, 1975) and in maize beer samples from South Africa (IARC Annual Report, 1976) and it was concluded that this is probably a general background level of contamination of little significance for cancer of the oesophagus. (The Chinese findings of nitrosamines seem to have been established so far only on the basis of gas chromatography (Kaplan and Tsuchitani, 1978) and without the final confirmation of analysis by mass spectrometry.) A case-control study in Normandy and Brittany has shown that the excess risk there can best be accounted for by a multiplicative effect of drinking and smoking (Tuyns and Jensen, 1976).

AETIOLOGICAL SUMMARY

The oddities of the pattern of incidence for cancer of the oesophagus can be accounted for only by assuming that a multiplicity of factors are involved in its causation. At present the items in the multifactorial package would seem to be as follows:

1. A conditioning of individual susceptibility (either from the effect of a very poor diet from infancy or by the harmful effect of alcohol on nutri-

tional status. Animal experiments have shown both that vitamin A and riboflavin can inhibit tumour development and that riboflavin deficiency can produce squamous metaplasia in the epithelium of the oesophagus in mice (Wynder and Klein, 1965; Wynder and Chan, 1970; overviews, Berg, 1975; Day and Muños, 1980).
2. A further heightening of susceptibility from repeated irritation of the oesophageal mucosa. Extreme mechanical trauma, as has been described after the swallowing of lye, gives an increased risk for oesophageal cancer. It seems likely that repeated small-scale trauma (caused, for example, by the ingestion of hot food and drinks or of dryish, scratchy bread) could also result in heightened individual susceptibility.
3. The action of some carcinogenic agent. Tobacco smoke which is mostly inhaled rather than swallowed, or grains of opium dross swallowed swiftly with tea (to avoid the bitter taste) can offer only a weakly carcinogenic stimulus to the oesophagus. This and the failure (except perhaps in China) to find any potent carcinogens at high levels in the highest-incidence areas suggest that perhaps a variety of weak carcinogenic agents may be acting on susceptible oesophageal tissue. These could occur, for example, in mouldy bread, or opium residues, in maize beer or apple brandy or tobacco or in a wealth of other substances.
4. The possibility that alcohol (Doll, 1971) or hot tea (Day and Muños, 1980) might act as solvents facilitating the passage of carcinogens to the basal layers of the oesophagus.

PATHOLOGY

There has been a recent surge of interest in the premalignant changes which occur in oesophageal tissue. For Western investigators this became possible with the invention of the fibrescope; in China it grew from the overriding concern to find effective treatment through early detection which in turn led to the invention of the simple balloon technique for taking cytological specimens.

Table 2. *Oesophageal lesions diagnosed by cytological screening in China*

Region	No. examined	mild dysplasia	marked dysplasia	cancer
N. Linhsien	4377	25.5	2.2	1.3
S. Linhsien	2835	18.3	0.7	0.7

The enormous screening programmes undertaken in the highest-incidence areas have also given an insight into the sequence of premalignant changes (Coordinating Committee, Chinese, 1974b). Table 2 shows the proportion of the population found to have mild amd marked dysplasia in the higher- and slightly-lower-incidence areas of north and south Linhsien.

Table 3 gives the results of repeated screening tests on the same individuals. The 27 per cent with marked dysplasia whose lesions progressed to carcinoma represent a 140-fold increase in risk compared with the 0.2 per cent developing cancer among 11 011 persons who had normal cytology at the first screening. (It has been suggested that the term 'hyperplasia', rather than 'dysplasia', would more accurately describe the conditions observed in China (Day and Muños, 1980).)

Table 3. *Progression of oesophageal lesions diagnosed at successive screening surveys in China*

	Persons with dysplasia follow-up 2, 3 and 4 + years after initial diagnosis of:	
	mild dysplasia (105 cases)	marked dysplasia (79 cases)
	Percentages	
Progressing to carcinoma	0.0	26.6
Progressing to marked dysplasia/recurring marked dysplasia	15.2	17.7
No change	40.0	15.2
Regressing to mild dysplasia or to normal	44.8	40.5

Table 4 summarizes the results of endoscopic examination and of histological diagnosis of oesophageal biopsies from 430 individuals over the age of 15 in the highest-incidence areas of Iran. The high rate of oesophagitis was observed at all ages although it increased in severity with age. It apparently

Table 4. *Results of a survey in Iran of premalignant changes in the oesophagus of 430 subjects from the regions of highest incidence for cancer of the oesophagus*

Endoscopic diagnoses	Males	Females	Histological diagnoses	Males	Females
	Percentages			Percentages	
Normal	11.0	10.4	Normal	2.8	5.9
Oesophagitis			Oesophagitis		
mild	37.6	59.9	mild	58.7	57.6
moderate	36.7	23.1	moderate	21.6	17.6
severe	11.0	4.7	severe	2.8	1.0
Varices			Acanthosis	66.2	64.9
single	5.9	6.1			
multiple	7.3	12.3			
Incompetent cardia	7.3	8.5	Atrophy	12.7	8.3
Hiatal hernia	0.9	0.9	Dysplasia	4.7	2.9
Cancer			Cancer	2.8	2.0
suspected	0.5	0.4			
malignant	2.3	0.9			

differed in appearance from oesophagitis which is observed in the West in association with reflux and this was borne out by the low frequency of incompetent cardia found in Iran (Crespi et al, 1979).

The Chinese have concentrated both on curing and on preventing cancer of the oesophagus. There is some indication that their massive early detection programmes and skill at surgery have been rewarded by higher five-year survival rates after radical treatment than are common in the West— some 41 per cent in Linhsien compared with 10 per cent in Birmingham, UK* (Waterhouse, 1974). Prevention in China has been approached by an aggressive Public Health attack on all suspected aetiological factors but sufficient time has not yet elapsed to assess whether the variables truly involved have indeed been included in the prevention package.

In Iran it had been planned to mount controlled intervention trials, and it is hoped that these can soon be implemented.

REFERENCES

Ahmed, N. & Cook, P. (1969) The incidence of cancer of the oesophagus in West Kenya. *British Journal of Cancer*, **23**, 302-312.

Audigier, J.C., Tuyns, A.J. & Lambert, R. (1975) Epidemiology of oesophageal cancer in France. *Digestion*, **13**, 209-219.

Berg, J.W. (1975) Diet. In *Persons at High Risk for Cancer* (Ed.) Fraumeni, J.F. pp. 201-224. New York and London: Academic Press.

Berman, C. (1935) Malignant disease in the Bantu. *South African Journal of Medical Sciences*, **1**, 12-30.

Bohdal, M., Gibbs, N.E. & Simmons, W.K. (1969) Report to Ministry of Health of Kenya, Nutrition Survey.

Boyd, J.T., Doll, R. & Gurd, C.H. (1973) Cancer incidence in Fiji. *International Journal of Epidemiology*, **2**, 177-187.

Bradshaw, E. & Schonland, M. (1969) Oesophageal and lung cancer in Natal African males in relation to certain socio-economic factors. *British Journal of Cancer*, **23**, 275-284.

Bradshaw, E. & Schonland, M. (1974) Smoking, drinking and oesophageal cancer in African males of Johannesburg, South Africa. *British Journal of Cancer*, **30**, 157-163.

Burkitt, D.P., Hutt, M.S.R. & Slavin, G. (1968) Clinico-pathological studies of cancer distribution in Africa. *British Journal of Cancer*, **22**, 1-6.

Burrell, R.J.W. (1957) Oesophageal cancer in the Bantu. *South African Medical Journal*, **31**, 401-409.

Burrell, R.J.W. (1962) Oesophageal cancer among Bantu in the Transkei. *Journal of the National Cancer Institute*, **28**, 495-514.

Burrell, R.J.W. (1969) Distribution maps of oesophageal cancer among Bantu in the Transkei. *Journal of the National Cancer Institute*, **43**, 877-888.

Burrell, R.J.W., Roach, W.A. & Shadwell, A. (1966) Oesophageal cancer in the Bantu of the Transkei associated with mineral deficiency in garden plants. *Journal of the National Cancer Institute*, **36**, 201-209.

Collis, C.H., Cook, P.J., Foreman, J.K. & Palframan, J.F. (1971) A search for nitrosamines in East African spirit samples from areas of varying oesophageal cancer frequency, *Gut*, **12**, 1015-1018.

Cook, P. (1971) Cancer of the oesophagus in Africa. *British Journal of Cancer*, **25**, 853-880.

Cook, P.J. & Burkitt, D.P. (1971) Cancer in Africa. *British Medical Bulletin*, **27**, 14-20.

---

*In Birmingham some 28 per cent of patients are deemed suitable for radical treatment (surgery or radiotherapy). In Linhsien only around 20 per cent agree to undergo surgery (Muños, 1980, personal communication).

Cook-Mozaffari, P. (1979) The epidemiology of cancer of the oesophagus. *Nutrition and Cancer*, **1**, 51-61.
Cook-Mozaffari, P.J., Azordegan, F., Day, N.E., Ressicaud, A., Sabai, C. & Aramesh, B. (1979) Oesophageal cancer studies in the Caspian littoral of Iran: results of a case-control study. *British Journal of Cancer*, **39**, 293-309.
Coordinating Group for Research on the Aetiology of Oesophageal Cancer of North China (1974a) *The Epidemiology of Oesophageal Cancer in North China and Preliminary Results in the Investigation of its Aetiological Factors*. Peking.
Coordinating Group for Research on the Aetiology of Oesophageal Cancer of North China (1974b) *Studies of the Relationship Between Epithelial Dysplasia and Carcinoma of the Oesophagus*. Peking.
Crespi, M., Muñoz, N., Grassi, A., Aramesh, B., Amiri, G., Mojtabai, A. & Casale, Z. (1979) Oesophageal lesions in northern Iran: a premalignant condition? *Lancet*, **ii**, 217-221.
Davies, S. (1924) Cancer in China. *British Medical Journal*, **i**, 131.
Day, N.E. & Muños, N. (1980) Cancer of the oesophagus. In *Cancer Epidemiology and Prevention* (Ed.) Schottenfeld, D. & Fraumeni, J.F. New York: W.B. Saunders.
de Jong, U.W., Breslow, N., Goh Ewe Hong, J., Sridharan, M. & Shanmugaratnam, K. (1974) Aetiological factors in oesophageal cancer in Singapore Chinese. *International Journal of Cancer*, **13**, 291-303.
Doll, R. (1967) *Prevention of Cancer; Pointers from Epidemiology*. Nuffield Provincial Hospitals Trust.
Doll, R. (1969) The geographical distribution of cancer. *British Journal of Cancer*, **23**, 1-8.
Doll, R. (1971) Oesophageal cancer: a preventable disease? In *International Seminar on the Epidemiology of Oesophageal Cancer*. Indian Cancer Society and UICC.
Doll, R. & Cook, P. (1967) Summarizing indices for comparison of cancer incidence data. *International Journal of Cancer*, **2**, 269-279.
Doll, R., Muir, C. & Waterhouse, J. (Ed.) (1970) *Cancer Incidence in Five Continents*. Vol. II. Berlin: Springer-Verlag.
Doll, R., Payne, P. & Waterhouse, J. (Ed.) (1966) *Cancer Incidence in Five Continents*. Vol. I. Berlin: Springer-Verlag.
Elgood, C.A. (1951) *A Medical History of Persia*. London: CUP.
Fernandez, N.A. (1975) Nutrition in Puerto Rico. *Cancer Research*, **35**, 3272-3291.
Gear, H.S. (1935) The incidence of tumours, benign and malignant, in hospital patients in China. *Chinese Medical Journal*, **49**, 261-272.
Hewer, T., Rose, E., Ghadirian, P., Castegnaro, M., Bartsch, H., Malazeille, C. & Day, N. (1978) Ingested mutagens from opium and tobacco pyrolysis products and cancer of the oesophagus. *Lancet*, **ii**, 494-496.
Higginson, J. & Oettlé, A.G. (1960) Cancer incidence in the Bantu and Cape Coloured Races of South Africa: report of a cancer survey in the Transvaal (1953-1955). *Journal of the National Cancer Institute*, **24**, 589-671.
Hirayama, T. (1971) An epidemiological study of cancer of the oesophagus in Japan, with special reference to the combined effect of selected environmental factors. In *International Seminar on the Epidemiology of Oesophageal Cancer*. Indian Cancer Society and UICC.
Hormozdiari, H., Day, N.E., Aramesh, B. & Mahboubi, E. (1975) Dietary factors and oesophageal cancer in the Caspian littoral of Iran. *Cancer Research*, **35**, 3493.
IARC (1968) *Internal Report*. Conference held to discuss future plans for research into the aetiology of cancer of the oesophagus.
IARC (1970) *Annual Report*. Lyon, France: World Health Organization.
IARC (1975) *Annual Report*. Lyon, France: World Health Organization.
IARC (1976) *Annual Report*. Lyon, France: World Health Organization.
IARC (1978) *Annual Report*. Lyon, France: World Health Organization.
Iran-IARC, Joint Study Group (1977) Oesophageal cancer studies in the Caspian littoral of Iran: results of population studies— a prodrome. *Journal of the National Cancer Institute*, **59**, 1127-1138.
Kaplan, H.S. & Tsuchitani, P.J. (Ed.) (1978) *Cancer in China*. New York: Alan R. Liss.
Keen, P. (1971) An apparent epidemic of oesophageal cancer in southern Africa. In *International Seminar on the Epidemiology of Oesophageal Cancer*. Indian Cancer Society and UICC.

Kmet, J. & Mahboubi, E. (1972) Oesophageal cancer in the Caspian littoral of Iran: initial studies. *Science*, **175**, 846-853.

Kmet, J., McLaren, D.S. & Siassi, F. (1980) Epidemiology of oesophageal cancer with special reference to nutritional studies among the Turkoman of Iran. In *Advances in Modern Human Nutrition*, in press.

Macrae, S.M. & Cook, B.V. (1975) A retrospective study of the cancer patterns among hospital in-patients in Botswana 1960-72. *British Journal of Cancer*, **32**, 121-133.

Macvicar, N. (1925) *South African Medical Record*, **23**, 315.

Magee, P.N. & Barnes, J.M. (1967) Carcinogenic nitroso compounds. *Advances in Cancer Research*, **10**, 168-193.

Mahboubi, E., Kmet, J., Cook, P., Day, N.E., Ghadirian, P. & Salmasizadeh, S. (1973) Oesophageal cancer studies in the Caspian littoral of Iran: the Caspian Cancer Registry. *British Journal of Cancer*, **28**, 197-214.

Martinez, I. (1969) Factors associated with cancer of the oesophagus, mouth and pharynx in Puerto Rico. *Journal of the National Cancer Institute*, **42**, 1069-1094.

McGlashan, N.D. (1969) Oesophageal cancer and alcoholic spirits in central Africa. *Gut*, **10**, 643-650.

McGlashan, N.D., Patterson, R.L.S. & Williams, A.A. (1970) *N*-Nitrosamines and grain-based spirits. *Lancet*, **ii**, 1138.

McGlashan, N.D., Walters, C.L. & McLean, A.E.M. (1968) Nitrosamines in African alcoholic spirits and oesophageal cancer. *Lancet*, **ii**, 1017.

Miller, R.W. (1978) Epidemiology. In *Cancer in China* (Ed.) Kaplan, H.S. & Tsuchitani, P.J. New York: Alan R. Liss.

Oettlé, A.G. (1963) Regional variations in the frequency of Bantu oesophageal cancer cases admitted to hospitals in South Africa. *South African Medical Journal*, **37**, 434-439.

Prates, M.D. & Torres, F.O. (1965) A cancer survey in Lourenco Marques. *Journal of the National Cancer Institute*, **35**, 729-757.

Robertson, M.A., Harington, J.S. & Bradshaw, E. (1971) The cancer pattern in Africans at Baragwanath Hospital, Johannesburg. *British Journal of Cancer*, **25**, 377-384.

Rose, E.F. (1968) Carcinogenesis and oesophageal insults. *South African Medical Journal*, **42**, 334-336.

Rose, E.F. (1967) A study of oesophageal cancer in the Transkei. *National Cancer Institute Monograph*, No. 25, 83-96.

Rose, E.F. (1973) Oesophageal cancer in the Transkei: 1955-69. *Journal of the National Cancer Institute*, **51**, 7-16.

Rose, E.F. (1978) The interplay of factors determining a cancer pattern. *Progress in Experimental Tumour Research*, **12**, 95-101.

Rose, E.F. (1979) The role of demographic risk factors in carcinogenesis. In *Prevention and Detection of Cancer* (Ed.) Nieburgs, H.E. pp. 25-45. New York: Marcel Dekker.

Rose, E.F. & McGlashan, N.D. (1975) The spatial distribution of oesophageal carcinoma in the Transkei, South Africa. *British Journal of Cancer*, **31**, 197-206.

Rose, E.F. & Procter, D.S.C. (1970) The Butterworth Diagnostic Clinic for oesophageal cancer. *Suid-Afrikaanse Mediese Tydskrip*, **44**, 1199-1203.

Schoenberg, B.S., Bailar, J.C. & Fraumeni, J.F. (1971) Certain mortality patterns of oesophageal cancer in the United States, 1930-1967. *Journal of the National Cancer Institute*, **46**, 63-73.

Schonland, M. & Bradshaw, E. (1968) Cancer in the Natal African and Indian 1964-66. *International Journal of Cancer*, **3**, 304-316.

Schonland, M. & Bradshaw, E. (1969) Oesophageal cancer in Natal Bantu: a review of 516 cases. *South African Medical Journal*, **43**, 1029-1031.

Schuyler, A. (1876) *Turkistan*. London: Sampson, Low, Marston, Searle and Rivington.

Sutherland, J.C. (1968) Cancer in a Mission Hospital in South Africa. *Cancer*, **22**, 471-481.

Templeton, A.C. (Ed.) (1973) *Tumours in a Tropical Country*. Berlin, Heidelburg and New York: Springer-Verlag.

Tuyns, A. (1970) Cancer of the oesophagus: further evidence of the relation to drinking habits in France. *International Journal of Cancer*, **5**, 152-156.

Tuyns, A. & Jensen, O.M. (1976) Aetiological factors in oesophageal cancer in France. In *IARC Annual Report*. Lyon: IARC.

Uganda Government (1963) *Report of the Spiritous Liquor Commission*. Uganda: Government Printer.
Vambery, A. (1869) *Travels in Central Asia*. London: John Murray.
Vint, F.W. (1935) Malignant disease in the natives of Kenya. *Lancet*, **ii**, 628-630.
Waterhouse, J.A.H. (1974) *Cancer Handbook of Epidemiology and Prognosis*. Edinburgh and London: Churchill Livingstone.
Waterhouse, J., Muir, C., Correa, P. & Powell, J. (Ed.) (1976) *Cancer Incidence in Five Continents*. Vol. III. Lyon: IARC Scientific Publications.
Wynder, E.L. & Bross, I.J. (1961) *Cancer*, **14**, 389.
Wynder, E.L. & Chan, P.C. (1970) The possible role of riboflavin deficiency in epithelial neoplasia. II. Effect on skin tumour development. *Cancer*, **26**, 1221-1224.
Wynder, E.L. & Klein, U.E. (1965) The possible role of riboflavin deficiency in deficiency in epithelial neoplasia. I. Epithelial changes in mice in simple deficiency. *Cancer*, **18**, 167-180.

17
Epidemiology and Pathology of Gastric Cancer

D.W. DAY

EPIDEMIOLOGY

On a global scale gastric cancer results in more deaths than any other form of malignant disease. In England and Wales it is the third most common fatal cancer behind those of the lung and colorectum and in 1973 there were 12 191 deaths from malignant neoplasms of the stomach, the vast majority of which were adenocarcinomas. This total accounted for just over 10 per cent of all deaths from malignant disease. The remainder of this discussion will be confined to adenocarcinoma of the stomach.

The facts which have emerged from epidemiological studies and which provide the clues to the aetiology of this important disease are as follows:

Age and sex incidence. Stomach cancer incidence and mortality rates rise steeply with age, showing a constant rate of increase. Men are more often affected by the disease than women, the ratio varying from approximately one in young adults to a maximum of two or more around the age of 60 and falling thereafter to approach unity again at advanced ages. It has been suggested that allowing for a latent interval this corresponds to differences in total calorie consumption between the sexes (Griffith, 1968).

This sex ratio shows little variation in different countries, unlike that of oesophageal carcinoma. When malignant tumours are subdivided according to their location within the stomach, however, there is more variation in the sex ratio and adenocarcinoma occurring at the cardia appears to have a higher male to female predominance than tumours at other sites (Sterup and Mosbech, 1971; MacDonald, 1972).

Geographical variation. There are large differences in the incidence of cancer in different countries. Thus there is an approximately 30-fold increase in the disease incidence in Japan and several Asian republics of the USSR, compared to large parts of rural Africa south of the Sahara. Within the continent of South America the frequency is high in Argentina, Brazil, Chile and Puerto Rico and relatively low in Guatemala, Mexico and Peru. Even inside countries, where reporting and classification of gastric cancer incidence and mortality can be assumed to be uniform, wide variations occur from area to area. For example, there are considerable differences in age-adjusted death rates within Japan (Hirayama, 1971), and in the countries of Latin America there is a tendency for populations in the central Andean region to be at higher risk than residents of the tropical zones. Similar differences have been reported from low-incidence countries (Wynder et al, 1963; Segi and Kurihara, 1966).

Variations of incidence and mortality with time. Striking reductions in the incidence and mortality of the disease with time have occurred in many developed countries (Haenszel, 1958; Hakama, 1972; Clemmesen, 1977), apparently unaccounted for by such factors as more precise diagnosis, changes in age distribution of the population or in the ratio of foreign-born to indigenous groups. The decline has been most marked in the United States where gastric cancer was the major cancer 45 years ago and where the age-adjusted mortality rate in males dropped from 28 per 100 000 in 1930 to 9.7 per 100 000 in 1967. In Japan the decline has occurred more recently, the decrease in stomach cancer in males varying from 19 to 35 per cent in age-specific death rates between the years 1955 and 1973. Some, but not all, of this reduction can be attributed to the nationwide programme of early detection of stomach cancer (Hirayama, 1975).

Studies in migrants. Important recent advances in the epidemiology of stomach cancer have resulted from investigations of migrant populations. Thus studies of Japanese who have moved to the United States of America have shown a relatively slow fall in mortality from gastric cancer in the first generation, but the rate drops sharply in their offspring born in the USA (Buell and Dunn, 1965). In first-generation Japanese living in Hawaii those born in high-risk prefectures in Japan had a significantly higher risk of gastric cancer than those born in low-risk prefectures. This difference was not apparent in the next generation (Haenszel et al, 1972). On the other hand, the risks for large bowel cancer among these same migrants rose during their lifetime to approach the risk characteristic of the United States white host population. These findings highlight the importance of environmental factors in determining the incidence of gastric cancer. The fact that the migrants continue to have the high rates of their country of origin suggests either that they are exposed in young life to an exogenous agent which determines the later development of gastric cancer or alternatively that they retain their former way of life and in particular their dietary habits in the new country, whereas their offspring adopt the life-style of their birth place. It appears from analysis of these groups and from studies in Colombia, where migrants from high- to low-risk areas retain a high risk of gastric cancer (Correa et al, 1976), that factors acting in early life are important in determining the onset of disease later.

Variation with social class. A number of epidemiological investigations from different countries have shown a relationship of socioeconomic factors to gastric cancer mortality. In general, the lower the income, social class or living standard the higher the mortality from gastric cancer (Cohart, 1954; Stukonis and Doll, 1969). Studies have shown an increased number of deaths from gastric cancer associated with specific occupations. These include coal-mining (Matolo et al, 1972), working with asbestos fibres (Selikoff, Hammond and Churg, 1968; Enterline, DeCoufle and Henderson, 1972), and workers in the rubber industry (McMichael, Andjelkovic and Tyroler, 1976). However, it is probable that socioeconomic status is more important than specific occupational risk factors (Creagan, Hoover and Fraumeni, 1974) in accounting for excess risk of cancer in these groups.

Dietary influences. An obvious environmental influence and one subject to worldwide variation is food, and numerous studies have been made in an attempt to explain the peculiarities of gastric cancer distribution. The possible effects of diet in the causation of gastric cancer are:

1. the presence of carcinogens occurring naturally in food or of precursors which in vivo are converted into carcinogens;
2. the introduction of carcinogens in the preparation of food;
3. the absence of a protective factor or factors.

Dietary studies have tended to give confusing results since the long interval between exposure and onset of disease complicates the collection of reliable and relevant histories of food practices. It is known that the total calorie intake does not account for differences between countries with low and high gastric cancer mortalities.

General conclusions which have been reached from epidemiological studies on diet show an association of gastric cancer with a high consumption of starches and a reduced consumption of fat, fresh fruits and green, leafy vegetables. In Hawaii, Japanese stomach cancer patients drank significantly less milk than matched controls and ate a greater amount of pickled vegetables and dried, salted fish, the elevated risk being roughly proportional to the quantity of these foods eaten (Haenszel et al, 1972).

The possible importance of food preparation is also suggested by the studies of Dungal (1961) and Sigurjonsson (1967) in Iceland who found high levels of various polycyclic hydrocarbons in home-smoked mutton and trout eaten by farmers in whom the prevalence of gastric cancer was very high. In rats which were fed this smoked food tumours were induced, although not in the stomach. Merliss (1971) put forward the view that the high incidence of stomach cancer in Japanese could be explained by their consumption of rice to which commercial talc has been added to improve its flavour, the latter contaminated by asbestos. Talc crystals, but not asbestos fibres, have been demonstrated in the tumour cells of Japanese gastric cancer patients (Matsudo, Hodgkin and Tanaka, 1974).

Despite these associations between certain foods and increased risk no single item has been identified which is common to all high-risk areas. More consistent results have been obtained for foods associated with a decreased risk, such as lettuce or celery. It therefore seems likely that it is the interplay of dietary factors which is important, with protective as well as antagonistic effects.

There is current interest in the role which N-nitroso compounds may play in the aetiology of gastric carcinoma. In experimental animals, nitrosamines and nitrosamides are carcinogens in at least ten species (Sander, Burkle and Schweinsberg, 1972) and the stomach is among the organs affected. N-nitroso compounds may be formed in vivo by the interaction of nitrites and secondary amines or amides. Nitrosatable compounds occur naturally in many foods, particularly in fish and meat, or may be ingested as drugs (Lijinsky, 1974). The nitrosating nitrite and more importantly nitrate are present in vegetables, drinking water, and cured meat products to which nitrate or nitrite has been added as a preservative. It has been shown that considerable proportions of either endogenous nitrate or added nitrate are converted by bacteria to nitrite in food kept at room temperature for 24 hours, whereas at 2 °C nitrite formation is completely prevented for up to 72 hours (Weisburger and Raineri, 1975).

The N-nitrosation reaction is acid catalysed, but can be catalysed by bacteria at neutral pH values. It is inhibited by ascorbic acid. Bacterial colonization of the stomach may occur in chronic gastritis or following partial gastrectomy and gastroenterostomy (Drasar and Shiner, 1969). There are several reports of carcinoma developing in the gastric stump many years after gastric resection, and increased nitrite levels in the gastric juice have been found in post-gastrectomy patients (Jones, Davies and Savage, 1978). Urinary tract infections also result in the production of N-nitrosamines in the bladder and these could act secondarily on the stomach (Hicks et al, 1977).

As well as endogenous production, preformed N-nitroso compounds have been found in a wide range of foodstuffs, including cured meat products and fish, and in particular fried or grilled bacon. Epidemiological studies in Chile (Zaldivar and Robinson, 1973; Armijo and Coulson, 1975) have found a correlation between gastric cancer mortality and per capita usage of nitrogen fertilizer. An increased incidence of gastric cancer has been associated with high levels of nitrate in the drinking water supply in Narino, Colombia (Correa, Cuello and Duque, 1970), and Worksop, England (Hill, Hawksworth and Tattersall, 1973). The significance of these findings awaits precise measurements of the levels of exposure to nitrate and total nitrate intake in such populations.

Endogenous factors. Numerous studies have been carried out on the hereditary aspects of gastric carcinoma and an hereditary influence has been clearly demonstrated in the approximately 20 per cent increased liability of people of blood group A to have the disease compared with people of other blood groups (Aird and Bentall, 1953). There have been several reports of family aggregations of gastric cancer although most can be criticized on the basis of incomplete or inaccurate collection of the family data or the lack of suitable controls. Woolf (1961) studied both the blood relatives and the spouses of propositi with gastric cancer and found that there was a twofold increase in gastric cancer in blood relatives compared with controls, but no increase in spouses over their controls. Although this suggests that genetic factors are operating it does not exclude the possibility of environmental influences, since cancer patients and their spouses share a similar environment only during their married lives. The increased risk of gastric cancer in patients with pernicious anaemia is well established (Mosbech and Videbaek, 1950), as is the importance of heredity in pernicious anaemia.

PATHOLOGY

A lot of recent interest and research has involved epidemiological investigations of the histological patterns of stomach cancer. These investigations utilized the classification proposed by Laurén in 1965, and before the results of the studies are discussed a brief description of this classification will be given.

The Laurén classification. Based on a histological study of 1344 gastrectomy specimens collected at the University of Turku, Finland, between 1945 and 1964 this classification cuts across the classical descriptions and allocates gastric carcinoma into two main groups, intestinal type and diffuse type. The basis of this division is the histology and cytology, the secretion of mucus and the mode of growth of the two types.

In general terms, intestinal type carcinomas have a glandular pattern, usually accompanied by papillary formation or solid components, and are made up of rather large, pleomorphic cells with large, hyperchromatic nuclei often showing mitoses. Cells lining the glands are well polarized and columnar, and usually have a prominent brush border (Figure 1). Secretion, when present, tends to occur focally in the cytoplasm of scattered cells, or if extracellular, is located mostly in the gland lumens. Diffuse type carcinomas are composed of scattered solitary cells or small clusters of cells, and when of a more solid cellular appearance the individual cells are only loosely attached to each other (Figure 2). A glandular structure is uncommon and if present the glands are poorly formed. The individual cells are small and uniform with indistinct cytoplasm and regular, often pyknotic, nuclei without many mitoses. In the occasional tumours with a glandular structure the lining cells are unpolarized and when a surface brush border is present it is sparse and uneven. Nearly all these tumours show extensive areas where there is intracellular mucin and this is evenly distributed throughout the cytoplasm. If extracellular, secreted mucin is dispersed in the stroma.

The mode of growth in the two types of tumour varies. Intestinal carcinomas are mostly well defined and show variation in structure of the tumour between the centre and the periphery. Inflammatory cell infiltration is usually profuse. Diffuse carcinomas are more uniform in structure and not so well defined, with a tendency to spread widely in the submucosa. Connective tissue proliferation is more marked and inflammatory cell infiltration less prominent than in intestinal carcinomas.

In both groups solid and mucinous tumours occur but can be distinguished on structural grounds.

Of the total series of tumours, 53 per cent were intestinal, 33 per cent diffuse and the remaining 14 per cent unclassified.

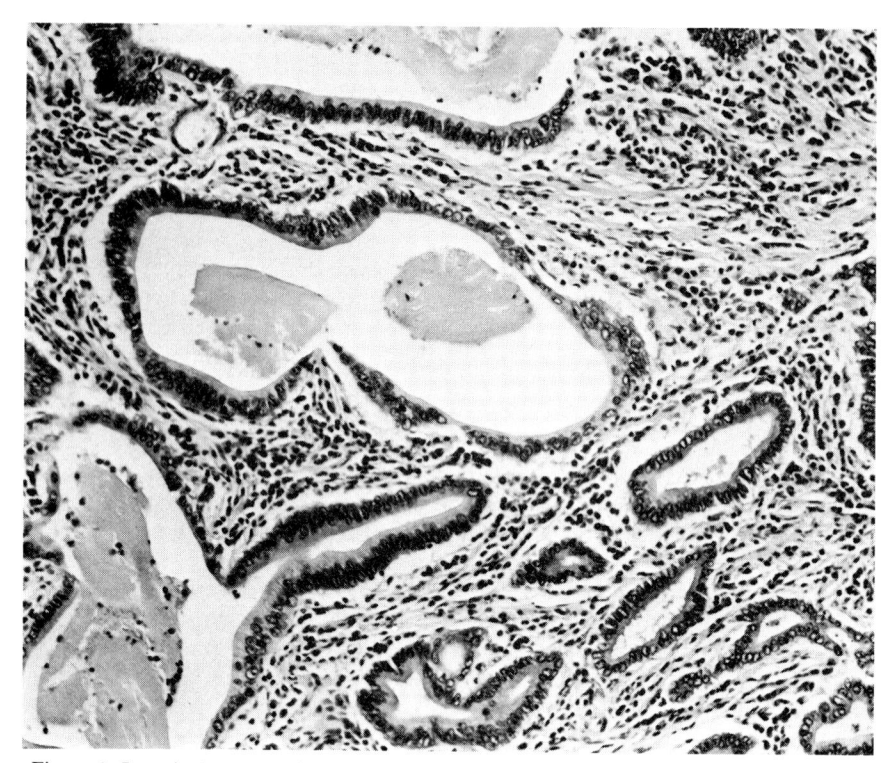

Figure 1. Intestinal type carcinoma. Glands lined by polarized columnar cells with a brush border. Inflammatory cell infiltration of the connective tissue stroma is a prominent feature. Haematoxylin and eosin, × 150.

Analysis of the two main groups showed a 2 to 1 male:female ratio in the intestinal group, the mean age of the patients being 55.4 years. With diffuse carcinomas the sex ratio was approximately one and the mean age of the patients 47.7 years. Macroscopically, 60 per cent of the intestinal type tumours were polypoid or fungating, 25 per cent excavated and 15 per cent infiltrating, whereas the corresponding figures for diffuse carcinoma were 31, 26 and 43 per cent. An important difference between the two groups was in the frequency of intestinal metaplasia, that is the change which occurs in association with chronic inflammation and glandular atrophy of the mucosa of the stomach and results in an epithelium which has the morphological, histochemical and ultrastructural characteristics of intestinal mucosa (Figure 3). It was present more often and was more extensive in the adjacent mucosa of intestinal type tumours than in diffuse carcinomas. Of the 153 patients who received curative treatment the prognosis was slightly better with intestinal type tumours where the three-year survival was 43 per cent compared with 35 per cent with diffuse tumours.

On the basis of these pathological and clinical differences Laurén suggested that the aetiology and pathogenesis of the two types of gastric carcinoma might be different.

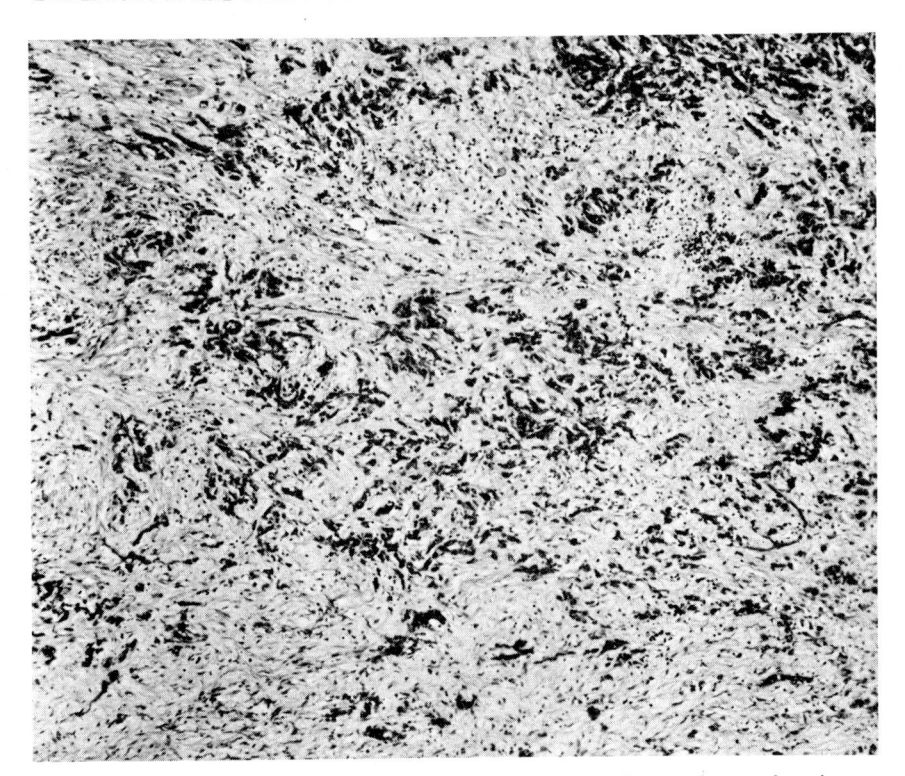

Figure 2. Diffuse type carcinoma. Individual and small loosely adherent clumps of carcinoma cells are dispersed in a connective tissue stroma. Only occasional inflammatory cells are present. Haematoxylin and eosin, × 50.

Epidemiology-pathology studies. Several investigations have been carried out exploring the possibility that variation in gastric cancer rates with place and time might be related to changes in the frequency of intestinal-type gastric cancers. Analysis of histological material from Cali in Colombia, where the incidence of gastric cancer is high, and from three low-risk cities in Colombia and Mexico showed that the proportion of gastric cancers of intestinal type was greatest in Cali (Muñoz et al, 1968). Subsequent study of stomach cancer deaths in Cali indicated that the intestinal type tumours accounted for most of the excess incidence among individuals who had migrated from rural areas in the South of Colombia (Correa, Cuello and Duque, 1970). A comparison of the pathology of stomach cancer in Miyagi prefecture in Japan and of Japanese Hawaiians showed that the estimated incidence rates for diffuse carcinoma differed little between the two areas and that the disparity in overall incidence was concentrated in the intestinal, mixed and other groups which were much reduced in Hawaii. Age-incidence slopes of the two main types were different and an association with blood group A was limited to diffuse type carcinomas (Correa et al, 1973). However, contradictory results have been obtained by Kubo (1973) in a study of material from the low-incidence areas of Minnesota, USA, and New Zealand,

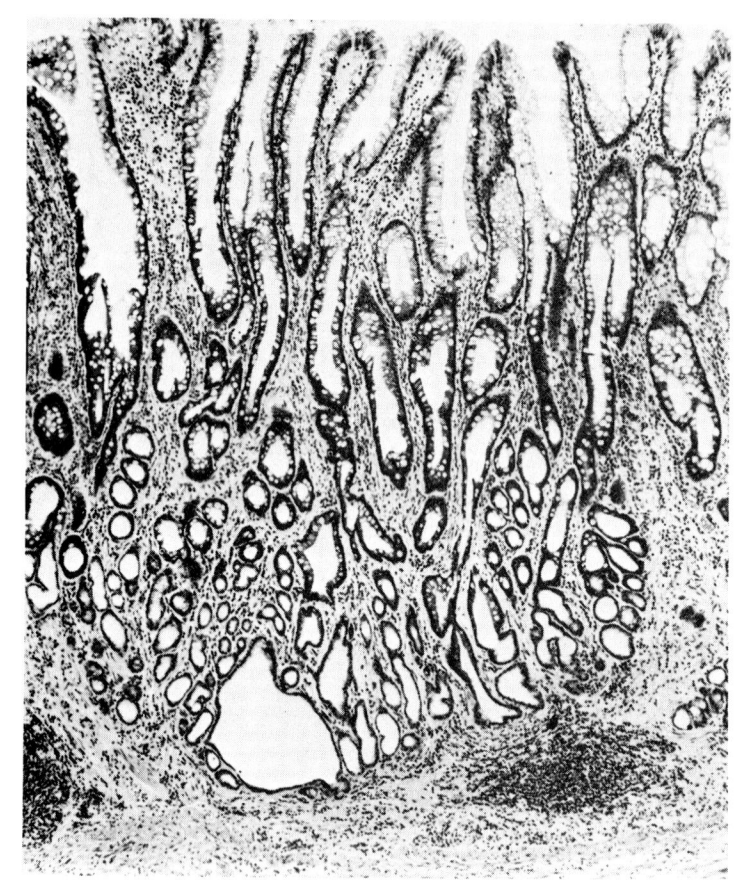

Figure 3. Atrophic gastritis with intestinal metaplasia. Haematoxylin and eosin, × 60.

and from the high-incidence areas of Korea and Kyushu, Japan, who found that the age-sex specific proportions of diffuse-type gastric cancer in these different populations did not vary. An investigation in Northern Nigeria, where gastric cancer is uncommon, showed a predominance of the intestinal type in all age groups and both sexes (Mabogunje, Subbuswamy and Lawrie, 1978).

This conflicting evidence indicates the need for further checks and standardization of criteria, particularly in interpopulation studies.

In summary, although epidemiological studies have provided many clues the principal causes of gastric cancer remain unknown. This is largely related to the fact that environmental influences which initiate carcinogenesis in a susceptible individual occur many years prior to diagnosis or death from the disease, at which time detection or measurement of exposure to such influences may not be possible. The link between cause and effect becomes less tenuous if precursor lesions can be identified. It is known that people with the histological appearance of atrophic gastritis, consisting of variable inflammation, atrophy of gastric glands and, often, associated intestinal metaplasia, are statistically at increased risk of developing gastric cancer (Siurala, Varis and Wiljasalo, 1966; Correa et al, 1976) and studies have been carried out in which these changes have been used as epidemiological markers for gastric cancer (Correa, Cuello and Duque, 1970; Correa et al, 1976; Haenszel et al, 1976). In high-risk areas, however, a large proportion of the population may be affected and more discrimination may be achieved by the histochemical identification of subgroups of intestinal metaplasia which have increased malignant potential (Teglbjaerg and Nielsen, 1978; Jass and Filipe, 1979) and by the detection and follow-up of people with epithelial dysplasia of the gastric mucosa (Ming, 1979; Morson et al, 1980).

REFERENCES

Aird, I. & Bentall, H.H. (1953) A relationship between cancer of stomach and ABO blood groups. *British Medical Journal*, **i**, 799-801.

Armijo, R. & Coulson, A.H. (1975) Epidemiology of stomach cancer in Chile — the role of nitrogen fertilisers. *International Journal of Epidemiology*, **4**, 301-309.

Buell, P. & Dunn, Jr, J.E. (1965) Cancer mortality among Japanese Issei and Nisei of California. *Cancer*, **18**, 656-664.

Clemmesen, J. (1977) Statistical studies in the aetiology of malignant neoplasma. Trends and risks — Denmark 1943-1972. *Acta Pathologica et Microbiologica Scandinavica* (Suppl.), **261**, 1-286.

Cohart, E.M. (1954) Socioeconomic distribution of stomach cancer in New Haven. *Cancer*, **7**, 455-461.

Correa, P., Cuello, C. & Duque, E. (1970) Carcinoma and intestinal metaplasia of the stomach in Colombian migrants. *Journal of the National Cancer Institute*, **44**, 297-306.

Correa, P., Sasano, N., Stemmermann, G.N. & Haenszel, W. (1973) Pathology of gastric carcinoma in Japanese populations: comparisons between Miyagi prefecture, Japan and Hawaii. *Journal of the National Cancer Institute*, **51**, 1449-1457.

Correa, P., Cuello, C., Duque, E., Burbano, L.C., Garcia, F.T., Bolanos, O., Brown, C. & Haenszel, W. (1976) Gastric cancer in Colombia. III. Natural history of precursor lesions. *Journal of the National Cancer Institute*, **57**, 1027-1035.

Creagan, E.T., Hoover, R.M. & Fraumeni, J.F. (1974) Mortality from stomach cancer in coal mining regions. *Archives of Environmental Health*, **28**, 28-30.

Drasar, B.S. & Shiner, M. (1969) Studies on the intestinal flora. Part II. Bacterial flora of the small intestine in patients with gastrointestinal disorders. *Gut*, **10**, 812-819.

Dungal, N. (1961) The special problem of stomach cancer in Iceland, with particular reference to dietary factors. *Journal of the American Medical Association*, **178**, 789-798.

Enterline, P., DeCoufle, P. & Henderson, V. (1972) Mortality in relation to occupational exposure in the asbestos industry. *Journal of Occupational Medicine*, **14**, 897-903.

Griffith, G.W. (1968) The sex ratio in gastric cancer and hypothetical considerations relative to aetiology. *British Journal of Cancer*, **22**, 163-172.

Haenszel, W. (1958) Variation in incidence of and mortality from stomach cancer, with particular reference to the United States. *Journal of the National Cancer Institute*, **21**, 213-262.

Haenszel, W., Kurihara, M., Segi, M. & Lee, R.K.C. (1972) Stomach cancer among Japanese in Hawaii. *Journal of the National Cancer Institute*, **49**, 969-988.

Haenszel, W., Correa, P., Cuello, C., Guzman, N., Burbano, L.C., Lores, H. & Muñoz, J. (1976) Gastric cancer in Colombia. II. Case control epidemiologic study of precursor lesions. *Journal of the National Cancer Institute*, **57**, 1021-1026.

Hakama, M. (1972) Trends in stomach cancer incidence for male cohorts in Finland. *Annals of Clinical Research*, **4**, 300-403.

Hicks, R.M., Walters, C.L., Elsebai, I., El Aasser, A.-B., El Merzabani, M. & Gough, T.A. (1977) Demonstration of nitrosamines in human urine: preliminary observations on a possible aetiology for bladder cancer in association with chronic urinary tract infections. *Proceedings of the Royal Society of Medicine*, 70, 413-417.

Hill, M.J., Hawksworth, G. & Tattersall, G. (1973) Bacteria, nitrosamines and cancer of the stomach. *British Journal of Cancer*, 28, 562-567.

Hirayama, T. (1971) Epidemiology of stomach cancer. In *Early Gastric Cancer* (Gann Monograph on Cancer Research 11) (Ed.) Murakami, T. p. 3. Tokyo: University of Tokyo Press.

Hirayama, T. (1975) Epidemiology of cancer of the stomach with special reference to its recent decrease in Japan. *Cancer Research*, 35, 3460-3463.

Jass, J.R. & Filipe, M.I. (1979) Variants of intestinal metaplasia associated with gastric carcinoma. A histochemical study. *Histopathology*, 3, 191-199.

Jones, S.M., Davies, P.W. & Savage, A. (1978) Gastric-juice nitrite and gastric cancer. *Lancet*, i, 1355.

Kubo, T. (1973) Gastric carcinoma in New Zealand. Some epidemiologic-pathologic aspects. *Cancer*, 31, 1498-1507.

Laurén, P. (1965) The two histological main types of gastric carcinoma: diffuse and so-called intestinal-type carcinoma. An attempt at a histo-clinical classification. *Acta Pathologica et Microbiologica Scandinavica*, 64, 31-49.

Lijinsky, W. (1974) Reaction of drugs with nitrous acid as a source of carcinogenic nitrosamines. *Cancer Research*, 34, 255-258.

Mabogunje, O.A., Subbuswamy, S.G. & Lawrie, J.H. (1978) The two histological types of gastric carcinoma in Northern Nigeria. *Gut*, 19, 425-429.

MacDonald, W.C. (1972) Clinical and pathological features of adenocarcinoma of the gastric cardia. *Cancer*, 29, 724-732.

Matolo, N.M., Klauber, M.R., Gorishek, W.M. & Dixon, J.A. (1972) High incidence of gastric carcinoma in a coal mining region. *Cancer*, 29, 733-737.

Matsudo, H., Hodgkin, N.M. & Tanaka, A. (1974) Japanese gastric cancer. Potentially carcinogenic silicates (talc) from rice. *Archives of Pathology*, 97, 366-368.

McMichael, A.J., Andjelkovic, D.A. & Tyroler, H.A. (1976) Cancer mortality among rubber workers: an epidemiologic study. *Annals of the New York Academy of Sciences*, 271, 125-142.

Merliss, R.R. (1971) Talc-treated rice and Japanese stomach cancer. *Science*, 173, 1141-1142.

Ming, S.-C. (1979) Dysplasia of gastric epithelium. *Frontiers of Gastrointestinal Research*, 4, 164-172.

Morson, B.C., Sobin, L.H., Grundmann, E., Johansen, A., Nagayo, T. & Serck-Hanssen, A. (1980) Precancerous conditions and epithelial dysplasia in the stomach. *Journal of Clinical Pathology*, in press.

Mosbech, J. & Videbaek, A. (1950) Mortality from and risk of gastric carcinoma among patients with pernicious anaemia. *British Medical Journal*, ii, 390-394.

Muñoz, N., Correa, P., Cuello, C. & Duque, E. (1968) Histologic types of gastric carcinoma in high- and low-risk areas. *International Journal of Cancer*, 3, 809-818.

Sander, J., Burkle, G. & Schweinsberg, F. (1972) Induction of tumours by nitrite and secondary amines or amides. In *Topics in Chemical Carcinogenesis* (Ed.) Nakahara, W., Takayama, S., Sujimura, T. & Odashima, S. pp. 292-312. Baltimore: University Park Press.

Segi, M. & Kurihara, M. (1966) *Cancer Mortality for Selected Sites in 24 Countries, No. 4 (1962-1963)*. Sendai: Department of Public Health, Tohoku University School of Medicine.

Selikoff, I.J., Hammond, E.C. & Churg, J. (1968) Asbestos exposure, smoking and neoplasia. *Journal of the American Medical Association*, 204, 104-110.

Sigurjonsson, J. (1967) Occupational variations in mortality from gastric cancer in relation to dietary differences. *British Journal of Cancer*, 21, 651-656.

Siurala, M., Varis, K. & Wiljasalo, M. (1966) Studies of patients with atrophic gastritis: A 10-15 year follow-up. *Scandinavian Journal of Gastroenterology*, 1, 40-48.

Sterup, K. & Mosbech, J. (1971) Sex ratio of gastric cancer related to site of the tumour. *Scandinavian Journal of Gastroenterology* (Suppl.), 9, 87-89.

Stukonis, M. & Doll, R. (1969) Gastric cancer in man and physical activity at work. *International Journal of Cancer*, 4, 248-254.

Teglbjaerg, P.S. & Nielsen, H.O. (1978) 'Small intestinal type' and 'colonic type' intestinal metaplasia of the stomach. *Acta Pathologica et Microbiologica Scandinavica*, **86**, 351-355.

Weisburger, J.H. & Raineri, R. (1975) Dietary factors and the etiology of gastric cancer. *Cancer Research*, **35**, 3469-3474.

Woolf, C.M. (1961) The incidence of cancer in the spouses of stomach cancer patients. *Cancer*, **14**, 199-200.

Wynder, E.L., Kmet, J., Dungal, N. & Segi, M. (1963) An epidemiological investigation of gastric cancer. *Cancer*, **16**, 1461-1496.

Zaldivar, R. & Robinson, H. (1973) Epidemiological investigation on stomach cancer mortality in Chileans: association with nitrate fertiliser. *Zeitschrift für Krebsforschung und Klinische Onkologie*, **80**, 289-295.

18

The Aetiology of Colorectal Cancer

M.J. HILL

Large bowel cancer has been described as a disease of Western civilization and is, indeed, common in Western countries and rare in black Africa, Asia, Central America and the Andean countries of South America. The epidemiology of the disease has been extensively reviewed elsewhere (Haenszel and Correa, 1973; Hill, 1975a, 1979, Wynder, 1975, Kassira, Parent and Vahouny, 1976). Although there are some voices to the contrary (e.g., Enstrom, 1975) most epidemiologists agree that diet is important in the aetiology of the disease; however, there is no agreement concerning which component of the diet is the most important. A summary of the components of the diet incriminated in the disease has been given by Hill (1979); it is an impressive list!

In order to explain this correlation there has been an extensive search for carcinogens preformed in the diet. This search has been successful in that many have been detected (e.g., polycyclic hydrocarbons, N-nitroso compounds, aflatoxins and other mycotoxins, harman, nor-harman and other such products of cooking); however, none of these correlates with the risk of colorectal carcinogenesis. In 1967, therefore, we commenced studies on our hypothesis that the carcinogen or promoter responsible for the disease was formed in situ in the colon by bacterial action on some benign substrate.

BACTERIAL PRODUCTION OF CARCINOGENS

In testing this hypothesis we have examined a wide range of bacterial metabolites (reviewed by Hill, 1977a, 1977b) and have concluded that the best evidence implicates metabolites of the bile acids.

Substrate

A considerable amount of work has been carried out on the possible role of bile acids in human colorectal carcinogenesis. In studies comparing populations in different countries or within a country there was a correlation between faecal bile acid (FBA) concentration and incidence of colorectal cancer (Table 1). There have been two exceptions to this. An IARC working

© 1980 W.B. Saunders Company Ltd.

Table 1. *The relationship between faecal bile acid concentration and large bowel cancer incidence in studies of various populations*

Populations studied	Relationships observed	Reference
England, Scotland, USA, India, Uganda, Japan	Good correlation with FBA concentration	Hill et al (1971)
Americans, Chinese, Japanese and 7th Day Adventists in New York	Good correlation with FBA concentration	Wynder and Reddy (1974)
Three income groups in Hong Kong	Good correlation with FBA concentration	Crowther et al (1976)
Kuopio, Finland, and New York	Good correlation with FBA concentration	Wynder and Reddy (1978)
Kuopio and Copenhagen	Poor correlation with FBA concentration	IARC Working Party (1977)
Rural and urban Finland and rural and urban Denmark	Good correlation with FBA concentration	IARC Working Party (1980, in preparation)
Japanese living in Hawaii and in Japan	Poor correlation with FBA concentration	Mower et al (1979)

party (1977) compared populations in Finland and Denmark with a fourfold difference in bowel cancer incidence and found only a small difference in FBA concentration; however, in a subsequent more extensive study a good correlation between FBA concentration and incidence of the disease was observed (IARC Working Party, 1980, in preparation). In the second, a comparison of Japanese living in Hawaii with those living in Japan again showed little difference in FBA concentration. A feature of this study was the high concentration of chenodeoxycholic acid reported. This is very unusual since this acid is readily degraded to lithocholic acid and so is normally present only in very small amounts.

There have been several case-control studies. In our own study (Hill et al, 1975) we compared persons with large bowel cancer with persons having non-malignant gastrointestinal disease and showed that the FBA concentration was greater in the persons with large bowel cancer. Reddy and Wynder (1977) obtained similar results when they compared colorectal cancer cases with healthy control persons (Table 2) but in three other studies no difference, or even a lower FBA concentration in the bowel cancer cases, was observed (Blackwood et al, 1978; Moskovitz, White and Floch, 1978; Mudd et al, 1978).

A possible clue to the reasons for this discrepancy was provided by Moskovitz, White and Floch who noted that, in their non-gastrointestinal cancer patients, the FBA concentration was very much lower in those with liver involvement. We have continued our study of bowel cancer cases and, following this observation, have re-analysed our cases on the basis of Dukes' classification and the subsite of the tumour (Table 3). In addition, we have compared our cases with normal healthy controls. We are following up these

Table 2. *Case control studies of the relation between faecal bile acids and bowel cancer*

Number and type of cases	Number and type of control	FBA in cases/controls	Reference
Colorectal (44)	Non-malignant bowel disease (99)	> 1	Hill et al (1975)
Colon	Normal controls	> 1	Reddy and Wynder (1977)
Colorectal	Normal controls	< 1	Blackwood et al (1978)
	Normal controls	~ 1	Mudd et al (1978)
Colorectal	Normal controls and non GI cancer cases	< 1	Moskowitz, White and Floch (1978)

patients postoperatively and, consequently, we have been rejecting those cases with a poor prognosis and so have only a small number of cases with liver metastases; these all had relatively low FBA concentrations. In contrast, 79 per cent of Dukes A and 60 per cent of Dukes B cases had high FBA concentrations (defined as the upper 20 per cent of the normal FBA range in healthy persons). It is possible, therefore, that a high FBA concentration can be observed only in relatively early cases.

In contrast to the studies on humans the experiments carried out using the animal model have unambiguously supported a role for FBAs in colorectal

Table 3. *FBA concentration and NDC carriage in patients with large bowel cancer by subsite and by Dukes' classification*

	Number assayed	FBA concentration (mg/g dry wt)	% carrying NDC	% with high FBA/NDC[a]
All colorectal cancers	84			
Dukes A	17	10.6	88	77
Dukes B	36	10.7	72	52
Dukes C	25	9.6	80	32
Dukes C2	6	7.7	50	0
All colon cancers	30	10.6	80	47
caecum + asc. + trans.	10	9.0	80	30
desc. + sigmoid	20	11.4	80	55
All rectal cancers	38	10.3	79	58
upper third	13	10.3	85	61
mid third	12	10.8	67	42
lower third	13	10.0	85	46
Normal healthy persons		7.9	35-40	8-10

[a] 'High FBA' is above the level of the 80th percentile in a normal healthy British population (this is currently 9.9 mg/g dry weight of faeces).
asc. = ascending; trans. = transverse; desc. = descending.

carcinogenesis following dimethylhydrazine initiation (Table 4). In this, I include only those studies in which either FBA concentrations were measured or the effect of dietary change on FBA concentration is known.

There has been a lot of discussion (Cruse et al, 1978; Cruse, Lewin and

Table 4. *Studies, using dimethylhydrazine-induced carcinogenesis in rats, on the role of FBA in colorectal carcinogenesis*

Manipulation	Effect on FBA concentration	Effect on colorectal carcinogenesis
Diet change		
added fat	Increase	Increase
added meat	Increase	Increase
added pectin	Increase	Increase
added bran	Decrease	Decrease
added lactulose	Decreased metabolism	Decrease
Vivonex diet	Decrease	Decrease
Administration of cholestyramine	Increase	Increase
Bile diversion to caecum	Increase	Increase
Diversion of faecal stream	Decrease	Decrease

Clark, 1979a, 1979b) of an experiment in which rats treated with dimethylhydrazine were fed an elemental diet alone or supplemented with cholesterol; those fed the cholesterol supplement had a higher incidence of tumours. On the basis of this single experiment (using highly artificial conditions even in the context of a highly artificial animal model) other hypotheses have been dismissed and cholesterol put forward as the major aetiological agent in colorectal carcinogenesis. Table 5 summarizes the evidence from human studies on the role of cholesterol or its metabolites in

Table 5. *The relationship between faecal neutral steroid (FNS) output and metabolism and the incidence of large bowel cancer (LBC)*

Type of study	Results	Reference
International comparison of six populations	Correlation between total FNS and LBC; no relation with metabolism	Hill et al (1971)
Four populations within New York	Correlation between LBC and total FNS; no relation with metabolism of FNS	Wynder and Reddy (1974)
Three income groups in Hong Kong	Little relation between LBC and FNS or metabolism of FNS	Crowther et al (1976)
Four populations in Scandinavia	Inverse relation with total FNS; no relation with metabolism of FNS	IARC Working Party (1980, in preparation)
Case-control study	No relation with total FNS or metabolism of FNS	Hill et al (1975)

the causation of colorectal cancer. It is far from overwhelming. The comparison of bowel cancer cases and controls is given in more detail in Table 6. The relationship between cholesterol metabolites and bowel cancer, suggested by Wilkins and Hackman (1974), has been discussed elsewhere (Hill, 1977b, 1977c).

In my opinion the evidence overwhelmingly favours a role for bile acids rather than neutral steroids.

Table 6. *Faecal neutral steroids in large bowel cancer cases compared with control patients*

	Faecal neutral steroid concentration (mg/g dry wt)	% as the bacterial metabolites
Large bowel cancer cases	22.4	64
Other large bowel disease	21.4	60
Controls with disease other than of the large bowel	19.5	62

Postulated product of bacterial metabolism

In our original postulate (Hill et al, 1971) we noted that in in vitro experiments deoxycholic acid may be converted to the very potent carcinogen 20-methylcholanthrene. Following the report by Coombs and Croft (1969) of the carcinogenicity of a range of substituted cyclopentaphenanthrenes I suggested a pathway, theoretically possible, by which intestinal bacteria might produce such a molecule using only four types of nuclear dehydrogenation reaction (Hill and Drasar, 1974). On further consideration, and in the light of further data on the carcinogenicity of partially unsaturated polycyclic compounds, I have modified my views even further and now favour a moiety with only one or two double bonds (Hill, 1975b, 1977c).

Only certain clostridia of the human gut bacterial flora are able readily under anaerobic conditions to introduce double bonds into the bile acid nucleus (Goddard et al, 1975) unless the bile acids are used as the sole carbon source (Barnes et al, 1975). By using a deliberately crude assay system we are able to divide persons into carriers or non-carriers of nuclear dehydrogenating clostridia (NDC). In our hands 35 to 50 per cent of populations in North West Europe carry NDC and this result has been confirmed by Blackwood et al (1978) and by Laurell and his co-workers (IARC Working Party, 1977). Populations in Japan, India, Uganda and Nigeria, which have a low incidence of colorectal cancer, contain very few NDC carriers. In our case-control study 83 per cent of our colorectal cancer cases carried NDC compared with only 43 per cent of control persons (see Table 3); a similar result has been obtained by Blackwood et al (1978).

There have been several reports in which groups have obtained different results from those described above by using different methods. Floch and his co-workers (Moskowitz, White and Floch, 1978) examined the numbers of all clostridia per gram of faeces in colorectal cancer cases and in controls and found no difference; we have obtained similar results when we, too, include the non-NDC together with the NDC, but this is hardly relevant. Moore and Holdeman (1975) and Finegold et al (1975) used classical bacteriological techniques to identify and quantitate large numbers of different species of clostridia and were unable to detect any difference between colorectal cancer or high risk cases and controls. We have not attempted to confirm these observations but unreservedly accept these findings; unfortunately, neither of these two groups attempted to assay the ability of any of their strains to desaturate the steroid nucleus. Hedges, Hedges and Reddy (1978) demonstrated that NDC could readily be demonstrated in faecal samples which had been first frozen then heat-shocked to activate spores when they appeared to be absent using classical techniques; if this is so then clearly the classical techniques are less efficient in detecting these clostridia and should therefore not be used in studies of these organisms.

We have assayed NDC in various groups of patients with diseases which put them at increased risk of developing LBC. Patients with intestinal polyps have a carriage rate of NDC similar to that in healthy control persons (Table 7); however, when classified by size and type of polyp, persons with small

Table 7. *Mean FBA concentration and rate of NDC carriage in various groups of patients and controls*

Description of polyp	Number of persons studied	Mean FBA concentration (mg/g dry wt)	% carriers of NDC
All colorectal polyps	98	8.1	36
non-adenomatous polyps	19	6.8	31
all adenomas	79	8.4	37
adenomas diameter < 5 mm	20	6.6	20
6-10 mm	7	7.4	28
11-20 mm	30	8.7	54
> 20 mm	22	10.1	67
Tubular adenomas	36	8.1	36
Tubulovillous adenomas	11	8.4	45
Villous adenomas	17	9.4	59
Persons with chronic ulcerative colitis	79	7.7	29
those who later developed carcinoma or severe dysplasia	9	10.0	63

adenomas (which have a low malignant potential) have a low carriage rate whilst those with large adenomas (which have a high malignant potential) have a high carriage rate of NDC similar to that in large bowel cancer (LBC) patients. Similarly, persons who have had chronic ulcerative colitis for more than 10 years (and who therefore have a risk of LBC higher than that of the general population) have a normal carriage rate of NDC; however, those who have actually developed LBC or have developed precancer have a relatively high carriage rate of these organisms.

The value of a FBA/NDC discriminant

We have attempted to develop a discriminant based on the faecal bile acid concentration and the presence of NDC. If NDC are able to produce a carcinogen or a promoter from the bile acids, then persons will be at high risk only if they carry NDC and if they also have a high FBA concentration (defined arbitrarily as above the 80th percentile point in the distribution of FBA concentrations in normal control persons).

We have analysed our large bowel cancer cases and controls in this way (see Table 3); we have also divided the bowel cancer cases by subsite and by Dukes' classification. Clearly our discriminant characterizes patients with cancer of the rectum and left colon but is relatively poor in characterizing those whose tumour is in the caecum, ascending or transverse colon. Furthermore, although the numbers are very small, our discriminant does not characterize those patients with liver metastases at all. We are now testing the discriminant prospectively in a large population of persons aged 45 to 75 years; this study has been briefly described by Hill (1977c).

We believe that the bile acid metabolite produced by NDC is probably a cancer promoter. The mode of action of cancer initiators is relatively well understood but there are few data on the mechanism by which compounds promote carcinogenicity. It has been noted by Hecker (1980) that irritant action is a necessary but insufficient property of cancer promoters. Incidentally, Cruse, Lewin and Clark (1979a) used the irritant properties of bile acids as evidence *against* their being colorectal cancer promoters; its lack of irritancy was cited as evidence in favour of cholesterol being a promoter. In order to try to determine more exactly the role of bile acid metabolites in colorectal carcinogenicity, we have attempted to combine the evidence from metabolic epidemiology with that from histopathology. This led to our postulated aetiology of the adenoma-carcinoma sequence (Hill, Morson and Bussey, 1978).

HISTOPATHOLOGY OF COLORECTAL CARCINOGENESIS

Although there are some with other opinions, most pathologists agree that the majority (if not all) of colorectal cancers arise in pre-existing adenomas. If such adenomas could be prevented then the subsequent carcinomas would also be prevented; in some senses, therefore, if we are attempting to prevent cancer of the large bowel it might be more sensible to study the aetiology of the precursor colorectal adenomas. This, however, is far from simple, because most colorectal adenomas are unrecognized and unreported.

There have been few good studies of the incidence of large bowel adenomas, and these have been summarized by Correa (1978) and Hill (1978). In summary, large bowel adenomas are common in persons living in Western countries and less common in persons living in Africa, Asia and the Andean and Central American countries. This is similar to the geographical distribution of large bowel carcinomas. Migrants from Japan to California soon achieve an incidence of adenomas similar to that of native-born

Americans, indicating that the major aetiological agent in adenogenesis is environmental. Thus in our postulated adenoma-carcinoma sequence we have an environmental agent E_1 causing adenomas to form in previously normal mucosa (Figure 1).

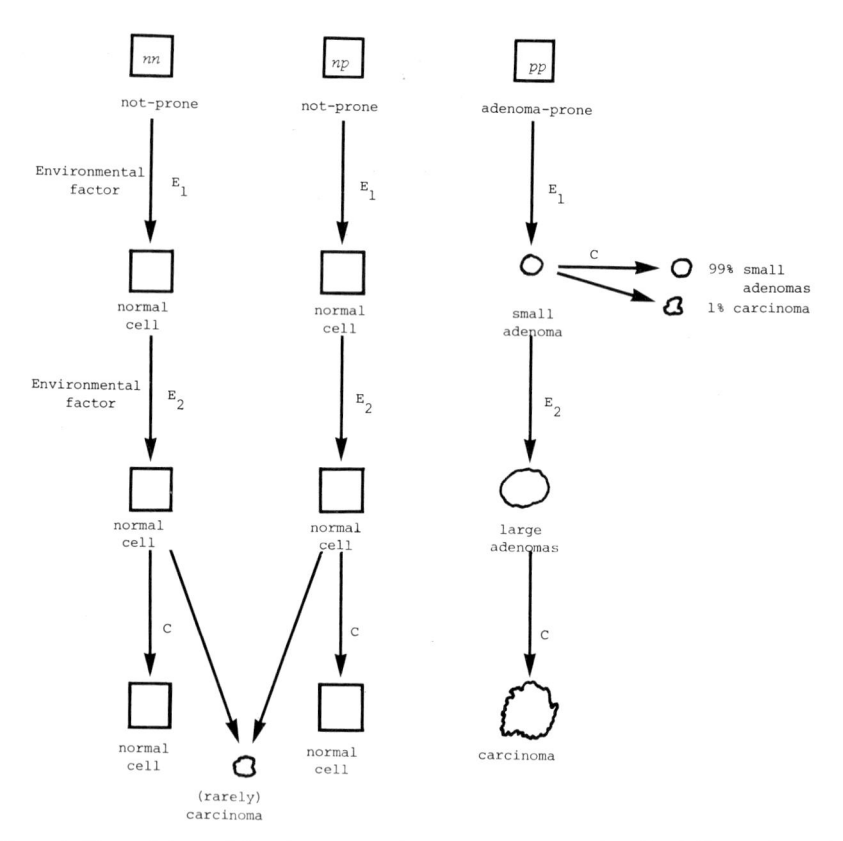

Figure 1. The aetiology of the adenoma-carcinoma sequence postulated by Hill, Morson and Bussey (1978).

In considering the next stage in the adenoma-carcinoma sequence, the evidence from the histopathogenesis of the disease (Table 8) is that carcinomas are very much more likely to arise in large adenomas than in small ones, and are much more likely to arise in villous than in tubular adenomas. Most other common types of polyps appear to have no malignant potential and need not be considered further. Consequently, in assessing the risk of an adenoma becoming malignant we need to consider its size and its 'villousness', and we need, therefore, a better understanding of the factors causing adenomas to grow and the factors determining their morphology. There is some evidence from epidemiology, Most Japanese, Iranian or Colombian adenomas are very small and adenomas greater that 2 cm in diameter are

THE AETIOLOGY OF COLORECTAL CANCER

Table 8. *The relationship between the malignant potential of an adenoma and size and histopathology*

Size and histopathology of the adenoma	Proportion of the total sample (%)	Proportion with a malignant component (%)
Diameter > 20 mm	17.3	46
10-20 mm	23.3	9.5
< 10 mm	59.4	1.3
Histological classification		
villous adenoma	9.7	40.7
intermediate type	15.3	22.5
tubular adenoma	75	4.8

Data from Morson (1974).

rare; in contrast, such large adenomas are relatively common in Western persons (Table 9). From the evidence of post-mortem studies large adenomas have a distribution along the colorectum similar to that of carcinomas and different from that of small adenomas. This difference in

Table 9. *Relative size distribution of adenomas studied by Muto et al (1977) in British and in Japanese persons*

	Size distribution of colorectal adenomas			
	Average	< 1 cm	1-2 cm	> 2 cm
England		59.4	23.3	17.3
Japan		80.8	14.9	4.3

distribution of carcinomas and adenomas along the colorectum indicates that the factor causing adenomas to become malignant differs from that which causes adenomas to arise in previously normal mucosa. This conclusion is supported by the difference in the incidence of adenomas in populations with a similar low incidence of colorectal cancer (Table 10). In our hypothesis, therefore, we postulate a factor E_2 which causes small adenomas (with a low malignant potential) to grow to a large size and with a high malignant potential; this factor differs from E_1.

Table 10. *The incidence of adenomas and of carcinomas in the large bowel of persons living in various countries*

Country	Prevalence of adenomas (%)	Incidence of carcinomas (per 100 000/year; age adjusted persons 35-64)
South Africa (blacks)	0	4.0
Iran	1	low
Colombia (Cali)	8.6	5.7
Japan	9	5.0

Data summarized by Hill (1978).

The final stage in carcinogenesis is rather more problematical. The malignant potential of large adenomas in various countries is similar (Table 11), indicating that the factor causing malignancy in adenomas is widespread and is as common in countries with a low incidence of colorectal cancer as in

Table 11. *The malignant potential of adenomas (by size) in three countries*

Diameter of adenoma	% of adenomas with a malignant component in various countries		
	England	Japan	Sweden
< 10 mm	1.7	1.7	3.6
10-20 mm	9.5	10.5	59.0
> 20 mm	46.1	41.7	

those countries with a high incidence. Furthermore, the malignant potential appears to be roughly related to the volume of the adenoma. It is known that there is a normal mutation rate in cells; perhaps a constant proportion of these give rise to malignancy, so that the risk of malignancy would be dependent on the number of adenomatous cells (i.e., the volume of the adenoma). If this is so, than we would need to postulate that the cells in an adenoma are very much more likely to undergo a malignant mutation than are normal mucosal cells, and that the cells in a villous adenoma are more likely to undergo such a mutation than are cells in a tubular adenoma. In our hypothesis we have called this final agent 'C' (for 'chance').

It has been noted that the relatives of an index case of colorectal cancer have an above-average risk of developing the disease (Lovett, 1974), indicating that there is a familial component to the aetiology of the disease. This component could be due to a shared environment (e.g., familial dietary tastes or recipes) or could be due to genetic factors. Veale (1965) postulated that there is an autosomal recessive gene, designated p, which confers 'adenoma proneness' on a person; on this hypothesis persons will be 'adenoma prone' (i.e., sensitive to agent E_1) only if they are pp, whilst persons who are pn or nn (n being the normal alternative to p) will not develop adenomas regardless of their level of exposure to E_1. This has been incorporated into Figure 1 although it has still to be demonstrated; in post-mortem series it is normally difficult to determine the blood relationships of persons because of the limited personal data collected. If true, however, it would mean that, although the incidence of colorectal adenomas is determined by the amount of E_1 in the environment, genetic factors determine which persons in a uniformly exposed population actually develop adenomas.

The nature of E_1 and E_2

There is a limited amount of data available which helps us to characterize factors E_1 and E_2. The geographical variation in the incidence of adenomas together with the increased incidence experienced by Japanese who migrate to California indicate that E_1 is an environmentally determined agent. The relatively even distribution of adenomas along the colorectum indicates that

E_1 is either delivered to the colorectal mucosa by the vascular system or else enters the large bowel in a form that requires little or no further metabolism (e.g., the enterohepatically circulated conjugates of polycyclic aromatic hydrocarbons, which merely require the action of bacterial β-glucuronidase — a very potent enzyme present in the caecum at high activity). Furthermore, it has been demonstrated that diversion of the faecal stream causes small adenomas to regress or disappear (Cole and Holden, 1959), indicating that the agent causing adenomas to form is luminal and also needs to be supplied continuously. There is preliminary evidence that a similar regression of adenomas can be achieved by the administration of ascorbic acid in a form which allows it to be released in the large bowel; this indicates that E_1 is sensitive to antioxidant. All of this is consistent with E_1 being the faecal mutagen described by Bruce and his colleagues (Wang et al, 1978).

In most countries outside of black Africa there is a very much greater incidence of adenomas than of carcinomas, indicating that most adenomas do not become malignant (although of course they all have a malignant potential). Under these circumstances, the rate-limiting step in the adenoma-carcinoma sequence is the rate of growth of adenomas (i.e., the availability of E_2). Consequently, the deductions made from the epidemiology of colorectal cancers will apply to E_2 and so we have much more information about this factor than we have about E_1. Thus, a high exposure to E_2 is associated with a Western diet rich in fat and meat; from the distribution of large adenomas and of carcinomas along the colorectum we can deduce that there is a concentration gradient of E_2 consistent with its being the bacterial metabolite of the bile acids already described in the first half of this paper. This conclusion is supported by the results of our studies of patients with colorectal adenomas (see Table 7). When the patients with adenomas were considered as a group, their mean FBA concentration (8.1 mg/g dry weight) and their carriage rate of NDC (36%) was little different from that of a normal healthy population of persons aged 45 to 75 years studied by us as part of our prospective study of large bowel cancer (described briefly by Hill, 1977c). This indicates clearly that our bacterial metabolite of the bile acids has no role in the pathogenesis of colorectal adenomas and is not E_1. However, when subdivided into groups on the basis of the diameter of the adenoma both the percentage who carried NDC and the mean FBA concentration increased with adenoma size; persons with an adenoma greater than 20 mm diameter had faecal analyses little different from those of persons with a Dukes A carcinoma. Similarly, persons with a villous adenoma had a carriage rate of NDC and a mean FBA concentration higher than those in persons with tubular adenomas. Thus there was a good correlation between the FBA/NDC discriminant in faeces of a person and the malignant potential of his adenoma.

Dysplasia is clearly one of the factors to be taken into account in assessing the malignant potential of an adenoma; in our study we were unable to subdivide our patients on the basis of the severity of dysplasia in their adenomas (because very few had severe dysplasia). However, we have been able to relate our FBA/NDC discriminant to dysplasia in a group of patients who have had chronic ulcerative colitis with total involvement of the large bowel for at least 10 years, and so are at increased risk of developing a carcinoma. These patients have elected to retain their colon and visit the out-patients department at St Mark's Hospital at least annually; we have obtained faecal samples from these patients at each visit and so are able to calculate a 'running mean' value for their FBA concentration and also to check the consistency of their NDC carriage status. In general, the patients have not changed their NDC carriage status during the time that we have followed them (up to five years). As with the adenoma patients, when these colitics were treated as a group their faecal analyses were little different from those of a normal healthy population (see Table 7). To date, nine of these patients have developed severe dysplasia and, on resection, five were found to have adenocarcinoma of the colon. Their mean FBA concentration was much higher than that of the group as a whole, as was their carriage rate of NDC. The prospective study of colitics and the study of patients with colorectal adenomas are continuing.

CONCLUSIONS

We initially developed a postulate for the causation of large bowel cancer and attempted to test it by metabolic epidemiological techniques and then to fit those results into the context of the observations of histopathologists. This has led to the formulation of a more refined postulate for the aetiology of the adenoma-carcinoma sequence.

The next stage of our work will be directed towards testing this more refined and more complex postulate. What is clear is that there is no simple and single mechanism for the causation of this very common cancer. Nevertheless, there are grounds for thinking that considerable progress has been made in recent years and that there is a good chance that we will be able to begin taking steps to reduce the incidence of colorectal cancer by public health measures in the foreseeable future.

ACKNOWLEDGEMENTS

This work is financially supported by the Cancer Research Campaign.

REFERENCES

Barnes, P., Bilton, R., Mason, A., Fernandez, F. & Hill, M.J. (1975) The coupling of anaerobic steroid dehydrogenation to nitrate reduction in *Pseudomonas* NC1B 10590 and *Clostridium paraputrificum*. *Transactions of the Biochemical Society*, **3**, 299-301.

Blackwood, A., Murray, W.R., Mackay, C. & Calman, K. (1978) Faecal bile acids and clostridia in the aetiology of colorectal cancer and breast cancer. *British Journal of Cancer*, **38**, 175.

Cole, J.W. & Holden, W.D. (1959) Postcolectomy regression of adenomatous polyps in the human colon. *Archives of Surgery*, **79**, 385-392.

Coombs, M.M. & Croft, C.J. (1969) Carcinogenic cyclopenta[a]phenanthrenes. *Progress in Tumour Research*, **11**, 69-80.

Correa, P. (1978) Epidemiology of polyps and cancer. In *The Pathogenesis of Colorectal Cancer* (Ed.) Morson, B. pp. 126-152. London: W.B. Saunders.

Crowther, J.S., Drasar, B.S., Hill, M.J., MacLennan, R., Magnin, D., Peach, S. & Teoh-Chan, C.H. (1976) Faecal steroids and bacteria and large bowel cancer in Hong Kong by socio-economic groups. *British Journal of Cancer*, 34, 191-198.

Cruse, P., Lewin, M. & Clark, C.G. (1979a) Dietary cholesterol is co-carcinogenic for human colon cancer. *Lancet*, i, 752-755.

Cruse, P., Lewin, M. & Clark, C.G. (1979b) Cholesterol and colon cancer. *Lancet*, ii, 43-44.

Cruse, P., Lewin, M., Ferulano, G. & Clark, C.G. (1978) Co-carcinogenic effects of dietary cholestrol in experimental colon cancer. *Nature*, 276, 822-824.

Enstrom, J.E. (1975) Colorectal cancer and the consumption of beef and fat. *British Journal of Cancer*, 32, 432-439.

Finegold, S.M., Flora, D., Attebury, H. & Sutter, V. (1975) Fecal bacteriology of colonic polyp patients and control patients. *Cancer Research*, 35, 3407-3417.

Goddard, P., Fernandez, F., West, B., Hill, M.J. & Barnes, P. (1975) The nuclear dehydrogenation of steroids by intestinal bacteria. *Journal of Medical Microbiology*, 8, 429-435.

Haenszel, W. & Correa, P. (1973) Cancer of the large intestine. Epidemiological findings. *Diseases of the Colon and Rectum*, 16, 371-377.

Hecker, E. (1980) Diterpene ester type modulators of carcinogenesis — new findings in the mechanism of chemical carcinogenesis and in the aetiology of human tumours. In *Naturally Occurring Carcinogens-Mutagens and Modulators of Carcinogenesis* (Ed.) Miller, E.C., Miller, J.A., Hirono, I., Sugimura, T. & Takayama, S. pp. 263-286. Tokyo: Japanese Scientific Press.

Hedges, A.R., Hedges, K. & Reddy, B.S. (1978) Effect of freezing of human fecal specimens upon the isolation of Nuclear Dehydrogenating Clostridia (39998). *Proceedings of the Society for Experimental Biology and Medicine*, 157, 94-96.

Hill, M.J. (1975a) The etiology of colon cancer. *CRC Critical Reviews in Toxicology*, 4, 31-82.

Hill, M.J. (1975b) The role of colon anaerobes in the metabolism of bile acids and steroids, and its relation to colon cancer. *Cancer*, 36, 2387-2400.

Hill, M.J. (1977a) Bacterial metabolism. In *Topics in Gastroenterology* (Ed.) Truelove, S.C. & Lee, E. 5th edn. Oxford: Blackwell.

Hill, M.J. (1977b) The aetiology of colonic cancer. In *The Gastrointestinal Tract* (Ed.) Yardley, J., Morson, B. & Abell, M. pp. 124-132. Baltimore, MD: Williams and Wilkins.

Hill, M.J. (1977c) The role of unsaturated bile acids in the aetiology of large bowel cancer. In *Origins of Human Cancer* (Ed.) Hiatt, H., Watson, J. & Winsten, J. pp. 1627-1640. New York: Cold Spring Harbor Laboratory.

Hill, M.J. (1978) Aetiology of the adenoma-carcinoma sequence. In *The Pathogenesis of Colorectal Cancer* (Ed.) Morson, B. pp. 153-162. London: W.B. Saunders.

Hill, M.J. (1979) Bacterial metabolism and colon cancer. *Nutrition and Cancer*, 1, 46-49.

Hill, M.J. & Drasar, B.S. (1974) Bacteria and the aetiology of cancer of the large intestine. In *Anaerobic Bacteria: Role in Disease* (Ed.) Balows, A., DeHaan, R.M., Dowell, V. & Guze, L. pp. 119-133. Springfield, Ill.: Thomas.

Hill, M.J., Morson, B.C. & Bussey, H.J.R. (1978) Aetiology of adenoma-carcinoma sequence in large bowel. *Lancet*, i, 245-247.

Hill, M.J., Drasar, B.S., Aries, V.C., Crowther, J.S., Hawksworth, G.M. & Williams, R.E.O. (1971) Bacteria and aetiology of cancer of the large bowel. *Lancet*, i, 95-100.

Hill, M.J., Drasar, B.S., Williams, R.E.O., Meade, T.W., Cox, A.G., Simpson, J.E.P. & Morson, B.C. (1975) Faecal bile acids and clostridia in patients with cancer of the large bowel. *Lancet*, i, 535-538.

IARC Working Party (1977) Dietary fibre, transit time, faecal bacteria, steroids and colon cancer in two Scandinavian populations. *Lancet*, ii, 207-211.

Kassira, E., Parent, L. & Vahouny, G. (1976) Colon cancer: an epidemiological survey. *American Journal of Digestive Diseases*, 21, 205-214.

Lovett, E. (1974) Familial factors in the etiology of carcinoma of the bowel. *Proceedings of the Royal Society of Medicine*, 67, 751-752.

Moore, W.E.C. & Holdeman, L.V. (1975) Discussion of current bacteriological investigations of the relationships between intestinal flora, diet and colon cancer. *Cancer Research*, 35, 3418-3420.

Morson, B. (1974) The polyp cancer sequence in the large bowel. *Proceedings of the Royal Society of Medicine*, **67**, 451-457.

Moskovitz, M., White, C. & Floch, M. (1978) Bile acid and neutral steroid excretion in carcinoma of the colon, other cancers and control subjects. *Gastroenterology*, **75**, 1071.

Mower, H.F., Ray, R.M., Shoff, R., Stemmermann, G.N., Normura, A., Glober, G.A., Kamiyama, S., Shimada, A. & Yamakawa, H. (1979) Faecal bile acids in two Japanese populations with different colon cancer risks. *Cancer Research*, **39**, 328-331.

Mudd, D.G., McKelvey, S.T., Sloan, J.M. & Elmore, D.T. (1978) Faecal bile acid concentrations in patients at increased risk of large bowel cancer. *Acta Gastroenterologica Belgica*, **41**, 241-244.

Muto, T., Ishikawa, K., Kino, I., Nakamura, K., Sugano, H., Morson, B.C. & Bussey, H.J.R. (1977) Comparative histological study of large bowel adenomas in Japan and England with special reference to malignant potential. *Diseases of the Colon and Rectum*, **20**, 11.

Reddy, B.S. & Wynder, E.L. (1977) Metabolic epidemiology of colon cancer. Faecal bile acids and neutral sterols in colon cancer patients and patients with adenomatous polyps. *Cancer*, **39**, 2533-2539.

Veale, A.M.O. (1965) *Intestinal Polyposis*. Eugenits Laboratory Memoirs Series, 40. London: Cambridge University Press.

Wang, T., Kakizoe, T., Dion, P., Furrer, R., Varghese, A.J. & Bruce, W.R. (1978) Volatile nitrosamines in normal human faeces. *Nature*, **276**, 280-282.

Wilkins, T.D. & Hackman, A.S. (1974) Two patterns of neutral steroid conversion in the faeces of normal North Americans. *Cancer Research*, **34**, 2250-2254.

Wynder, E.L. (1975) The epidemiology of large bowel cancer. *Cancer Research*, **35**, 3388.

Wynder, E.L. & Reddy, B.S. (1974) Metabolic epidemiology of colorectal cancer. *Cancer*, **34**, 801-806.

Wynder, E.L. & Reddy, B.S. (1978) Etiology of cancer of the colon. In *Colon Cancer* (Ed.) Grundmann, E. pp. 1-14. Stuttgart: Gustav Fischer Verlag.

19

Screening for Colorectal Cancer

J.D. HARDCASTLE

In 1972, 19 561 new cases of cancer of the large intestine and rectum were registered in England and Wales, compared with 30 132 cases of carcinomas of the lung and 19 512 cases of carcinoma of the breast. Colorectal cancer is therefore the second commonest epithelial cancer in England and Wales. The registration of new cases in England and Wales has remained relatively constant over the last few years (Registrar General Statistics Review, 1972-73), the United Kingdom remaining one of the high-risk areas.

The results of treatment over large areas of the country can be obtained from the Regional Cancer Registries. In the Birmingham region (Slaney, 1971), in the decade 1950-61 the five-year survival rate of carcinoma of the rectum was 22 per cent and carcinoma of the colon 21 per cent. Only 52 per cent of the patients with carcinoma of the rectum and 46 per cent of patients with carcinoma of the colon had a curative tumour operation. The five-year survival rate has remained unchanged during the subsequent decade (Slaney, 1978). Similar results have been found in other parts of the country, for example the South Western Cancer Registry (Walker, 1968) and the Trent Regional Cancer Registry 1968-69.

Results of treatment in specialist centres give a biased view of the effectiveness of treatment due to selection of cases. For example, at St Mark's hospital in London, 80 per cent of the patients are referred by general practitioners, some for second opinion, and 17 per cent from consultants in other hospitals. Fifty per cent of referrals come from the London postal district, 44 per cent from other parts of the United Kingdom, and 5 per cent from abroad. Less than 5 per cent of colon cancers are admitted as an emergency (Hawley, 1977). The overall five-year survival rate of 516 patients between 1948 and 1967 was 52.5 per cent with a corrected figure of 62.9 per cent for carcinoma of the colon, and a corrected figure of 63.8 per cent for carcinoma of the rectum.

The survival of patients admitted to a regional hospital resembles more closely the cancer registry figures. Of 391 patients admitted in the Oxford region over a six-year period from 1966 to 1971 the corrected five-year survival was 37.2 per cent (Gill and Morris, 1978).

© 1980 W.B. Saunders Company Ltd.

FACTORS AFFECTING PROGNOSIS

Pathological Stage and Histological Grading

Prognosis in colorectal cancer is directly related to the degree of spread. Tumours limited to the bowel wall (Dukes' stage A) have a corrected survival rate of over 90 per cent (Bussey, 1963; Gill and Morris, 1978), whereas those tumours that have spread beyond the bowel wall to the regional lymph nodes are associated with a corrected five-year survival rate of only 27 per cent.

There is also a good correlation between the histological grade of the tumour and the extent of spread. The majority of the Stage A tumours are well differentiated whilst those that have spread distally are usually poorly differentiated (Goligher, 1975).

Unfortunately, in a regional hospital the majority of patients (58.8 per cent) present with tumours that have already spread into the regional nodes or liver, 35.5 per cent having spread through the bowel wall and only 5.7 per cent localized to the bowel (Stage A) (Gill and Morris, 1978). In 200 consecutive admissions to the Nottingham hospitals, only 3.5 per cent were Stage A (Holliday and Hardcastle, 1979).

Delay in Treatment After Symptomatic Diagnosis

At the Massachusetts General Hospital, there has been a steady reduction in the patient delay before presenting to hospital for treatment, from six to seven months in 1950 to just over two months in 1976 (Welch and Donaldson, 1974). During this time there has been no change in the number of disseminated tumours and no increase in the survival following curative surgery. Keddie and Hargreaves (1968) found no relation between the pathological stage and the duration of symptoms, and this has been confirmed from a recent study in Nottingham (Holliday and Hardcastle, 1979). Indeed, Slaney (1971) found that the longer the delay the better the prognosis, indicating that the more malignant tumours present because of rapidly progressive symptoms whereas in slowly growing tumours minimal symptoms may have been present for many months.

It would appear that once symptoms develop the tumour has advanced to such a degree that the outcome is determined by the malignant nature of the tumour and its ability to spread to distant organs. This, however, does not mean that earlier diagnosis would not improve the survival of the individual patient. The hospital mortality of patients admitted as an emergency with colonic obstruction or perforation is greater than those patients treated electively. In the Oxford region the hospital mortality of emergency treatment was 24 per cent, compared with only 3.6 per cent in patients admitted for elective surgery (Till, 1977). In the Nottingham area, 42 per cent of colonic cancers are admitted as an emergency (Holliday and Hardcastle, 1979), 76 per cent of these patients having seen a general practitioner on at least one, and often several occasions. A greater awareness of the colonic symptoms could result in more patients being admitted earlier and their operation carried out as an elective procedure with a consequently lower hospital mortality rate. Symptoms of colonic cancer are, however, very common in the population. In a group of healthy adults, Jones (1976) found 70 per cent suffered from periodic diarrhoea and 38 per cent had passed blood in the stool, and in a more recent study of apparently healthy subjects Thompson and Heaton (1978) found that in 30 per cent functional bowel symptoms occurred. Most patients, therefore, suffer symptoms suggestive of colonic cancer from time to time and consult their doctor only when the symptoms persist. Greater awareness of the significance of these symptoms by health education programmes could lead to considerable anxiety and overload of the facilities available.

Diagnosis in the Asymptomatic Stage

The five-year survival rate of 58 persons found to have colorectal cancer following proctosigmoidoscopic screening at the Strang Clinic and Memorial Sloan Kettering Cancer Center was 88 per cent and further follow-up indicates that the 15-year survival is maintained at this level (Sherlock and Winawer, 1977). Seventy-two per cent of these patients were diagnosed at the time of their first visit at a time when tumours of all stages would be present, from small malignant polyps to large carcinomas about to become symptomatic, and it is unlikely that the latter would have a prognosis better than patients presenting with symptoms. In a study undertaken by Gilbertsen and Nelms (1978), 27 adenocarcinomas were found at the first sigmoidoscopic examination in 21 150 participants. The observed five-year survival rate was 65 per cent. In 22 per cent of the patients the tumour was shown to have spread distally compared with 55 per cent in a group of symptomatic patients. In the subsequent annual follow-up, 13 adenocarcinomas of the rectum were detected. All the tumours were confined to the bowel wall, eight confined to the mucosa; only one cancer had invaded the muscle. The five-year survival rate of this group was 85 per cent which included one operative death.

In a study currently in progress to evaluate haemoccult faecal occult blood testing, 75 colorectal cancers have been detected in the asymptomatic stage; 65 per cent were found to be in Stage A, 13 per cent in Stage B, 16 per cent in Stage C and only 5 per cent had spread to the liver (Gilbertsen, 1979).

In other published series (Glober and Peskoe, 1974; Hastings, 1974; Miller and Knight, 1977), five of nine asymptomatic cancers were found to be Stage A and in the Sloan Kettering Cancer Center series, where the detailed pathological stage was not given, six of seven asymptomatic cancers were said to be localized Stage A and B (Sherlock and Winawer, 1977).

Greegor (1978) quotes a similar experience. In 62 symptomless cancers 86 per cent were confined to the bowel wall whilst in a group presenting with symptoms only 60 per cent were so localized.

It would thus appear that the pathological stage of asymptomatic tumours diagnosed either by proctosigmoidoscopy or following the detection of faecal occult blood is similar and that these tumours are at a more localized stage of growth and thereby possibly have a better prognosis than symptomatic cancer.

RISK FACTORS IN COLORECTAL CANCER

Age

The incidence of colorectal cancer rises rapidly after the age of 40 to 45 years (Falterman et al, 1974) and continues to increase approximately twofold in each subsequent decade, reaching a peak at the age of 75. Between 35 and 80 years of age, the age-specific rates of rectal and colonic cancer are practically equal, both rates increasing approximately in proportion to the sixth power of the age (Doll, 1977).

Genetic Factors

The cancer risk in familial polyposis which is inherited as an autosomal dominant is well recognized, with an almost 100 per cent risk of eventually developing carcinoma (Alm and Licznerski, 1973). There is a similar colon cancer risk in the rarer polyposis syndromes associated with other abnormalities, for example Gardner's syndrome (soft tissue and bony tumours), Turcot's syndrome (CNS tumours) and Oldfield's syndrome (multiple sebaceous cysts). Once symptoms develop, 50 per cent of new patients already have cancer of the large bowel whereas only 9 per cent of polyposis patients traced through family studies have developed cancer (Bussey, 1975).

Several authors have described families in which there is a high incidence of colorectal cancer but without evidence of familial polyposis (Dunstone and Knaggs, 1972; Lynch, Krush and Guirgis, 1973). In some cases there appears to be an association with carcinoma of the breast and endometrium and an increased likelihood of cancer of the proximal colon (Lynch et al, 1977). Detailed analysis of family histories of patients undergoing treatment for colorectal cancer has shown that in first-degree relatives the number of deaths from cancer of the bowel is three times that expected from a comparable group in the population (Lovett, 1976). The early age of onset of the cancer and the presence of multiple adenomas in the resected specimen lead to an even greater risk that other members of the family will develop cancer of the large bowel.

Benign Adenomas and Previous Colorectal Cancer

The role of polyps as a cancer precursor has been a controversial subject for a number of years, partly because there are many different histological types of polyps, but only those classified as neoplastic polyps or adenomas have a malignant potential (Morson and Dawson, 1972).

The prevalence of adenomatous polyps based on post-mortem studies is closely related to the frequency of colorectal cancer (Correa et al, 1977). Adenomas present in higher-risk areas such as the United States are larger and show greater cellular atypia compared with those occurring in low-risk regions such as Japan (Arminski and McLean, 1964; Correa et al, 1972). In the African Bantu, in whom the risk of colorectal cancer is very low, in

14 000 autopsies studied no adenomatous polyps were discovered (Bremner and Ackerman, 1970). An increase in the incidence of colorectal cancer in the United States has been documented since 1940 (Axtel and Chiazze, 1966), during which time the prevalence of adenomatous polyps has also steadily increased (Helwig, 1947; Blatt, 1961; Arminski and McLean, 1964).

The increased rate of developing cancer in the presence of pre-existing adenomas has been shown in a number of studies. It is well known that patients who have had a cancer resected have a greater chance of developing a further colorectal malignant tumour (Heald and Lockhart-Mummery, 1972), the risk reaching 10 per cent in 25 years if adenomatous polyps were present in the resected specimen, but only 4 per cent if they were absent (Morson, 1976). In an eight-year follow-up of patients found to have adenomatous polyps, 2.7 per cent developed cancer, whereas in a number of persons free of adenomas at the first examination, no cancer developed (Brahme et al, 1974). In a 15-year study of patients with adenomatous polyps removed during sigmoidoscopy, the risk of developing colon cancer was doubled (Prager et al, 1974).

There is increasing evidence that the majority of colorectal tumours arise within pre-existing adenomas. In a series of malignant tumours examined at St Mark's hospital, 14.2 per cent of the tumours showed evidence of contiguous benign tumour. In tumours with invasion of the submucosa only, 60 per cent were associated with adenomatous tissue, whereas of those tumours that invaded through the bowel wall only 7 per cent had evidence of benign origin (Morson, 1966), suggesting that as cancer spreads through the bowel wall it expands on the mucosal surface to destroy surviving benign tissue. Malignant potential of adenomatous polyps increases with size (Grinnell and Lane, 1958). The risk of malignant change is greater in villous adenomas and appears to be related to the degree of mucosal dysplasia (Grinnell and Lane, 1958; Kaneko, 1972).

Familial polyposis provides a good model to study the development of cancer from pre-existing adenomas (Bussey, 1975). In the St Mark's series the average age of diagnosis of polyposis without cancer is 27 years, and of polyposis with cancer 39 years. The 12 years' difference is likely to be an underestimate of the time taken to develop malignant change, as is shown by observation of patients not treated surgically; 11 per cent developed cancer between 0 and five years, rising to 55 per cent between 15 and 20 years. Solitary adenomatous polyps appear to behave in a similar manner. Of four patients seen at the St Mark's Hospital, three developed cancer within 12.5 years (Morson, 1976). At the Mayo Clinic, a single adenomatous polyp in the sigmoid colon developed malignant change after 15 years of observation (Mayo and de Castro, 1956). From these figures it would appear that the development of colorectal cancer from an adenomatous polyp may take between 10 and 15 years. However, the great majority of colorectal adenomas appear to remain quiescent and do not grow and develop invasive features.

Inflammatory Bowel Disease

Ulcerative colitis is associated with a five to ten times increased risk of colorectal cancer. The risk of developing cancer is dependent upon the extent of the disease and the length of history. Careful studies by MacDougall (1964), De Dombal et al (1966) and Hinton (1966) have shown that carcinoma generally develops only when the colitis has involved most of the large intestine. The risk of developing cancer within 10 years of the onset of the disease is small (one in 860 patient years of follow-up), rising to one in 200 patient years in the 10-to-20 years decade and one in 60 patient years when the disease has been present for more than 20 years (Lennard-Jones et al, 1977). The presence of epithelial dysplasia (Morson and Pang, 1967) can be used as a means of selecting patients for prophylactic colectomy. In a group of 229 patients with long-standing colitis followed by regular mucosal biopsies colectomy was recommended in seven patients because of severe mucosal dysplasia. Carcinoma confined to the bowel wall (Dukes' Stage A) was found in four (Lennard-Jones et al, 1977). Mucosal dysplasia can, however, only be used as a guide as it was not present in 12 per cent of patients with colonic cancer complicating ulcerative colitis (Dobbins, 1977).

In Crohn's disease there is a slightly increased incidence of colonic malignancy, especially with the early onset of the disease (Weedon et al, 1973), and this may affect by-passed segments and fistulous tracts (Greenstein et al, 1978).

SCREENING METHODS IN ASYMPTOMATIC COLORECTAL CANCER

Examination of Faeces for Occult Blood

Examination of faeces for occult blood has had a poor reputation in the past because of the high incidence of false positive reactions (Irons and Kirsner, 1965). In normal medical students on an unrestricted diet, false positive reactions were obtained in 61 per cent using a saturated guaiac reagent and in 32 per cent using an orthotoluidine tablet test (Ostrow et al, 1973). These false positive reactions are due to a combination of factors. In normal individuals radiochromium studies have shown a blood loss of 1 to 2 ml per 24 hours (Ebaugh et al, 1958). Meat and other blood-containing food in the diet increase the frequency of false positive reactions; with saturated guaiac reagent, this increases from 39 per cent to 61 per cent and with the orthotoluidine test from 23 per cent to 32 per cent (Ostrow et al, 1973). Many of the chemical tests depend upon the peroxidase-like activity of haematin. Vegetable and bacterial peroxidases may, therefore, interfere with the reaction, particularly after storage of faeces, and in some vegetables (e.g., yellow turnip) the activity may persist even after cooking (Illingworth, 1965).

For screening purposes, a faecal occult blood test must have a very low false positive rate. It must be easy to perform with little or no error. It should be applicable to persons on an unrestricted diet and not affected by the storage of faeces for up to five days. It should also be sufficiently insensitive so as not to detect the loss of blood which occurs in normal individuals.

Until 1969 the most widely used occult blood tests in the United Kingdom were the benzidine and orthotoluidine tests. In 1969 the Department of Health advised against the use of both these tests because of the possible carcinogenic effect of benzidine and orthotoluidine.

The haemoccult test has been widely used for colorectal screening in America and in Germany and is based on the guaiac reaction. This depends upon the oxidation of α-guaiaconic acid to a quinone structure which has a blue colour. It is thought that the haematin part of haemoglobin catalyses the oxidation process in the presence of hydrogen peroxide. The haemoccult slide test differs from the saturated guaiac test in that the guaiac reagent is stabilized on filter paper. The test is much less sensitive than the standard guaiac reagent. Ostrow et al (1973) have shown that 50 per cent of the stools containing 5 to 10 mg of haemoglobin per gram stool are positive and uniformly positive reactions are obtained only with stools containing 10 mg or more of haemoglobin per gram of stool.

Similar results were obtained by Stroehlein et al (1976) using ^{51}Cr method to measure gastrointestinal blood loss. They found that with a loss of 10 ml of blood per day, 67 per cent of haemoccult tests were positive and with a loss of 30 ml per day, 93 per cent were positive.

On an unrestricted diet radioactive chromium studies have shown that 8 to 12 per cent false positive results are obtained with haemoccult (Morris et al, 1976; Stroehlein et al, 1976). It is possible that some of these false positive reactions are due to other peroxidases in the stool, and may be diluted by the larger volume of stool induced by laxatives (Morris et al, 1976). Bleeding from colorectal cancer is reduced on a bland diet (Greegor, 1971), and therefore it has been recommended that a high-bulk diet should be taken whilst the specimens are collected although there is little direct evidence that this increases the rate of bleeding from colonic neoplasms. There is also evidence that large amounts of vitamin C may interfere with the haemoccult slide test, resulting in a false negative result even in the presence of a significant amount of blood in the stool (Jaffe et al, 1975). The haemoccult slide test may convert during storage from positive to negative, especially in the presence of low concentrations of haemoglobin (Winawer et al, 1977). This may be prevented by rehydration of the slide before testing (Wells and Pagano, 1977); however, this is not now recommended as it was found to increase the number of false positive reactions and reduce the predictive value of the test from 50 to 44 per cent (Winawer, 1979).

Colorectal cancers bleed intermittently and the blood is not uniformly dispersed in the stool specimen (Ebaugh et al, 1958). It is therefore recommended that two different parts of the stool should be tested on three consecutive days, the patient being thoroughly investigated if only one of the six tests proves to be positive.

More specific and sensitive tests of occult bleeding have been developed: for example, an immunodiffusion method (Barrows et al, 1978) and one involving extraction of haem and degradation to the peroxide (Jaffe and

Zierdt, 1979). Both tests are, however, more complicated and are unlikely to replace the simpler chemical test as a screening test.

Acceptability of the haemoccult slide test

The acceptability of the haemoccult test as collected from the published literature is shown in Table 1 and varies with the degree of motivation of the

Table 1

Reference	Number offered test	Number accepted	% Acceptance	% Positive	Number of cancers detected	Number of polyps
Miller and Knight (1977)	2332	2205	94.5	2.8	3	7
Gnauck (1977)	—	8000	—	3.8	32	45
Ross and Johnson (1976)	1187	1103	93.0	7.0	4	—
Richardson (1977)	1038	885	85.0	6.1	0	4
Winawer et al (1977)	6597	5607	85.0	1.0	7	23
Hastings (1974)	2272	1835	80.0	6.2	5	—
Helfrick and Petrucci (1979)	49157	19707	40.0	4.6	15	18
Glober and Peskoe (1974)	1682	1539	91.5	23.7	3	3
Frühmorgen and Demling (1978)	6007	5015	83.5	2.7	13	83
Spinnelli et al (1979)	5954	5015	—	1.75	10	9
Hardcastle and Balfour (1980)	1638	713	45.0	3.8	2	4
Otto, Bunnemann and Hans-Joachim (1979)	8727	—	—	3.2	27	35
Bralow (1979)	3798	—	79.0	10.9	7	11
Gilbertsen (1979)	32000	—	—	—	72	458
Samec (1979)	5323	3887	73.0	4.12	12	23
Durst, Neumann and Schmidt (1976)	4000	1125	28.0	5.8	4	4

screened group. Some of the studies relate to highly motivated groups in the population who attend diagnostic clinics for health checks and are obviously likely to accept this further investigation. For example, 85 per cent of 6597 men and women attending the Strang clinic in New York accepted the invitation of haemoccult screening in addition to sigmoidoscopy (Winawer et al, 1977) and 83.5 per cent of 6007 attending the Erlangen diagnostic clinic in Germany returned the completed slides (Frühmorgen and Demling, 1978).

In the United States the offer of free rectal examination and occult blood screening resulted in 3450 registering for the study, of which 2625 (76 per cent) returned the test (Hastings, 1974). Eighty per cent of those who availed themselves of the physical examination returned the test compared with only 39 per cent of those who accepted the haemoccult test kit alone. In Hawaii a group of men examined as part of a heart study volunteered for colorectal screening and 91.5 per cent of the 1682 men receiving the test packages returned them (Glober and Peskoe, 1974). Both these studies have high compliance rates and obviously someone would not register for the test if he were unlikely to return it. A study undertaken in a United States airforce base (Miller and Knight, 1977) resulted in a compliance rate of 94.5 per cent and this also clearly does not represent the population as a whole. When haemoccult slides are distributed at meetings at which the problem of colorectal cancer and its early diagnosis were explained, 85 per cent of those who agreed to participate returned the completed slides (Richardson, 1977). A similar compliance (79 per cent) was obtained in Florida where public awareness was obtained by newspaper, radio and television advertisements and doctors in the area were informed by meetings and detailed letters (Bralow, 1979). However, an American Cancer Society screening programme in Washington DC resulted in only 20 per cent of 41 975 tests being returned (Helfrick and Petrucci, 1979). Durst, Neumann and Schmidt (1976) in Germany found that only 28 per cent of persons invited for screening accepted the invitation, and indeed when test kits were distributed randomly to the adult population in the United States James (1977) found that only 15 per cent were returned. When the participants' homes were visited, 20 per cent accepted the invitation.

Thus the compliance rate for haemoccult slide testing is dependent upon many factors: for example, public awareness and education in respect of colorectal cancer, the motivation of the screened group, the methods in which the test kits are presented and the financial consequences of the test. All these factors vary from country to country and care should be taken in using compliance data obtained in the United States in Great Britain. In Great Britain a Pilot Study has been undertaken in the East Midlands to study the response of persons over the age of 45 years in a single general practice to the offer of colorectal screening by the haemoccult test. A total of 1638 invitations were sent and 45 per cent of the test kits were completed and returned. The compliance rate was low (25 per cent) in those over 75 years and varied between 41 and 56 per cent in the other decades (Hardcastle and Balfour, 1980). The health centre studied serves a middle-class rural area where the standard of medical care is excellent. This method of invitation may produce an entirely different result in an area of different social class and where the medical service is not provided on such a personal basis.

In the majority of studies the number of positive results varies from 7 to 1 per cent, depending partly upon the degree of dietary restrictions (see Table 1). Glober and Peskoe (1974) reported an initial 25.7 per cent positive reaction which may be due to local dietary habits. Of persons found to be positive on an unrestricted diet 30 per cent and 80 per cent revert to negative after dietary restrictions (Glober and Peskoe, 1974; Ross, 1976; Miller and Knight, 1977). The importance of avoiding red meat and blood-containing foods is confirmed by the work of Goulston (1979) who found that on an unrestricted Australian diet the false positive rate was 11 per cent and fell to 2 per cent after restriction of the above foods. Severe dietary restrictions can, however, reduce the acceptability of the test and the need for them may vary from country to country.

In studies where blood loss in the stool has been measured by the ^{51}Cr method, the haemoccult test has been found to give 8 to 12 per cent false positive results (Morris et al, 1976; Stroehlein et al, 1976).

Number of cancers detected and missed by haemoccult screening

The number of cancers detected varies considerably from study to study (see Table 1), depending upon the number of symptomatic persons included in the screened group. The diagnostic clinics in Germany from which large series have been reported (Gnauck, 1977; Frühmorgen and Demling, 1978) provide an investigative service for symptomatic persons and under these circumstances 4 to 2.6 per 1000 cancers are detected.

When there is good evidence that at least 90 per cent of the group are truly asymptomatic, the detection rate would appear to be seven in 5607 (Winawer et al, 1977), three in 1539 (Glober and Pescoe, 1974); that is, approximately 1.4 per 1000. In a number of the studies, however, many of those found to be positive have not been completely investigated because of difficulties of follow-up and control in the private health care system of the United States (Bralow, 1979; Helfrick and Petrucci, 1979). Adenomatous polyps are detected more frequently than carcinoma (see Table 1) but in some series details of histological examination are not given.

The false negative rate of the haemoccult test in colorectal cancer is unknown and would require total colonoscopy on all haemoccult negative asymptomatic persons.

Rigid sigmoidoscopy has, however, been done in addition to haemoccult screening. Winawer et al (1977) found two cancers and 15 adenomas in 5607 asymptomatic haemoccult negative persons. Additional lesions missed in the colon will be detected only after several years of follow-up. However, Greegor (1971) did not find any significant false negativity in his personal experience if patients had followed the prescribed diet and slide preparation instructions.

In a study conducted by Miller, sigmoidoscopy was performed prior to distribution of haemoccult slides. In 2332 persons registering for the test, two cancers and four adenomatic polyps were discovered on the rectal examination and sigmoidoscopy, the haemoccult testing adding only one further cancer and three polyps. Whether the four polyps and two cancers detected on sigmoidoscopy would have been detected by haemoccult screening is unknown. Using three haemoccult slide tests per patient, Gnauck (1977) found seven out of 96 colorectal cancers were negative. Deyhle (1976) reported three out of 32 colorectal cancers negative and Samec (1979) found four cancers and 51 polyps (27 over 5 mm in size) in 540 haemoccult negative persons.

It would thus appear that at least 10 per cent of colorectal cancers are missed by the haemoccult test. The number of undetected adenomatous polyps appears to be even greater; in a group of patients known to have polyposis coli only 32 per cent were positive (Parlides et al, 1977) and in 98 large polyps, 27 were negative (Gnauck, 1977).

Sigmoidoscopy in the Detection of Asymptomatic Colorectal Cancer

Approximately 42 per cent of all colorectal cancers occur within the range of the rigid 25 cm sigmoidoscope (Falterman et al, 1974). The risk of the procedure is small. Gilbertsen (1974) reports a perforation rate of one in 20 600 examinations.

In the 1950s many cancer screening centres were started in the United States for sigmoidoscopic screening of asymptomatic persons. In presumed asymptomatic persons over the age of 40 years invasive cancers are detected in approximately 0.12 per cent (Moertel, Hill and Dockerty, 1966). In the University of Minnesota Cancer Detection Center, Gilbertsen (1978) found on initial procto-sigmoidoscopic examination of 21 150 participants 27 carcinomas (0.13 per cent). Seventy-eight per cent were localized to the bowel and 22 per cent had spread either to the regional lymph nodes or more distally. At the Strang Preventive Medicine Institute, of 47 091 procto-sigmoidoscopic examinations, in mostly asymptomatic persons, 58 cancers of the colon and rectum were detected (0.12 per cent); 56 of these patients were considered curable at surgery and the five-year survival rate was 88 per cent, in contrast to the national average five-year survival rate of about 40 per cent (Sherlock and Winawer, 1977). Of the 21 150 participants in the University of Minnesota Screening Programme (Gilbertsen, 1978) who underwent regular annual follow-up examinations, a total of 92 650 subsequent examinations were carried out, during which any polypoid lesion was removed, but the number found and histological details of the resected polyps are not available (Gilbertsen, 1979). Thirteen adenocarcinomas were detected; all were at an early stage of development and confined to the bowel wall. Eight of the 13 had malignant change confined to the mucosa and four had minimal invasion of the submucosa. Epidemiological data would suggest that in 92 560 patient years of observation, between 78 and 97 cancers should have been detected. That only 13 adenocarcinomas were detected suggests that the policy of removing polyps during the follow-up examinations had reduced the subsequent development of rectal cancer.

When sigmoidoscopy was included in a multiphasic screening study of 5156 persons, a reduction in mortality was demonstrated compared with a control group, two deaths occurring from colorectal cancer in the screened group whilst there were 10 deaths in the control group (Dales et al, 1973).

The cost of sigmoidoscopic screening is high. In 1971 Bolt estimated that the cost of discovering, through sigmoidoscopy, a potentially curable lesion was in the order of 70 000 dollars if the investigation had been carried out by trained doctors. However, the value of procto-sigmoidoscopy in the diagnosis and prevention of colorectal cancer cannot be related to the rate of detection of frank cancer alone. Adenomatous polyps are much commoner findings than cancer. The incidence of polyps on procto-sigmoidoscopy in persons over the age of 40 years has been reported to vary from 3.1 per cent (Moertel, Hill and Dockerty, 1966) to 12.3 per cent (Christianson and Turner, 1951). The apparently high rates in some of the series may be due to a failure to examine all polypoid lesions removed histologically, or to the incorrect interpretation of histological findings. In England, 27 adenomatous polyps (3.8 per cent) were found during sigmoidoscopy examination of 704 persons over the age of 40 years (Payne, 1976).

A higher incidence is found in post-mortem studies. Hughes and Aust (1968) found that 20 per cent of persons over 50 years had polyps greater than 3 mm in size in the rectum and colon. Arminski and McLean (1964), in a similar post-mortem study, found adenomatous polyps in the rectum in 8.3 per cent and in the colon in 33 per cent, and from their data they estimate that 4 per cent of the population harbour adenomatous polyps over 1 cm in diameter.

The value of rigid sigmoidoscopy is limited by the frequent failure to pass the instrument to its full length. In 50 per cent of 20 847 examinations, it was impossible to pass the instrument beyond 20 cm (Wilson, Dale and Brines, 1955). Even when it is apparently passed to its full extent the instrument often merely stretches the rectosigmoid region and only a small part of the sigmoid colon is visualized (Madigan and Hall, 1968).

The use of the fibreoptic flexible sigmoidoscope as an out-patient procedure after only minimal bowel preparation and without sedation is likely to prove extremely valuable. In a comparison of rigid and flexible sigmoidoscopy in 120 patients the flexible instrument was advanced on average 55 cm compared with 20.4 cm with the rigid sigmoidoscope. The examination took longer (9.4 minutes compared with 5.9 minutes) but more patients preferred the flexible instrument (Bohlman et al, 1977). More polyps are found with the flexible instrument. In a recent study in which 200 asymptomatic men over 40 years were examined, polyps greater than 0.5 mm were found in 10 per cent (Lipshuty et al, 1979). Fifty-five per cent of the polyps were proximal to 25 mm and in only 18 per cent were the lesions within the usual range of the rigid instrument.

Colonoscopy

Total colonoscopy should not be considered as an initial screening procedure in colorectal cancer. Considerable training is necessary before safe colonoscopy is possible. The colonoscope has a limited life-span and only three or four examinations can be carried out at each session.

Total colonoscopy is indicated in the following situations: (1) patients found to have persistently positive occult blood in the stool where barium enema examination has been found to be normal; in such cases Teague, Salmon and Read (1973) found 7 per cent of unsuspected cancers; (2) patients with doubtful lesions or stricture on barium enema examination; (3) to search for additional synchronous lesions in patients known to have colorectal cancer or adenomatous polyps. In 182 patients an additional 118 polyps were found, half of these missed by radiology, being 1 cm or larger (Wolff et al, 1974); (4) assessment of patients with inflammatory bowel disease, particularly in patients with long-standing ulcerative colitis, multiple mucosal biopsies being used to assess a degree of mucosal dysplasia (Morson and Pang, 1967); (5) endoscopic polypectomy has improved the management of adenomatous polyps, morbidity being greatly less than that of operative colotomy, which has a complication rate of 20 per cent (Kleinfield and Gump, 1960). In 300 endoscopic polypectomies (Williams et al, 1974) only one localized perforation occurred. In the collected series from the Southern Californian Society for gastrointestinal endoscopy, in 3850 colonoscopies and 901 polypectomies, 10 perforations occurred with one death, the overall morbidity rate of colonoscopy being 0.42 per cent (Berci et al, 1974).

Barium Enema Examination

Barium enema examination is too costly and time-consuming to be considered as a routine screening test. Good bowel preparation is essential as faecal residues can cause difficulties in interpretation. An air contrast technique is necessary to detect small polypoid lesions as conventional barium enema techniques can miss as many as 40 per cent of polypoid lesions and 10 per cent of carcinomas (Miller, 1974). Williams et al (1974) found that conventional barium enema detected 74 per cent of polyps over 5 cm in size whilst a Malmo air contrast technique was successful in 95 per cent.

Cytological Examination of Colonic Washings

Cytological examination of fluid obtained by colonic lavage has, in specialized centres, proved of value in the diagnosis of colon cancer (Raskin and Pletucka, 1970; Sherlock, Ehrlick and Winawer, 1972). However, in general it has remained unpopular. Cleansing enemas are time-consuming and unpleasant for the patient, highly trained cytopathologists are necessary and the time taken for the procedure is considerable. The usefulness of the cytological lavage method is greatest in those patients with underlying premalignant disease such as extensive ulcerative colitis or familial polyposis. Marked inflammation can, however, lead to problems in diagnosis and misinterpretation, even by experienced cytopathologists. Most patients with long-standing colitis can be more easily followed by colonoscopy and multiple mucosal biopsies (Lennard-Jones et al, 1977).

Tumour-associated Antigens in Colonic Washings

High levels of carcinoembryonic antigen (CEA) have been found in the lavage specimens of patients with adenocarcinoma or adenomatous polyps greater than 1 cm in size (Schwartz, 1977). CEA is probably associated with mucus produced in excess by these tumours (Molnar, Vandervoorde and Gitnich, 1976). The interesting feature about this work is that large adenomatous polyps known to have a high malignant potential (Grinnell and Lane, 1958) were associated with levels of CEA equivalent to those found in the presence of adenocarcinoma. As adenomatous polyps bleed relatively infrequently (Parlides et al, 1977) and are usually asymptomatic, the identification of CEA in colonic washings could be used as a diagnostic method. Further evaluation is needed together with a search for other tumour-associated products in the lavage washings.

CEA can be detected in the faeces (Freed and Taylor, 1972) of patients with colorectal cancer but in this qualitative study it was also found in faeces of five of ten healthy volunteers. Quantification of CEA in stool specimens has not been performed.

Tumour Markers in Blood and Urine

Unfortunately, all the recognized tumour markers are related to the tumour mass: for example, blood CEA levels are raised in only about 20 per cent of patients with Dukes' Stage A cancer compared with 50 to 65 per cent of Dukes' Stage C, and in almost all patients with extensive metastatic disease (Zamacheck, 1975) the main value of blood CEA estimations lies in the follow-up of patients following curative surgery when persistently elevated levels indicate recurrent tumour.

There are also no enzyme changes that are diagnostic of early colorectal cancer. A number of enzymes have been found to be raised, for example, sialyltransferase (Kessel and Allen, 1975) and urinary arylsulfatase (Morgan et al, 1975), but as in the case of CEA the blood or urine level is related to the amount of malignant tissue present. High urinary levels of polyamines (e.g., putrescine) have also been found in colorectal cancer (Russell, Durrie and Salmon, 1975) but, as with the enzymes discussed above, are of little value in the diagnosis of early cancer (Lipton, Sheehan and Harvery, 1975).

CONCLUSIONS

The prevalence of colorectal cancer over the age of 40 years is difficult to determine. It is, however, fairly accurately known for the rectum and rectosigmoid region in asymptomatic persons over the age of 40 years, where a conservative estimate would be 1.2 cancers per 1000 of the population. If it is assumed that approximately 50 per cent of all colorectal cancers occur within range of the rigid sigmoidoscope, then the prevalence of colorectal cancer is at least 2.4 per 1000, and this is likely to be an underestimate of the true figure.

The results of treatment of colorectal cancer have not improved over the last two decades (Slaney, 1978) and it seems unlikely that further improvement in surgical technique will lead to significantly longer survival. Adjuvant chemotherapy up to the present time has proved disappointing (Higgins, 1976). Although there are reports of improved survival with adjuvant radiotherapy in the rectum it has not proved helpful in the colon (Roswit, Higgins and Keehan, 1975). It therefore seems likely that earlier diagnosis is the best hope for future improvement, particularly as there is mounting evidence that the majority of colorectal cancers pass through a premalignant adenomatous stage, the treatment of which has been greatly improved by endoscopic polypectomy.

There is evidence that rectal cancer diagnosed in the asymptomatic stage by procto-sigmoidoscopy is at a more favourable pathology stage and the long-term survival is better than in symptomatic cancer (Sherlock and Winawer, 1977; Gilbertsen and Nelms, 1978). Both these studies were, however, uncontrolled and the persons screened were self-selected attendees at screening clinics.

Faecal occult blood screening by the haemoccult method has been shown to result in the detection of approximately 1.4 cancers per 1000 asymptomatic persons screened. Tumours appear to be detected at an earlier pathological stage than symptomatic cancer but whether survival is improved is unknown. It is, however, the only method at the present time that could be applied to population screening in the United Kingdom.

The method is acceptable to approximately 50 per cent of the population and the load on hospital investigative facilities is likely to be small, particularly if the flexible sigmoidoscope is used to investigate all those found to be positive before resorting to barium enema or total colonoscopy (Hardcastle and Balfour, 1980).

REFERENCES

Alm, J. & Licznerski, G. (1973) The intestinal polyposes. *Clinics in Gastroenterology*, 2, 577-602.

Arminski, T.C. & McLean, D.W. (1964) Incidence and distribution of adenomatous polyps of the colon and rectum based on 1000 autopsy examinations. *Diseases of the Colon and Rectum*, 7, 249-261.

Axtell, L.M. & Chiazze, L. (1966) Changing relative frequency of cancers of the colon and rectum in the United States. *Cancer*, 19, 750-754.

Aylett, S.O. (1968) Rectal bleeding with special reference to cancer of the large intestine. *British Medical Journal*, iii, 103-106.

Barrows, G.H., Burton, R.M., Jarrett, D.D., Russell, G.G., Alford, D. & Songster, C.L. (1978) Immunological detection of human blood in feces. *American Journal of Clinical Pathology*, 69, 342-346.

Berci, G., Panish, J.F., Schopiro, M. & Corlin R. (1974) Complications of colonoscopy and polypectomy, report of the Southern Californian Society for Gastrointestinal Endoscopy. *Gastroenterology*, 67, 584-585.

Blatt, L.J. (1961) Polyps of the colon and rectum: incidence and distribution. *Diseases of the Colon and Rectum*, 4, 277-282.

Bohlman, T.W., Katon, R.M., Lipshuty, G., McCool, M.F., Frederick, W.S. & Melnyk, C.S. (1977) Alimentary tract fiberoptic pansigmoidoscopy: an evaluation and comparison with rigid sigmoidoscopy. *Gastroenterology*, 72, 644-649.

Bolt, R.J. (1971) Sigmoidoscopy in detection and diagnosis in the asymptomatic individual. *Cancer*, 28, 121-122.

Brahme, F., Ekelund, G.R., Norden, J.R. & Wackest, A. (1974) Metachronous colo-rectal polyps: comparison of development of colo-rectal polyps and carcinomas in persons with and without histories of polyps. *Diseases of the Colon and Rectum*, 17, 166-171.

Bralow, S.P. (1979) Colo-rectal cancer screening program in Serasota, Florida. *Symposium on Colo-rectal Cancer, New York.*

Bremner, C.G. & Ackerman, L.V. (1970) Polyps and carcinoma of the large bowel in the South African Bantu. *Cancer*, 26, 991-999.

Bussey, H.J.R. (1963) The long term results of surgical treatment of cancer of the rectum. *Proceedings of the Royal Society of Medicine*, 56, 494.

Bussey, H.J.R. (1975) Familial polyposis coli. Baltimore: Johns Hopkins University Press.

Christianson, W.H. & Turner, R.J. (1951) Results of sigmoidoscopic examinations at a cancer detection centre. *American Journal of Surgery*, 81, 14-17.

Correa, P., Duque, E., Cuello, C. & Haenszel, W. (1972) Polyps of the colon and rectum in Cali, Colombia. *International Journal of Cancer*, 9, 86-96.

Correa, P., Strong, J.P., Reif, A. & Johnson, W.D. (1977) The epidemiology of colo-rectal polyps. *Cancer*, 39, 2258-2264.

Dales, L.G., Friedman, G.D., Ramcharan, S., Siegelaub, A.B., Campbell, R.F. & Morris, F.C. (1973) Outpatient clinic utilization, hospitalization and mortality experience after seven years. *Preventive Medicine*, 2, 221-223.

De Dombal, F.T., Watts, J.M., Watkinson, G. & Goligher, J.C. (1966) Local complications of ulcerative colitis; stricture, pseudopolyposis and carcinoma of the colon and rectum. *British Medical Journal*, i, 1442-1447.

Deyhle, P. (1976) Vorsorgeuntersuchung bein dickdarmkarzinom. *Deutsche Medizinische Wochenschrift*, **101**, 1226-1228.
Dobbins, W.O. (1977) Current status of the precancer lesion in ulcerative colitis. *Gastroenterology*, **73**, 1431-1433.
Doll, R. (1977) General epidemiology: an analysis of 1000 cases. *Topics in Gastroenterology*, **5**, 3-13.
Dukes, C.E. (1940) Cancer of the rectum. *Journal of Pathology and Bacteriology*, **50**, 527.
Dunstone, G.H. & Knaggs, T.W.L. (1972) Familial cancer of the colon and rectum. *Journal of Medical Genetics*, **9**, 451-456.
Durst, J., Neumann, G. & Schmidt, K. (1976) Okkultes Blut im Stuhl. *Deutsche Medizinische Wochenschrift*, **101**, 440-443.
Ebaugh, F.G., Clemens, T., Rodnan, G. & Peterson, R.E. (1958) Quantitative measurement of gastrointestinal blood loss. *American Journal of Medicine*, **25**, 169-181.
Falterman, K.W., Hill, C.B., Markey, J.C., Fox, J.W. & Cohn, I. (1974) Cancer of the colon, rectum and anus: a review of 2313 cases. *Cancer*, **34**, 951-959.
Freed, D.L.J. & Taylor, G. (1972) Carcinoembryonic antigen in faeces. *British Medical Journal*, **i**, 85-87.
Frühmorgen, P. & Demling, L. (1978) Erste ergebnisse einer prospektiven Feldstudie mit einem modifizierten Guajak-Test zum Nachweiss von okkultem blut im stuhl. In *Kolorektale Krebsvorsorge*. pp. 68-72. Nürnberg: Verlag Wachholz.
Gilbertsen, V.A. (1974) Proctosigmoidoscopy and polypectomy in reducing the incidence of rectal cancer. *Cancer*, **34**, 936-939.
Gilbertsen, V.A. (1979) University of Minnesota program in screening with fecal blood testing and with sigmoidoscopy. *Symposium on Colo-rectal Screening, New York*.
Gilbertsen, V.A. & Nelms, J.M. (1978) The prevention of invasive cancer of the rectum. *Cancer*, **41**, 1137-1139.
Gill, P.G. & Morris, P.J. (1978) The survival of patients with colo-rectal cancer treated in a regional hospital. *British Journal of Surgery*, **65**, 17-20.
Glober, G.A. & Peskoe, S.M. (1974) Outpatient screening for gastrointestinal lesions using guaiac impregnated slides. *Digestive Diseases*, **19**, 399-403.
Gnauck, R. (1977) Dickdarmkarzinom — screening mit haemoccult. *Leber Magen Barm*, **7**, 32-35.
Goligher, J.C. (1975) Surgical anatomy and physiology of the colon, rectum and anus. *Surgery of the Anus, Rectum and Colon*, London: Baillière Tindall.
Goulston, K. (1979) Effect of diet on fecal occult blood test. *Symposium on Colo-rectal Cancer, New York*.
Greegor, D.H. (1971) Occult blood testing for detection of asymptomatic colon cancer. *Cancer*, **28**, 131-134.
Greegor, D.H. (1978) Über entstehung, durchführung und folgen des modifizierten Guajak-Tests. In *Kolorektale Krebsvorsorge*. pp. 61-67. Nürnberg: Verlag Wachholz.
Greenstein, A.J., Sachar, D., Pucillo, A., Kreel, I., Geller, S., Ianowitz, H.D. & Aufses, A. (1978) Cancer in Crohn's disease after discovery surgery: a report of seven carcinomas occurring in excluded bowel. *American Journal of Surgery*, **135**, 86-90.
Grinnell, R.S. & Lane, N. (1958) Benign and malignant adenomatous polyps and papillary adenomas of the colon and rectum. An analysis of 1856 tumours in 1335 patients. *Surgery*, **106**, 519-538.
Hardcastle, J.D. & Balfour, T.W. (1980) Evaluation of the haemoccult faecal occult blood test in the diagnosis of asymptomatic colo-rectal cancer — a feasibility study in general practice. *Communication to the British Medical Association Clinical Meeting, Nottingham.*
Hastings, J.B. (1974) Mass screening for colo-rectal cancer. *American Journal of Surgery*, **127**, 228-233.
Hawley, P.R. (1977) The results of surgery in a specialized hospital. *Topics in Gastroenterology*, **5**, 65-75.
Heald, R.J. & Lockhart-Mummery, H.E. (1972) The lesion of the second cancer of the large bowel. *British Journal of Surgery*, **59**, 16-19.
Helfrick, G.B. & Petrucci, P. (1979) Public screening with fecal occult blood testing. *Symposium on Colo-rectal Cancer, New York*.
Helwig, E.B. (1947) The evaluation of adenomas of the large intestine and their relation to carcinoma. *Surgery, Gynecology and Obstetrics*, **84**, 36-49.

Higgins, G.A. (1976) Chemotherapy, adjuvant to surgery, for gastrointestinal cancer. *Clinics in Gastroenterology*, **5**, 795-808.
Hinton, J.M. (1966) Risk of malignant change in ulcerative colitis. *Gut*, **7**, 427-432.
Holliday, H. & Hardcastle, J.D. (1979) Delay in diagnosis and treatment of symptomatic colo-rectal cancer. *Lancet*, **i**, 309-311.
Hughes, L.E. & Aust, N.Z.J. (1968) The incidence of benign and malignant neoplasms of the colon and rectum: a post-mortem study. *Surgery*, **38**, 30-36.
Illingworth, D.G. (1965) Influence of diet on occult blood tests. *Gut*, **6**, 595-598.
Irons, G.V. & Kirsner, J.B. (1965) Routine chemical tests of the stool for occult blood; an evaluation. *American Journal of the Medical Sciences*, **249**, 247-259.
Jaffe, R.M. & Zierdt, W. (1979) A new occult blood test not subject to false-negative results from reducing substances. *Journal of Laboratory and Clinical Medicine*, **93**, 879-886.
Jaffe, R.M., Kasten, B., Young, D.S. & MacLowry, J.D. (1975) False-negative stool occult blood tests caused by ingestion of ascorbic acid (vitamin C). *Annals of Internal Medicine*, **83**, 824-826.
James, W.G. (1977) *Communication to a meeting of the American Society of Preventive Oncology, New York.*
Jones, I.S.C. (1976) An analysis of bowel habit and its significance in the diagnosis of carcinoma of the colon. *American Journal of Proctology*, **27**, 45-56.
Kaneko, M. (1972) On pedunculated adenomatous polyps of colon and rectum with particular reference to their malignant potential. *Mt Sinai Journal of Medicine*, **39**, 103-111.
Keddie, N. & Hargreaves, A. (1968) Symptoms of carcinoma of the colon and rectum. *Lancet*, **ii**, 749-750.
Kessel, D. & Allen, J. (1975) Elevated plasma sialyltransferase in cancer patients. *Cancer Research*, **35**, 670-672.
Kleinfield, G. & Gump, F.E. (1960) Complications of colotomy and polypectomy. *Surgery, Gynecology and Obstetrics*, **111**, 726-728.
Lennard-Jones, J.E., Morson, B.C., Ritchie, J.K., Shove, D.C & Williams, C.B. (1977) Cancer in colitis: assessment of the individual risk by clinical and histological criteria. *Gastroenterology*, **73**, 1280-1289.
Lipshuty, G.R., Katon, R.M., McCool, M.F., et al (1979) Flexible sigmoidoscopy as a screening procedure for neoplasia of the colon. *Surgery, Gynecology and Obstetrics*, **148**, 19-22.
Lipton, A., Sheehan, L. & Harvery, H.A. (1975) Urinary polyamine levels in patients with gastrointestinal malignancy. *Cancer*, **36**, 2351-2354.
Lovett, E. (1976) Family studies in cancer of the colon and rectum. *British Journal of Surgery*, **63**, 13-18.
Lynch, H.T., Krush, A.J. & Guirgis, H. (1973) Genetic factors in families with combined gastrointestinal and breast cancer. *American Journal of Gastroenterology*, **59**, 31-40.
Lynch, H.T., Harris, R.E., Bardawil, W.A., Lynch, P.M., Guirgis, H.A., Swartz, M.G. & Lynch, J.F. (1977) Management of hereditary site-specific colon cancer. *Archives of Surgery*, **112**, 170-174.
Madigan, M.R. & Hall, J.M. (1968) The extent of sigmoidoscopy shown on radiographs with special reference to the rectosigmoid junction. *Gut*, **9**, 355-362.
MacDougall, I.P.M. (1964) The cancer risk in ulcerative colitis. *Lancet*, **ii**, 655-658.
Mayo, C.W. & de Castro, C.A. (1956) Carcinoma of the sigmoid arising from a polyp first visualized fifteen years previously; report of case. *Proceedings of the Mayo Clinic*, **31**, 597-598.
Miller, R.E. (1974) Detection of colon carcinoma and the barium enema. *Journal of the American Medical Association*, **230**, 1195-1198.
Miller, S.F. & Knight, A.R. (1977) The early detection of colo-rectal cancer. *Cancer*, **40**, 945-949.
Moertel, C.G., Hill, J.R. & Dockerty, M.B. (1966) The routine proctoscopic examination: a second look. *Proceedings of the Mayo Clinic*, **41**, 368-374.
Molnar, I.G., Vandevoorde, J.P. & Gitnich, G.L. (1976) CEA levels in fluids bathing gastrointestinal tumours. *Gastroenterology*, **70**, 513-515.
Morgan, L.R., Samuels, M.S., Thomas, W., et al (1975) Incidence, mortality or prevalence as indicators of the cancer problem. *Cancer*, **36**, 2227-2345.
Morris, D.W., Hansell, J.R., Ostrow, J.D., Chuan-Shur Lee (1976) Reliability of chemical tests for fecal occult blood in hospitalized patients. *Digestive Diseases*, **21**, 845-852.

Morson, B.C. (1966) Factors influencing the prognosis of early cancer of the rectum. *Proceedings of the Royal Society of Medicine*, **59**, 607-608.

Morson B.C. (1976) Genesis of colo-rectal cancer. *Clinics in Gastroenterology*, **5**, 505-524.

Morson, B.C. & Dawson, I.M.P. (1972) *Gastrointestinal Pathology*. Oxford: Blackwell Scientific.

Morson, B.C. & Pang, L.S.C. (1967) Rectal biopsy as an aid to cancer control in ulcerative colitis. *Gut*, **8**, 423-434.

Ostrow, J.D., Mulvaney, C.A., Hansel, J.R. & Rhodes, R.S. (1973) Sensitivity and reproducibility of chemical tests for fecal occult blood with an emphasis on false-positive reactions. *American Journal of the Digestive Diseases*, **18**, 930-940.

Otto, P., Bunnemann, H. & Hans-Joachim, X. (1979) Screening and diagnosis in colo-rectal neoplasia. *Symposium on Colo-rectal Cancer, New York*.

Parlides, G.P., Mulligan, F.D., Clarke, D.N., et al (1977) Hereditary polyposis coli. I. The diagnostic value of colonoscopy, barium enema and fecal occult blood. *Cancer*, **40**, 2632-2639.

Payne, R.A. (1976) The incidence and clinical significance of rectal polyps. *Annals of the Royal College of Surgeons of England*, **58**, 241-242.

Prager, E.D., Swinton, N.M., Young, J., et al (1974) Follow-up study of patients with benign mucosal polyps discovered by procto-sigmoidoscopy. *Diseases of the Colon and Rectum*, **17**, 322-324.

Raskin, H.F. & Pletucka, S. (1964) The cytologic diagnosis of cancer of the colon. *Acta Cytologica*, **8**, 131-140.

Raskin, H.F. & Pletucka, S. (1970) Exfoliative cytology of the colon. *Cancer*, **28**, 127-130.

Richardson, J.L. (1977) Colo-rectal cancer: a mass screening and education program. *Geriatrics* (February), 123-131.

Ross, T.H. & Johnson, J.C.M. (1976) Detecting colo-rectal cancer. *Arizona Medicine*, **33**, 445-448.

Roswit, B., Higgins, G.A. & Keehan, R.J. (1975) Preoperative irradiation for carcinoma of the rectum and rectosigmoid colon: report of a national veterans administrative randomized study. *Cancer*, **35**, 1597-1602.

Russell, D.H., Durrie, B.G.M. & Salmon, S.E. (1975) Polyamines as predictors of success and failure in cancer chemotherapy. *Lancet*, **ii**, 797-799.

Samec, H.J. (1979) Hemoccult in colonrectal carcinoma in Austria. *Colo-rectal Symposium, New York*.

Schwartz, M.D. (1977) An evaluation of markers in the early detection of large bowel cancer. *Cancer*, **40**, 2620-2624.

Sherlock, P. & Winawer, S.J. (1977) The role of early diagnosis in controlling large bowel cancer. *Cancer*, **40**, 2609-2615.

Sherlock, P., Ehrlick, A.N. & Winawer, S.J. (1972) Diagnosis of gastrointestinal cancer; current status and recent progress. *Gastroenterology*, **63**, 672-700.

Slaney, G. (1971) Results of treatment of carcinoma of the colon and rectum. *Modern Trends in Surgery*, **3**, 69-89.

Slaney, G. (1978) *Communications of the British Society of Gastroenterology, Edinburgh*.

Spinelli, P., Bertario, L. & Berrino, F. (1979) Guaiac test — our experience and evaluation program of efficacy. *Symposium on Colo-rectal Cancer, New York*.

Stroehlein, J.R., Fairbanks, V.F., McGill, D.B. & Vay, L.W. (1976) Hemoccult detection of fecal occult blood quantitated by radioassay. *Digestive Diseases*, **21**, 841-844.

Teague, R., Salmon, P.R. & Read, A.E. (1973) Fiberoptic examinations of the colon; a review of 255 cases. *Gut*, **14**, 139-142.

Thompson, W.G. & Heaton, K.W. (1978) *Communication to the British Society of Gastroenterology, Edinburgh*.

Till, A.S. (1977) The results of treatment in district general hospitals. *Topics in Gastroenterology*, **5**, 77-85.

Walker, M.R. (1968) Cancer in South-West England. *Annals of the Royal College of Surgeons*, **42**, 145.

Weedon, D.D., Shorter, R.G., Ilstrup, D.M., Huizenga, K.A. & Taylor, W.F. (1973) Crohn's disease and cancer. *New England Journal of Medicine*, **289**, 1099-1102.

Welch, C.E. & Donaldson, G.A. (1974) Recent experiences in the management of cancer of the colon and rectum. *American Journal of Surgery*, **127**, 258-266.

Wells, H.J. & Pagano, J.E. (1977) 'Hemoccult' test — reversal of false-negative results due to storage. *Gastroenterology*, **72**, 1148.

Williams, C.B. & Teague, R. (1973) Progress report — colonoscopy. *Gut*, **14**, 990-1003.

Williams, C.B., Hunt, R.H., Loose, H., Sakai, Y. & Swarbrick, E.T. (1974) Colonoscopy in the management of colon polyps. *British Journal of Surgery*, **61**, 673-682.

Wilson, G.S., Dale, E.H. & Brines, O.A. (1955) An evaluation of polyps detected in 20 847 routine sigmoidoscopic examinations. *American Journal of Surgery*, **90**, 834-840.

Winawer, S.J. (1979) Validity of screening for colo-rectal cancer. *Symposium on Colo-rectal Cancer, New York*.

Winawer, S.J., Miller, D.G., Schottenfield, D., Leidner, S.D., Sherlock, P., Befler, B. & Stearns, M.W. (1977) Feasibility of faecal occult blood testing for detection of colo-rectal neoplasia. *Cancer*, **40**, 2616-2619.

Wolff, W.I., Shinya, H., Giffer, A., et al (1974) Comparison of colonoscopy and the contrast enema in five hundred patients with colo-rectal disease. *American Journal of Surgery*, **129**, 181-186.

Zamacheck, N. (1975) The present status of CEA in diagnosis, prognosis and evaluation of therapy. *Cancer*, **36**, 2460-2468.

20

Dysplasia in the Colorectum

B.C. MORSON
F. KONISHI

The concept of epithelial dysplasia as the main, if not the only, precursor lesion for colorectal cancer is an unfamiliar one and yet there is evidence that this is perhaps the best nomenclature for describing precancerous lesions in the large bowel. Currently, the persons at increased risk for colorectal cancer are those with the genetically predetermined condition known as familial polyposis, members of colorectal cancer families (in which the mode of inheritance is poorly documented), certain patients with a long history of chronic ulcerative colitis, individuals who have already had a partial resection of bowel for cancer and that large population of patients with adenomas of the colorectum. It is possible at the present time to give only a very approximate estimate of the magnitude of cancer risk in the last three clinical groups but it is certainly much lower than in the first two categories. The main object of this paper is to present the evidence that epithelial dysplasia is the common histological and cytological precursor change for all these groups and that the magnitude of risk varies with the grade of epithelial dysplasia as well as other factors.

This concept becomes clearer if we remember that the colorectal adenoma is by definition a focus of dysplasia and that familial polyposis is a condition in which enormous numbers of adenomas cover the mucosal surface of the large intestine. The evidence that most, if not all, colorectal cancers seen in polyposis patients, colorectal cancer families, so-called metachronous or second primary cancers, and in isolated or solitary malignant growths have evolved through the adenoma-carcinoma sequence is well established. A new approach would be to think in terms of the *dysplasia-carcinoma sequence* for these categories of patients, rather than adenoma-carcinoma, or polyp-cancer sequence. The latter can be confusing because not all 'polyps' are adenomas. The concept of dysplasia as the precursor lesion for cancer in chronic ulcerative colitis is already well documented (Morson and Pang, 1967; Lennard-Jones et al, 1977; Riddell and Morson, 1979).

© 1980 W.B. Saunders Company Ltd.

DEFINITIONS AND NOMENCLATURE

A *precancerous condition* as defined by the World Health Organization is a clinical state associated with a significantly increased risk of cancer, whereas a *precancerous lesion* is a histopathological abnormality in which cancer is more likely to occur than in its apparently normal counterpart (WHO, 1972). Precancerous conditions may also show precancerous lesions but the latter are sometimes found in the absence of any clinical condition.

Epithelial dysplasia of the colorectal epithelium, whether in the form of an adenoma or in ulcerative colitis, is a precancerous lesion which seldom gives rise to any clinical symptoms. The word 'dysplasia' should not be used synonymously with 'atypia' or, to be more accurate, 'cellular atypia' because the 'dysplasia' incorporates both structural as well as cytological abnormalities. A colorectal adenoma, by definition, always shows both structural and cytological abnormalities of dysplasia which vary in severity and can, therefore, be graded subjectively (see below). Adenomas can also be graded according to their structural appearance into tubular, tubulovillous and villous types (WHO, 1976), but the features of dysplasia are common to all three varieties.

Carcinoma-in-situ in adenomas is not a nomenclature favoured by us, but when used by others it would correspond to severe dysplasia. Likewise, we do not use such expressions as 'focal cancer' and 'intramucosal carcinoma' in the colorectum for dysplastic changes that are restricted to a line above the muscularis mucosae. It has been proven beyond doubt that only when invasion has occurred across this line does the disease have any potential for metastasis. We prefer to reserve the words 'cancer' and 'carcinoma' for lesions which have invaded across the muscularis mucosae into the submucosa. As long as the epithelial change is superficial to this line then it is best graded as mild, moderate or severe dysplasia which at least avoids the emotive and often misunderstood implications of 'cancer' or 'carcinoma' (Morson, 1978).

PRECANCEROUS CONDITIONS AND LESIONS OF THE COLORECTUM

There are five main categories: adenoma; familial polyposis, colorectal cancer families; patients who have had a colorectal cancer removed; chronic ulcerative colitis.

Adenoma. This is a precancerous lesion which can be regarded as a focus of epithelial dysplasia of varying severity which adopts three main structural variants, the tubular, tubulovillous and villous adenomas.

Familial polyposis. This is a precancerous condition in which the surface of the large bowel is covered by thousands of adenomas. It can be regarded as a condition in which visible and microscopic foci of dysplasia of variable severity are present in enormous numbers. It is, perhaps, this massive and extensive dysplasia of the colorectal epithelium which gives patients with familial polyposis their very high cancer risk.

Colorectal cancer families. These families are prone to colorectal cancer but do not have polyposis. However, it has been shown that affected members have rather more adenomas than are found in patients without a familial history of cancer. The adenoma-carcinoma (dysplasia-carcinoma) sequence has been demonstrated in colorectal cancer family members (Bussey, Ritchie and Morson, 1980).

Patients who have had a colorectal cancer removed. Statistically these patients are at increased risk of developing a second or metachronous cancer in any remaining large bowel, especially if adenomas were present in the first operation specimen (Bussey, Wallace and Morson, 1967).

Chronic ulcerative colitis. This is a precancerous condition, but only when patients have had extensive disease of the colorectum for more than ten years. They are then prone to develop the lesions of dysplasia of the colorectal epithelium (Lennard-Jones et al, 1977). If this dysplasia becomes severe then the patient is at high risk of developing one or more invasive carcinomas. Epithelial dysplasia in ulcerative colitis is essentially no different from the dysplasia seen in isolated adenomas or in familial polyposis except that it is diffuse and can occur in a flat as well as a polypoid mucosa. Moreover, there are some additional criteria for grading dysplasia in ulcerative colitis which are important (Lennard-Jones et al, 1977).

HISTOLOGY AND GRADING OF DYSPLASIA IN COLORECTAL ADENOMAS

The epithelial dysplasia in colorectal adenomas is a neoplastic change which is characterized by cytological and structural changes. The cytological changes include hyperchromatism, increased size, stratification, pleomorphism and loss of polarity of the nuclei with increased numbers of mitotic figures and depletion of mucin. The structural change is the disorganization of the epithelial crypts by branching, budding and bridging.

The degree of epithelial dysplasia is a continuous spectrum from mild change, which is closest to the normal epithelium, to severe changes which approximate to those seen in invasive carcinoma. It is customary to divide the changes into three categories of mild, moderate and severe. It is common to see different grades of dysplasia in one adenoma. Sometimes an area with one grade of dysplasia has a distinct boundary with an adjacent area showing a different grade but often there is a gradual transition between areas with different grades of dysplasia. All grades of epithelial dysplasia can be seen in adenomas of the histological types which are categorized as tubular, tubulovillous and villous.

Mild dysplasia (Figure 1). The nuclei are elongated, larger than normal and slightly hyperchromatic with a fine chromatin pattern. They are arranged regularly at the base of the cells. The amount of mucin is decreased and is confined to the lumenal border of the cells. The number of mitotic figures is slightly increased. Pleomorphism and loss of polarity of the nuclei are not typical features of this category. The glandular arrangement is irregular with some branching. The distinction from moderate dysplasia becomes blurred when the nuclei begin to become stratified with some loss of polarity and the amount of mucin is further decreased. Occasional reversed goblet cells (intra-epithelial goblet cells) may be seen.

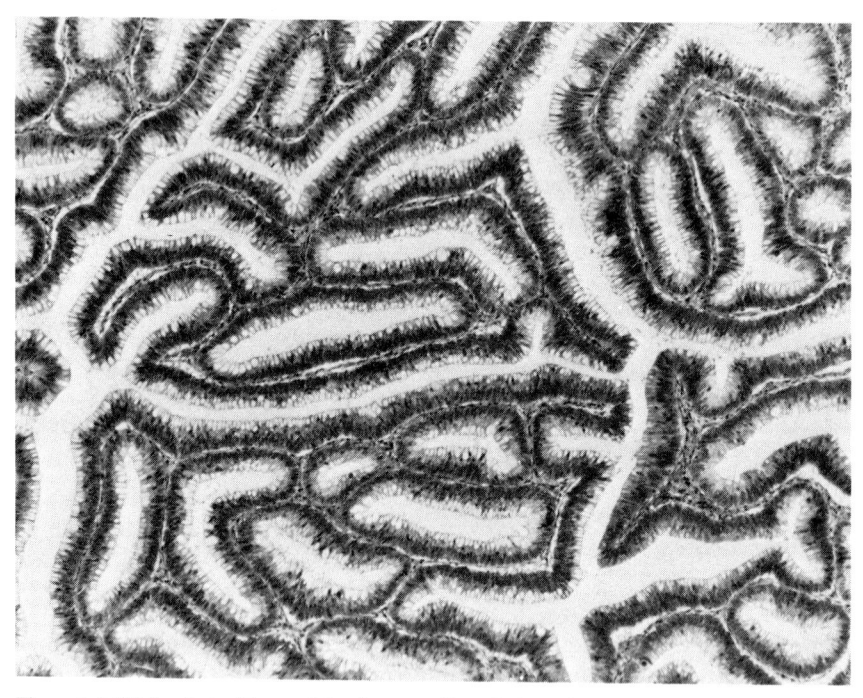

Figure 1. Mild dysplasia. The nuclei are arranged regularly at the base of the cells. The amount of mucin is slightly decreased. Haematoxylin and eosin, × 90.

Moderate dysplasia (Figure 2). This category can be defined as intermediate between mild dysplasia and severe dysplasia. The nuclei are round rather than elongated and the chromatin tends to show a clumping pattern. There is nuclear stratification and obvious loss of polarity with some increase in the nuclear-cytoplasmic ratio. The amount of mucin is further decreased and reversed goblet cells are seen more often. An important change is the tendency towards pleomorphism of the nuclei. Structural distortion of the crypts is more manifest, with folding of epithelial cells into the glandular lumen. This is different from the true intraglandular budding and bridging which is a feature of severe dysplasia.

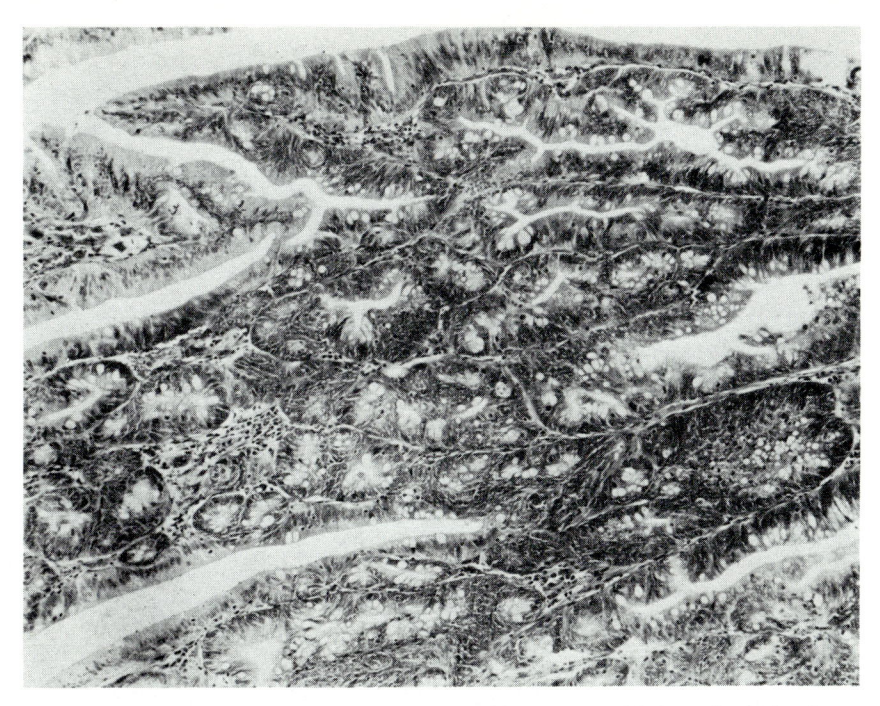

Figure 2. Moderate dysplasia. There is nuclear stratification and slight loss of polarity. Structural distortion of the crypts is more manifest. Haematoxylin and eosin, × 90.

Severe dysplasia (Figure 3). The changes are very similar to those of invading adenocarcinoma. The nuclei are large and pleomorphic with an obvious increase in the nuclear-cytoplasmic ratio. The chromatin pattern is either diffusely dark or open with clumping of the chromatin and one or more nucleoli can often be seen. The marked pleomorphism is associated with loss of polarity of the nuclei and an obvious increase in the number of mitotic figures. Little mucin is present and cannot be recognized as a clear droplet with haematoxylin and eosin staining. The glandular structure is very distorted, featuring frequent intraglandular bridging and budding, which gives the impression of glandular fusion. The condensed growth pattern shows the so-called 'glandular back-to-back' arrangement. In some cases, despite little evidence of intraglandular budding or bridging, the nuclei are large and show severe pleomorphism and loss of polarity. In many adenomas areas of severe dysplasia have a distinct boundary with adjacent less severe, even mild, dysplasia.

MALIGNANT POTENTIAL OF COLORECTAL DYSPLASIA

In Adenomas

The grading of adenomas into those showing mild, moderate or severe dysplasia has shown that, irrespective of histological growth pattern, their

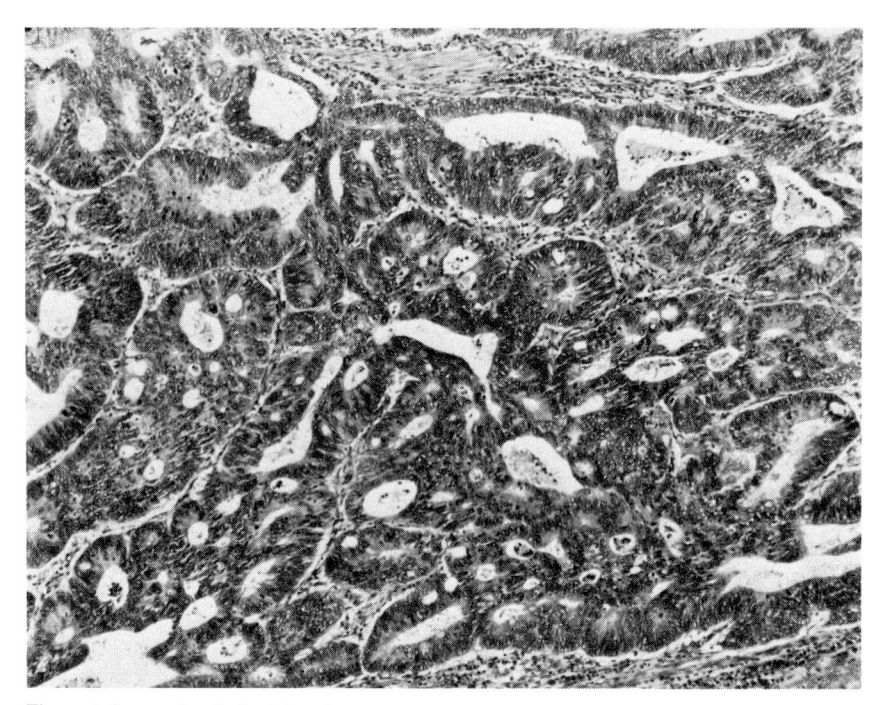

Figure 3. Severe dysplasia. There is marked pleomorphism of the nuclei associated with loss of polarity. The glandular structure shows frequent intraglandular bridgings and buddings. Haematoxylin and eosin, × 90.

malignant potential increases with an increasing degree of dysplasia (Table 1). The severity of dysplasia is also related to the size of the tumour. From Table 2 it can be seen that small adenomas under 1 cm in diameter, which make up the majority of tumours in this study, usually show mild dysplasia

Table 1. Grade of dysplasia in adenomas and percentage of carcinoma

Grade of dysplasia	Total no.	No. with malignancy	Percentage
Mild	1734	99	5.7
Moderate	549	99	18.0
Severe	223	77	34.5

Modified from Muto, Bussey and Morson (1975).

only and have a very low malignant potential. The malignancy rate rises to 27 per cent if severe dysplasia is present, but this is very rare in a polyp of this size. A similar relationship is seen in polyps 1 to 2 cm in diameter; those with mild dysplasia have a low malignant potential, whereas those with moderate and severe dysplasia are increasingly likely to contain invasive foci. In adenomas over 2 cm in size the malignancy rate is high but shows little relation to the degree of dysplasia. This could be due to sampling error, but it also shows again how, in practice, size is of major importance in the assessment of malignant potential. In Table 3 the cancer rates are charted according to the degree of dysplasia in the three histological variants of adenomas. The explanation for the high malignant potential in tumours with a villous

Table 2. *Percentage of carcinoma in relation to size and grade of dysplasia*

Grade of dysplasia	Size		
	Under 1 cm	1-2 cm	Over 2 cm
Mild	0.3% (1198)	3.0% (329)	42.3% (196)
Moderate	2.0% (244)	14.4% (167)	50.0% (134)
Severe	27.0% (37)	24.1% (83)	48.0% (100)

Modified from Muto, Bussey and Morson (1975).

Table 3. *Size, histological type and percentage of carcinoma*

Histological type	Size		
	Under 1 cm	1-2 cm	Over 2 cm
Tubular adenoma	1.0% (1382)	10.2% (392)	34.7% (101)
Tubulovillous adenoma	3.9% (76)	7.4% (149)	45.8% (155)
Villous adenoma	9.5% (21)	10.3% (39)	52.9% (174)

Modified from Muto, Bussey and Morson (1975).

component and mild or moderate dysplasia could be partly explained by a sampling error in the study of this group. Larger adenomas often show variable dysplasia in different parts of the same tumour and it is conceivable that the sections examined were not representative. It is also possible that sections of these larger tumours were taken from areas away from the malignant focus, which itself arose from a localized area of severe dysplasia. Kalus (1972) has shown that severe dysplasia in adenomas is found between seven and eight times more frequently when associated adenocarcinomas are also present than where there is no associated malignant lesion. Thus severe dysplasia would appear to be a more selective marker for cancer risk than other variables.

The demonstration of grades of epithelial dysplasia in adenomas is powerful support for the concept of the adenoma-carcinoma sequence (Lescher et al, 1967; Potet and Soullard, 1971; Kozuka, 1975) and suggests a gradual transition from a benign to a malignant tumour. It is probable that all carcinomas arising from epithelial surfaces have passed through stages of increasingly severe epithelial dysplasia before becoming invasive, and in the colon and rectum such a progression is seen only in adenomas. At any rate, no alternative mechanism for the histogenesis of large bowel carcinoma has yet been documented (Fenoglio and Lane, 1974; Muto, Bussey and Morson,

1975). Thus small areas of severe dysplasia other than those arising in long-standing ulcerative colitis (Morson and Pang, 1967; Riddell, 1976) have not been observed independent of adenomas, nor have very small invasive carcinomas without ulceration been seen. Small ulcerated invasive cancers without residual adenomatous tissue have been described (Weingarten and Turell, 1952; Spratt and Ackerman, 1962), but these could result from continued invasion plus surface ulceration in an adenoma, so that all adenomatous remnants and indeed the stalk, if present, would disappear, leaving an ulcerated plaque of carcinoma bordered by non-adenomatous mucosal epithelium. This course of events would be more likely in the case of tubular and tubulovillous adenomas, especially those on pedicles in the presence of advanced cancer, than it would in the typical broad-based sessile villous adenoma, which would logically be expected to retain adenomatous elements even with advanced invasive cancer (Enterline, 1976).

If carcinoma did arise on a background of normal mucosa, numerous examples of tiny independent carcinomas, under 0.5 cm in diameter, would have been encountered and reported. That this is not the case is strong presumptive evidence against a de novo origin of large bowel cancer.

Life history

Given that adenomas under certain circumstances may develop malignant change, how long does it take for the dysplasia-carcinoma sequence to evolve? In practice, the sequence is never less than five years, and averages 10 to 15 years, but may even cover a normal adult life-span (Muto, Bussey and Morson, 1975).

In patients with familial polyposis coli, the age distribution curves show a time interval of about 12 years between the average age at diagnosis of polyposis without cancer and of polyposis with cancer. This difference is likely to be an underestimation since determination of the age at onset of polyposis is inaccurate, although probably less so than for isolated adenomas. More information on the life history comes from an analysis of the time of onset of polyposis and cancer in patients with familial polyposis coli who were not operated on. Most of these patients come from the group who were under care at St Mark's Hospital before the operation of total colectomy and ileorectal anastomosis was established about 30 years ago. In Table 4 it can be seen that in 65 patients who did not have an operation, the likelihood of a carcinoma developing rose progressively as the period of observation increased. However, in the group of seven patients observed from 20 to 25 years, four did not develop carcinoma and one patient survived over 30 years before a malignant tumour supervened.

Epithelial Dysplasia in Ulcerative Colitis

There are two main histological varieties of epithelial dysplasia in ulcerative colitis, the adenomatous, which is probably the most common, and dysplasia in an entirely flat mucosa. Adenomatous dysplasia more often adopts a low villous pattern than a tubular type of proliferation, but in either case mani-

Table 4. *Length of dysplasia-carcinoma sequence in familial polyposis coli*

Period (years)	Number of patients observed	Number surviving period without cancer	Number developing cancer in period	Percentage developing cancer
0-5	65	59	6	9.2
5-10	45	35	10	22.2
10-15	23	16	7	30.4
15-20	12	8	4	33.3
20-25	7	4	3	42.6
25-30	3	1	2	66.6
30-35	1	—	1	100.0

Modified from Muto, Bussey and Morson (1975).

fests itself as a velvety or nodular macroscopic appearance. The resemblance to ordinary villous and tubular adenoma can be striking except that the lesions are poorly circumscribed, usually cover large areas of mucosa and are seldom raised up much above the adjacent flat mucous membrane, although large polypoid tumours do occur. Adenomatous dysplasia in colitis very rarely produces tumour on a stalk or pedicle. Small, isolated adenomas are occasionally discovered in the older patients with colitis and then consideration has to be given to whether they are the consequence of the inflammatory disease or a coincidental finding.

Some changes distinctive of dysplasia in flat mucosa have been described (Riddell, 1976). These include proliferation of enlarged, darkly-staining cells arranged in a line along the whole length of the crypt and accompanied by eosinophilic cytoplasm. Goblet cells are absent. This type of dysplasia often gives rise to a very poorly differentiated type of carcinoma in colitis. Another form closely resembles intramucosal carcinoma of the stomach and has been called in-situ anaplasia. Sometimes the dysplastic cells become vacuolated, stain poorly with mucin stains and resemble the clear cell type of carcinoma of the stomach and colon; the so-called nephrogenic carcinoma. Finally, a variety known as pancellular dysplasia has large hyperchromatic nuclei with loss of polarity and affects all cell lines including Paneth, argentaffin and goblet cells.

Dysplasia in colitis can be subjectively graded as mild, moderate and severe. Severe dysplasia can be regarded as synonymous with carcinoma-in-situ. Grading has been shown to have particular importance in the design of cancer prevention programmes for patients at increased risk. The term 'precancer' implies only an increased susceptibility to invasive carcinoma, but is used by us as a clinical counterpart for the grade of severe dysplasia.

A recent prospective study has shown that the detection of severe dysplasia by sequential rectal and colonic biopsy can detect those patients at special risk of developing cancer and that patients with mild to moderate dysplasia and those without biopsy evidence of dysplasia can safely continue under medical supervision (Lennard-Jones et al, 1977). Severe dysplasia is uncommon but is associated with a high risk of carcinoma (Morson and Pang, 1967; Myrvold, Kock and Ahren, 1974; Yardley and Keren, 1974) but if patients at increased risk, as judged by the length of history of symptoms and the extent of colitis, are identified and carefully followed up by sequential biopsies then any carcinomas will be detected at an early and curable stage of development.

Ideally, patients should be treated in the precancerous phase which puts a special responsibility on the pathologist who must screen all biopsies from patients with ulcerative colitis for dysplasia with especial care. Knowledge of whether the patient is clinically and statistically at increased risk may not always be available, so that it is essential to acquire experience in recognizing and grading dysplasia and differentiating it, in particular, from the much more common cellular changes which are reactive to the inflammation.

EPIDEMIOLOGY OF COLORECTAL DYSPLASIA

As yet very little study has been directly concentrated on the epidemiology of colorectal dysplasia. However, there is information on the epidemiology of adenomas which confirm that such an approach might be useful.

In populations with a high risk of colorectal cancer the incidence of large adenomas (over 1 cm diameter) is found to be greater than in countries with a low risk (Table 5). Large adenomas have a higher incidence of severe

Table 5. *Proportion of adenomas greater than 1 cm diameter in five populations*

Population	% of adenomas greater than 1 cm	Reference
England	39	Morson (1974)
Sweden	27	Berge et al (1973)
Colombia	2	Correa et al (1972)
USA	15	Arminski and McLean (1964)
Japan	5	Sato (1974)

dysplasia than small adenomas. In a comparison of the pathology of adenomas in England and Japan (Muto et al, 1977) it was found that villous tumours with their high malignant potential were much less common in Japan than England and that none of the Japanese villous tumours, in this study, exhibited severe dysplasia (Table 6). Moreover, the malignant poten-

Table 6. *Histology and malignant potential of adenomas in England and Japan*[a]

	% with severe dysplasia England	Japan	% with invasive cancer England	Japan
Tubular adenoma	4.4	4.6	4.8	2.1
Tubulovillous adenoma	9.7	15.8	22.5	5.3
Villous adenoma	11.1	Nil	40.7	75.5

Modified from Muto et al (1977).
[a] England 2506 cases; Japan 299 cases.

tial of severe dysplasia was much less in Japan than England (Table 7). There is one interesting comparison of the relative incidence of severe dysplasia in adenomas in two Japanese provinces (Table 8). The higher risk of colorectal cancer in Akita compared with Miyagi is matched by a greater incidence of severe dysplasia in the adenomas of the former compared with the latter.

Table 7. *Epithelial dysplasia and malignant potential of adenomas in England and Japan[a]*

	% of adenomas with invasive carcinoma		
	Mild	Moderate	Severe
England	5.7	18.0	34.5
Japan	1.0	7.9	13.0

Modified from Muto et al (1977).
[a]England 2506 cases; Japan 299 cases.

Table 8. *Incidence of structural and cytological atypia in two Japanese provinces*

Structural (%)	Mild	Moderate	Severe
Akita	77.1	20.8	2.1
Miyagi	87.3	12.1	0.6

Cytological (%)	0	I	II	III
Akita	67.7	22.9	7.3	2.1
Miyagi	65.9	26.6	6.4	1.2

Modified from Sato et al (1976).

Although these results show the importance of studying dysplasia on a population basis, comparing high-risk areas for colorectal cancer with low-risk areas, they are, as yet, insufficient for application to cancer prevention programmes. We can see the trend that severe dysplasia in adenomas might be a more selective marker for increased cancer risk than adenomas alone or even larger adenomas. But size is relatively simple to estimate in clinical or population studies whereas grading of dysplasia involves more exacting skills. More studies are required on the epidemiology of severe dysplasia in adenomas and correlation with the techniques of metabolic epidemiology and cytogenetics.

GENETIC FACTORS IN EPITHELIAL DYSPLASIA?

Adenomatosis (also known as familial polyposis coli) is undoubtedly a genetically determined disease, being due to a non-sex linked dominant gene transmitted on normal Mendelian lines. It has been suggested that in fact all adenomas have a genetic aetiology; that if the normal gene is designated +, and the gene for small numbers of adenomas is *p*, then persons with the combination + + will not carry adenomas; similarly, those who are *p* + will also appear normal and carry no adenomas, but that those who are *pp* will develop adenomas (Veale, 1965). To date this hypothesis has not been tested and so there is no direct evidence either to support or to refute it. However, this hypothesis must also be interpreted in the light of the concept that all adenomas, whether isolated lesions or in the enormous numbers found in familial polyposis, are foci of epithelial dysplasia. Is there a genetic factor in the aetiology of epithelial dysplasia? Current efforts in the field of the cytogenetics of familial polyposis may turn out to be important in the attempt to answer this question.

REFERENCES

Arminski, T.C. & McLean, D.W. (1964) Incidence and distribution of adenomatous polyps of the colon and rectum based on 1000 autopsy examinations. *Diseases of the Colon and Rectum*, **7**, 249.

Berge, T., Ekelund, G., Mellner, C., Pihl, B. & Wenckert, A. (1973) Carcinoma of the colon and rectum in a defined population. *Acta Chirurgica Scadinavica* (Suppl. 438).

Bussey, H.J.R., Ritchie, S. & Morson, B.C. (1980) The adenoma-carcinoma sequence in colorectal cancer families. *Gastroenterology*. In press.

Bussey, H.J.R., Wallace, M.H. & Morson, B.C. (1967) Metachronous carcinoma of the large intestine and intestinal polyps. *Proceedings of the Royal Society of Medicine*, **60**, 208.

Cook, M.G. & Goligher, J.C. (1975) Carcinoma and epithelial dysplasia complicating ulcerative colitis. *Gastroenterology*, **68**, 1127.

Correa, P., Duque, E., Cuello, C. & Haenszel, W. (1972) Polyps of the colon and rectum in Cali, Colombia. *British Journal of Cancer*, **9**, 86.

Enterline, H.T. (1976) Polyps and cancer of the large bowel. In *Current Topics in Pathology. Vol. 63. Pathology of the Gastrointestinal Tract* (Ed.) Morson, B.C. pp. 95-141. Berlin: Springer-Verlag.

Evans, D.J. & Pollock, D.J. (1972) In situ and invasive carcinoma of the colon in patients with ulcerative colitis. *Gut*, **13**, 566.

Fenoglio, G.M. & Lane, N. (1974) The anatomical precursor of colorectal carcinoma. *Cancer*, **34**, 819.

Hulten, L., Kewenter, J. & Ahren, C. (1972) Precancer and carcinoma in chronic ulcerative colitis. *Scandinavian Journal of Gastroenterology*, **7**, 663.

Isaacson, P. (1976) Tissue demonstration of carcinoembryonic antigen (CEA) in ulcerative colitis. *Gut*, **17**, 561.

Kalus, M. (1972) Carcinoma and adenomatous polyps of the colon and rectum in biopsy and organ tissue culture. *Cancer*, **30**, 972.

Kozuka, S. (1975) Premalignancy of the mucosal polyp in the large intestine. I. Histologic gradation of the polyp on the basis of epithelial pseudostratification and glandular branching. *Diseases of the Colon and Rectum*, **18**, 483.

Lennard-Jones, J.E., Morson, B.C., Ritchie, J.K., Shove, D.C. & Williams, C.B. (1977) Cancer in colitis: assessment of the individual risk by clinical and histological criteria. *Gastroenterology*, **73**, 1280.

Lescher, T.C., Dockerty, M.B., Jackman, R.J. & Beahrs, O.H. (1967) Histopathology of the larger colonic polyp. *Diseases of the Colon and Rectum*, **10**, 118.

Levin, R., Riddell, R.H. & Kirsner, J.B. (1976) Management of precancerous lesions of the gastrointestinal tract. *Clinics in Gastroenterology*, **5**, 827.

Morson, B.C. (Ed.) (1974) The poly-cancer sequence in the large bowel. *Proceedings of the Royal Society of Medicine*, **67**, 451.

Morson, B.C. (Ed.) (1978) *Pathogenesis of Colorectal Cancer*. Vol. 10 in series *Major Problems in Pathology*. Philadelphia, London and Toronto: W.B. Saunders.

Morson, B.C. & Pang, L. (1967) Rectal biopsy as an aid to cancer control in ulcerative colitis. *Gut*, **8**, 423.

Muto, T., Bussey, H.J.R. & Morson, B.C. (1975) The evolution of cancer of the colon and rectum. *Cancer*, **36**, 2251.

Muto, T., Ishikawa, K., Kino, I., Nakamura, K., Sugano, H., Bussey, H.J.R. & Morson, B.C. (1977) Comparative histologic study of adenomas of the large intestine in Japan and England, with special reference to malignant potential. *Diseases of the Colon and Rectum*, **20**, 11-16.

Myrvold, H.E., Kock, N.G. & Ahren, C. (1974) Rectal biopsy and precancer in ulcerative colitis. *Gut*, **15**, 301.

Potet, F. & Soullard, J. (1971) Polyps of the rectum and colon. *Gut*, **12**, 468.

Riddell, R.H. (1976) The precarcinomatous phase of ulcerative colitis. In *Current Topics in Pathology* (Ed.) Morson, B.C. Vol. 63, *Pathology of the Gastrointestinal Tract*. pp. 179-219. Berlin: Springer-Verlag.

Riddell, R.H. & Morson, B.C. (1979) Value of sigmoidoscopy and biopsy in detection of carcinoma and premalignant change in ulcerative colitis. *Gut*, **20**, 575.

Sato, E. (1974) Adenomatous polyps of large intestine in autopsy and surgical material. *Gann*, **65**, 295.

Sato, E., Ouchi, A., Sasano, N. & Ishidate, T. (1976) Polyps and diverticulosis of large bowel in autopsy population of Akita Prefecture, compared with Miyagi: high risk for colorectal cancer in Japan. *Cancer*, **37**, 1316-1321.

Spratt, Jr, J.S. & Ackerman, L.V. (1962) Small primary adenocarcinoma of the colon and rectum. *Journal of the American Medical Association*, **179**, 337.

Veale, A.M.O. (1965) *Intestinal Polyposis. Eugenics Laboratory Memoirs*, Series 40. London: Cambridge University Press.

Weingarten, M. & Turell, R. (1952) Carcinomatous mucosal excrescence of the rectum. *Journal of the American Medical Association*, **149**, 1467.

World Health Organization (1972) *Report of a WHO Meeting on the Histological Definition of Precancerous Lesions*. Geneva.

World Health Organization (1976) Histological typing of intestinal tumours. Vol. 15 in series *International Histological Classification of Tumours* (Ed.) Morson, B.C. & Sobin, L.H. Geneva: WHO.

Yardley, J.H. & Keren, D.F. (1974) 'Precancer' lesions in ulcerative colitis. A retrospective study of rectal biopsy and colectomy specimens. *Cancer*, **34**, 835.

21

Polyposis Syndromes

H.J.R. BUSSEY

The tissues forming the wall of the gastrointestinal tract are capable of producing a variety of tumours which are generally of a polypoid nature. Frequently these tumours are multiple and thus a number of polyposis conditions exist. These may be roughly classified into the following types:

1. Inflammatory. Usually secondary to non-specific chronic inflammatory bowel disease such as ulcerative colitis or parasitic infestation such as schistosomiasis.
2. Hamartomatous. Peutz-Jeghers syndrome, juvenile polyposis, neurofibromatosis, lipomatous polyposis.
3. Neoplastic. Adenomatous polyposis coli, lymphosarcomatous and leukaemic polyposis.
4. Miscellaneous. Hyperplastic (metaplastic) polyposis, polypoid lesions of Cronkhite-Canada syndrome and cystic pneumatosis.

Most of these conditions are exceedingly rare and even the more common types are only infrequently encountered, but among the latter group there are three syndromes whose similarities and differences are worth studying. These are (a) Peutz-Jeghers syndrome; (b) juvenile polyposis; (c) familial polyposis coli.

PEUTZ-JEGHERS SYNDROME

In this condition the polyps are hamartomas formed of gastrointestinal epithelium, together with smooth muscle derived from the muscularis mucosae, the latter mainly comprising the delicate stroma on which the epithelium is supported. Histologically, the epithelium is usually normal but occasionally a slight degree of mild hyperplasia may be present.

The polyps may be found in any part of the gastrointestinal tract but are most frequently present in the small intestine, followed by the stomach and the colorectum in that order. The number of polyps is usually small compared with the other two polyposis conditions to be discussed, often not exceeding 50 to 100 tumours. The polyps are usually between 1 and 2 cm in diameter, but may sometimes be as large as 5 cm in diameter. The size, coupled with the more common occurrence of the tumours in the small

© 1980 W.B. Saunders Company Ltd.

intestine, explains the principal symptom of intermittent episodes of abdominal colicky pain due to intussusception which may resolve spontaneously at first but, becoming more chronic, may result in obstruction and necrosis. This sequence of events usually begins in the first decade of life.

A more obvious aspect of the Peutz-Jeghers syndrome is the characteristic skin pigmentation. Small black or brown spots, 1 to 2 mm in diameter, are present on the lips, the perioral skin and buccal mucosa and are also frequently to be seen on the hands and feet. The spots are usually stated to have been noticed initially in the first year of life and gradually to fade away by early middle age.

The Peutz-Jeghers syndrome is a familial condition inherited as an autosomal dominant characteristic. As with all genetically derived conditions, solitary cases without any indication of the disease in other family members can be met with, presumably as the result of new gene mutation.

The possibility that an increased risk of gastrointestinal cancer is associated with the syndrome is still being argued. Although originally thought to be neoplastic lesions with a high incidence of associated malignancy, Peutz-Jeghers polyps are now considered to be hamartomas and as such to have little malignant potential. However, well-documented cases of gastrointestinal cancer in patients with the syndrome are recorded in the literature although they are not numerous (Achord and Proctor, 1963; Reid, 1965; Cochet et al, 1979). In most cases the cancers are situated in the stomach or duodenum and since most occur before the age of 40 years and, in a few instances, are said to have developed in a Peutz-Jeghers polyp, it is probable that there is a slightly increased risk of associated cancer. Colorectal cancers have been only rarely found in the condition. In one of two cases reported by Dodds et al (1972) adenomas were also present and the colonic cancer may have developed in one of these rather than in a Peutz-Jeghers polyp.

JUVENILE POLYPOSIS

Originally termed 'mucus retention polyps', juvenile polyps, singly or in small numbers, have been known to occur in young children for a considerable time. It is only since the early 1960s that a condition has been recognized in which juvenile polyps are present in large numbers (Veale et al, 1966). The tumours, whether found singly or multiple, are hamartomas in which there is an excess of lamina propria enclosing tubules lined with normal epithelium. Unlike the Peutz-Jeghers polyps, juvenile polyps contain no smooth muscle. The tumours are covered by a single cell layer of epithelium which is easily damaged, resulting in secondary inflammation. They are frequently passed during defaecation, auto-amputation being helped by the absence of muscle. This fragility gives rise to bleeding, often of a severe nature, which is the main symptom of the condition. Symptoms usually begin in the first decade of life and the average age at diagnosis is about 18 years. Tumours in juvenile polyposis, as with Peutz-Jeghers polyps, may be found in any part of the gastrointestinal tract but the distribution is different in that they are much less commonly found in the stomach and small intestine but are always present in the colorectum which is often the only region involved. The size distribution is similar to that of Peutz-Jeghers polyps but the number is generally much larger and may amount to several hundred. The histology may show considerable variation. About three-quarters of the polyps have the typical histology of juvenile polyps but the remainder differ in two respects. Firstly, the lamina propria may be decreased in amount, leaving the epithelium, which sometimes shows hyperplasia and a coarse villous pattern, as the dominant feature. Secondly, genuine epithelial dysplasia may be observed in about two-thirds of the atypical juvenile polyps. The dysplasia is usually of a mild character but very occasionally may be severe in nature.

Juvenile polyposis sometimes affects several members of a family and it almost certainly has a genetic origin, the nature of which still requires further investigation but which is likely to prove to be of a dominant character. It has also been found that the condition is accompanied by an increased incidence of other congenital abnormalities.

When first described it was thought that, as a hamartomatous lesion, juvenile polyposis had little malignant potential. However, as more cases have accumulated, it now appears that there is an increased risk of associated colorectal cancer. The overall incidence rate is about 10 per cent but it tends to be greater among those patients from families where several members have juvenile polyposis. This increased risk of colorectal cancer is almost certainly related to the epithelial dysplasia mentioned previously, particularly as there is a strong correlation between those patients who have polyps showing severe dysplasia and those who develop cancer.

FAMILIAL POLYPOSIS COLI

The main features of familial polyposis coli are the numerous adenomas in the colorectum, the extremely high incidence of associated colorectal cancer usually occurring in relatively young age groups, and its inheritance as a Mendelian dominant characteristic (Bussey, 1975).

The number of adenomatous polyps present in this condition greatly exceeds those present in the Peutz-Jeghers syndrome or in juvenile polyposis. They seldom number less than 500, average about 1000 and can exceed 5000. Although multiple adenomas occur in non-polyposis patients, the number rarely exceeds 50, giving a clear division between the two conditions. The adenomas of polyposis coli, which in no way differ from those found in smaller numbers in the non-polyposis patients, may start to develop towards the end of the first decade of life but are more commonly observed between the ages of 15 and 25 years. As the polyps grow in size and number, increased bowel movements and occasional episodes of slight rectal bleeding occur. Those symptoms are usually ignored until they get more severe, by which time malignancy has probably supervened. About two-thirds of the patients presenting for the first time with symptoms have already developed cancer. It is fairly certain that the remaining third would have followed a similar course had the patients not received surgical treatment. The average age at which colorectal cancer is diagnosed in polyposis patients is about 40 years.

Polyposis coli is treated in the individual by removing either the entire large intestine or only the colon with preservation of the rectum. The latter course requires biannual examinations for the purpose of discovering and destroying any new adenomas which have grown. Cancer of the rectum may subsequently develop but with regular surveillance this complication can be kept to a minimum. If it does occur the cancer should be at an early and, therefore, curable stage. Control of polyposis in the family is helped by constructing a detailed pedigree. This will indicate which members are at risk and these should be invited to attend for examination. Every child of a polyposis patient has a 50-50 chance of inheriting the disease and arrangements should be made for the children to be examined periodically from about the age of 14 years. If sigmoidoscopic examination is negative it should be repeated at about two-year intervals until middle age. Unless the propositus acquired his polyposis as the result of a new mutation, his sibs are also at risk and require investigation. The effect of this policy of family follow-up has been a marked decline in the incidence of colorectal cancer when affected members are first seen. It has already been stated that about 66 per cent of propositus cases have cancer when first seen. In relatives called up for examination because they are known to be at risk the proportion with cancer is currently about 5 per cent. Polyposis coli is the outstanding example of a precancerous condition in which cancer prevention methods have been applied with a considerable degree of success. However, a new problem has recently been reported in connection with familial polyposis coli. Since the condition was first described, it has been assumed that the polyps are confined to the large intestine, hence the general use of the term 'polyposis coli'. The few recorded examples of adenomatous polyps elsewhere in the gastrointestinal tract were considered to be incidental associations only (Chiat et al, 1962; Heald, 1967). In the last five years, however, there has been an increasing number of reports confirming a high incidence rate of adenomas in the small intestine and especially in the duodenum. Yao et al (1977) investigated 14 polyposis patients by duodenoscopy and found polyps in all 14, in each case confirming the polyps to be adenomas by histological examination. Adenomas are also being discovered more frequently in the ileum (Hamilton et al, 1979). Endoscopy has also revealed that some polyposis patients have multiple small polyps of the stomach. Histological examination has shown that these are probably hamartomas derived from the gastric mucosa. Although some adenomas of the stomach have also been recorded these seem to be confined mainly to the pyloric mucosa (Watanabe et al, 1978). Furthermore, there is an increasing number of reports of polyposis patients developing periampullary carcinoma. This is a general term covering malignancy in the region of the ampulla of Vater and including a miscellany of conditions such as adenocarcinoma of the duodenum, carcinoma of the pancreas and carcinoma of the common duct. This group of tumours has not been reported in sufficient detail to enable an incidence rate to be worked out for the different histological types but it is fairly certain that the majority of the periampullary malignancies are adenocarcinomas derived from the epithelium of the duodenum. It is also highly probable that these carcinomas develop from the adenomas now being increasingly observed in this region. How great a risk this poses for the polyposis patient has yet to be determined.

GARDNER'S SYNDROME

Gardner and Richards (1953) reported a family in which several members had polyposis coli and, in addition, multiple osteomas of the skull or mandible and multiple epidermoid cysts and fibromas of the skin. Other cases were subsequently published and the condition became known as 'Gardner's syndrome'. The exact relationship between polyposis and Gardner's syndrome has been a matter for debate which still continues. The idea that the two conditions were distinct entities, resulting from different gene mutations, seemed plausible and gained much support at first. As more cases accumulated, the division between polyposis with and without the extracolonic lesions became less well defined. The osteomas and cysts were sometimes few in number or one type of lesion might be absent. The syndrome was extended by the addition of dental abnormalities and desmoid tumours, usually of the abdominal wall but sometimes intra-abdominal (Gardner, 1962). Other workers made suggestions for further additions, not all of which are acceptable. The differential diagnosis between the two types was further eroded when it was shown that practically all polyposis patients had small subclinical osteomas when the mandible was examined radiologically (Utsunomiya and Nakamura, 1975). The general view now seems to be that a single gene mutation is accountable for both the intestinal polyps and the extracolonic lesions, the latter being more variable in their expressivity. What is certain is that there is little difference between the number, distribution or malignant potential of the adenomas in the two conditions and that these form the major threat to the patient's wellbeing. Among the extracolonic manifestations, the only one with serious clinical implications is the desmoid tumour when it occurs intra-abdominally. Several fatalities are known, caused by obstruction of the intestines or the ureter by desmoid tumours, usually after attempted surgical removal. On the other hand, patients with massive desmoid tumours, some of which have been found on laparotomy to be inoperable, are still living many years later without too much inconvenience from their desmoids.

Most of the periampullary malignancies which have been reported occurred in patients of the Gardner syndrome type, suggesting that these tumours were also part of the syndrome. With the recent observation of the high incidence of small intestinal adenomas, particularly in the duodenum, it is obvious that these tumours must be considered as part of the adenomatous component of the syndrome and not as another 'extracolonic' lesion.

FAMILIAL POLYPOSIS COLI AS AN EXPERIMENTAL MODEL

A discussion of familial polyposis coli would be incomplete without mention being made of its special role as a model for the study of the aetiology of colorectal cancer. As the one condition in which a practically 100 per cent malignant outcome can be guaranteed, it affords unrivalled opportunities for investigating the factors involved. For example, it is only from colectomy specimens removed for polyposis that a histological picture can be built up of the sequence of dysplastic changes starting from the involvement of a single epithelial tubule to the development of the mature adenomatous polyp (Bussey, 1979). Observations on patients with known polyposis for which either no, or only partial, surgery has been carried out have provided information about the time intervals involved both in the growth of adenomas and in the development of malignancy. The multiplicity of adenomas in the condition and the high incidence of colorectal cancer have supplied valuable evidence to support the adenoma-carcinoma sequence concept.

Knowledge acquired in the investigation may be profitably applied in other fields. Since the adenomas of polyposis coli have a genetic origin, it is natural to speculate on the possibility that the adenomas occurring in non-polyposis patients may also be inherited. Veale (1965) studied the evidence then available and decided that this was indeed a possibility but that, if so, the adenomas were likely to be inherited as a recessive character. Support for this view has come from the work of Lovett (1976) on family histories of patients with colorectal cancer which showed that there was an increased incidence of the same condition among the relatives. Since it is likely that the majority of colorectal cancers arise from adenomas, this implies an increased incidence of adenomas among the affected family members. An investigation has been carried out into the pathology of those members of the families studied by Lovett who were operated on at St Mark's Hospital. The results indicate a close relationship between the number of relatives in the family with colorectal cancer and the average number of adenomas found in the affected individuals. It may be that the taking of detailed family histories could identify those individuals who are at increased risk of intestinal cancer and that the application of a policy of periodic examination and removal of any polyps found could achieve a reduction in the incidence of colorectal cancer similar to that experienced in familial polyposis coli.

COMPARISON OF THE THREE GASTROINTESTINAL POLYPOSIS SYNDROMES

The three conditions discussed show both differences and similarities. With the wide variation in the clinical dangers of the syndromes correct diagnosis is vital and with this in mind the tendency has been to emphasize differences such as polyp distribution, symptoms and, especially, histology. From the academic aspect, however, it may be the similarities which have most interest. All three types of polyposis are inherited, probably in each case as a Mendelian dominant characteristic. Two are accompanied by associated extragastrointestinal lesions, also of a genetic nature (oral pigmentation in Peutz-Jeghers syndrome; osteomas and epidermoid cysts in Gardner's syndrome). Juvenile polyposis has an increased incidence of congenital malformations. Each produces mutiple polyps scattered throughout the gastrointestinal tract and in each at least some of the tumours are apparently of a hamartomatous nature. There is some blurring of the histological boundaries. Peutz-Jeghers-type polyps have been found among the juvenile polyps in at least one case of juvenile polyposis and not all lesions considered to be hamartomas can be assigned to a particular type. Epithelial dysplasia may be found in the polyps of each syndrome, although these is a wide variation in its extent and severity, being uncommon in Peutz-Jeghers polyposis, more frequent in juvenile polyposis and, of course, always present in polyposis coli. These different degrees of dysplasia are closely mirrored by the increased risk of gastrointestinal cancer associated with the three types. Widely as the three syndromes differ at the clinical level it is possible that at nuclear and chromosomal levels they are much closer together.

REFERENCES

Achord, J.L. & Proctor, H.D. (1963) Malignant degeneration and metastasis in Peutz-Jeghers syndrome. *Archives of Internal Medicine*, **111**, 498-502.
Bussey, H.J.R. (1975) *Familial Polyposis Coli*. 104 pp. Baltimore: Johns Hopkins University Press.
Bussey, H.J.R. (1979) Familial polyposis coli. In *Pathology Annual* (Ed.) Sommers, S.C. & Rosen, P.D. Part 1 (1979), pp. 61-81. New York: Appleton-Century-Crofts.
Chiat, H., Ross, S.T., Janelli, D.E. & Mandel, P.R. (1962) Familial polyposis of the colon with subsequent development of a duodenal polyp. Report of a case. *Diseases of the Colon and Rectum*, **5**, 444-445.
Cochet, B., Carrel, J., Desbaillets, L. & Widgren, S. (1979) Peutz-Jeghers syndrome associated with gastrointestinal carcinoma. *Gut*, **20**, 169-175.
Dodds, W.J., Schulte, W.J., Hensley, G.T. & Hogan, W.J. (1972) Peutz-Jeghers syndrome and gastrointestinal malignancy. *American Journal of Roentgenology*, **115**, 374-377.
Gardner, E.J. (1962) Follow-up study of a family group exhibiting dominant inheritance for a syndrome including intestinal polyps, osteomas, fibromas and epidermal cysts. *American Journal of Human Genetics*, **14**, 376-390.
Gardner, E.J. & Richards, R.C. (1953) Multiple cutaneous and subcutaneous lesions occurring simultaneously with hereditary polyposis and osteomatosis. *American Journal of Human Genetics*, **5**, 139-147.
Hamilton, S.R., Bussey, H.J.R., Mendelsohn, G., Diamond, M.P., Paylides, G., Hutcheon, D., Harrison, M., Shermata, D., Morson, B.C. & Yardley, J.H. (1979) Ileal adenomas after colectomy in nine patients with adenomatous polyposis coli/Gardner's syndrome. *Gastroenterology*, **77**, 1252-1257.
Heald, R.J. (1967) Gardner's syndrome in association with two tumours of the ileum. *Proceedings of the Royal Society of Medicine*, **60**, 914-915.
Lovett, E. (1976) Family studies in cancer of the colon and rectum. *British Journal of Surgery*, **63**, 13-18.
Reid, J.D. (1965) Duodenal carcinoma in the Peutz-Jeghers syndrome. *Cancer* (Philadelphia), **18**, 970-977.
Utsunomiya, J. & Nakamura, T. (1975) The occult osteomatous changes in the mandible in patients with familial polyposis coli. *British Journal of Surgery*, **62**, 45-51.
Veale, A.M.O. (1965) *Intestinal Polyposis. Eugenics Laboratory Memoirs, Series 40*. 104 pp. London: Cambridge University Press.
Veale, A.M.O., McColl, I., Bussey, H.J.R. & Morson, B.C. (1966) Juvenile polyposis coli. *Journal of Medical Genetics*, **3**, 5-16.
Watanabe, H., Enjoji, M., Yao, T. & Ohsato, K. (1978) Gastric lesions in familial adenomatosis coli; their incidence and histologic analysis. *Human Pathology*, **9**, 269-283.
Yao, T., Iida, M., Ohsato, K., Watanabe, H. & Omae, T. (1977) Duodenal lesions in familial polyposis of the colon. *Gastroenterology*, **73**, 1086-1092.

22

Spread of Rectal Cancer Within Veins and Mechanisms of Malignant Embolism

I.C. TALBOT

Despite the conventional view (Dukes, 1932) that cancer of the rectum spreads primarily by way of lymphatics patients rarely die from spread to lymph nodes alone (Taylor, 1962); it is metastatic spread to liver, as well as local recurrence, which principally determines the outcome of patients with this disease. Furthermore, patients often develop liver metastases when no lymph node deposits are found at operation. Could these apparent paradoxes be the result of a misconception about the relative importance of lymphatic spread as compared with direct invasion of veins by the primary growth? In order to try to answer this question a series of 703 cases of rectal cancer was reviewed, both histologically and clinically, with special emphasis on venous invasion and its various histological features, so that spread into veins could be related to the natural history of the disease.

MATERIALS AND METHODS

Occasional examples of grossly visible spread of carcinoma into the superior haemorrhoidal vein have been noticed for many years, but for meaningful clinicopathological correlation to be possible it is important that even relatively minor degrees of invasion of veins are not missed. Bussey and Morson (1974, personal communication) therefore devised a way of examining operation specimens of rectum removed in the treatment of cancer with the aim of increasing the chance of detecting venous invasion. Blocks for histology were taken from the formalin-fixed specimen (Figure 1) both from (A), the centre of the growth, and from (B), at multiple points tangential to the edge of the tumour, with the aim of including in histological sections transversely cut veins emerging from the periphery of the growth.

As an aid to the identification of venous invasion another series of operation specimens from 18 cases was examined in the above way after an injection technique (Talbot, 1979); 150 ml of 3 per cent aqueous silver nitrate solution was injected into the superior haemorrhoidal vein (SHV) of the fresh, unfixed specimen; after formalin fixation and preparation of histological sections the silver nitrate was reduced to metallic silver which

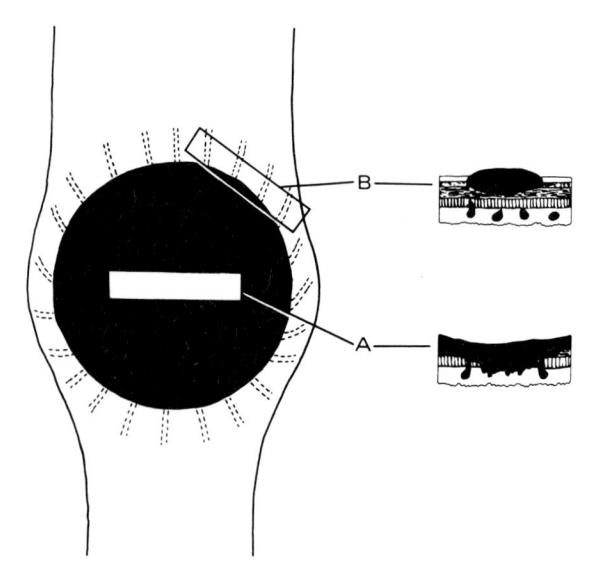

Figure 1. Diagram of the way blocks were taken from specimens of rectal cancer for histological examination.

formed a layer on the endothelial surface of the venous tributaries of the SHV (Figure 2). By using this technique tumour was recognized in a vein when the vessel was aneurysmally distended and even in some cases when the vein wall was destroyed. Recognition of these appearances enabled invasion of veins to be frequently detected in other specimens not injected with silver nitrate, when it might otherwise have been missed. Lesser degrees of damage to the vein wall were often found (partial damage), when there was a slight chronic inflammatory cell reaction around the vein (Figure 3), while in some cases there was no inflammatory reaction at all and the vein wall was intact (Figure 4).

Turning to the main series of 703 cases, the state of the vein wall, as described above, was determined in those cases in which venous invasion could be identified. Venous spread was quantified by observing whether invasion was limited to intramural veins (within the submucosa or muscularis of the rectum) or involved extramural veins (in perirectal adipose tissue). A further quantitative assessment was by the size of the veins invaded; these were divided into two categories: those with thick walls and a well-developed muscular coat (Figure 4) and those with only thin walls in which smooth muscle was inconspicuous (Figure 3).

Further histological observations were also made, concerning both the vein walls and the tumour within veins, all of which could possibly be relevant to the way venous permeation and embolism develop. Carcinomatous permeation of capillary channels within vein walls, with or without involvement of the lumen, was seen in a small number of cases (Figure 5), but most frequently carcinoma was found within the vein lumen, with a

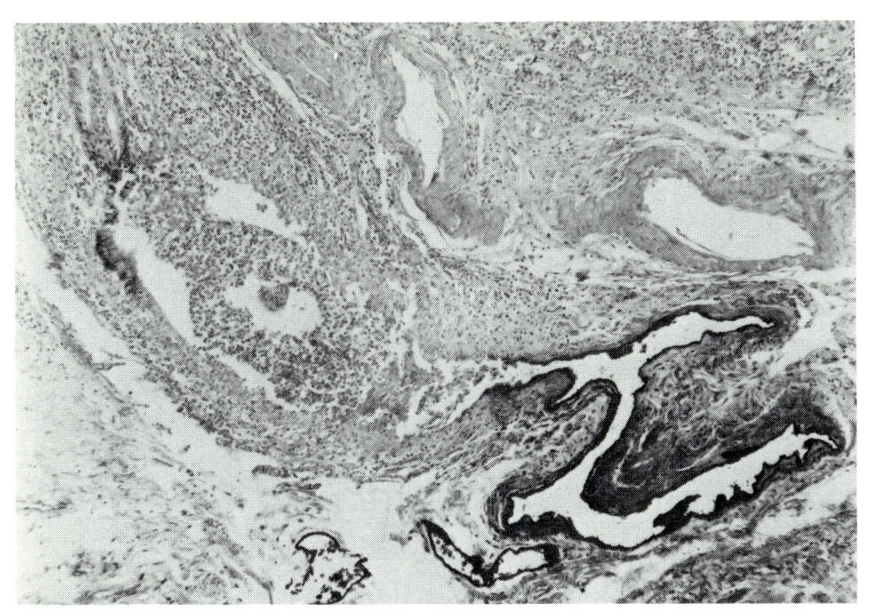

Figure 2. Section of specimen perfused with silver nitrate solution via the superior haemorrhoidal vein. Adenocarcinoma is seen invading the vein, although the vein wall is distended, inflamed and destroyed. Haematoxylin and eosin, × 100.

central zone of necrosis as shown in Figure 6. The nature of the point of contact between carcinoma and blood within a vein must obviously be important in the process of spread of tumour by the formation of malignant emboli, and the precise histological features of the tumour/blood interface were therefore determined in all cases with venous invasion; in some cases there was direct contact between tumour cells and venous blood (Figure 3), but in most cases there was a mantle of proliferated endothelial cells surrounding the intravenous growth, with or without an overlying cap of thrombus (Figure 6).

As well as the above features, the Dukes' stage of each tumour was, of course, also noted.

The clinical progress of all 703 patients was determined as a separate exercise, without knowledge of the histology, by reference to hospital case notes, correspondence with general practitioners and relatives and, occasionally, when all else failed, from death certificates.

RESULTS

Invasion of veins was found in 51.9 per cent of the 703 cases (Table 1) and, when present, the five-year survival rate, excluding patients who died within four weeks of operation and corrected to allow for deaths from all causes in an age-matched population, was only 43 per cent, whereas the five-year

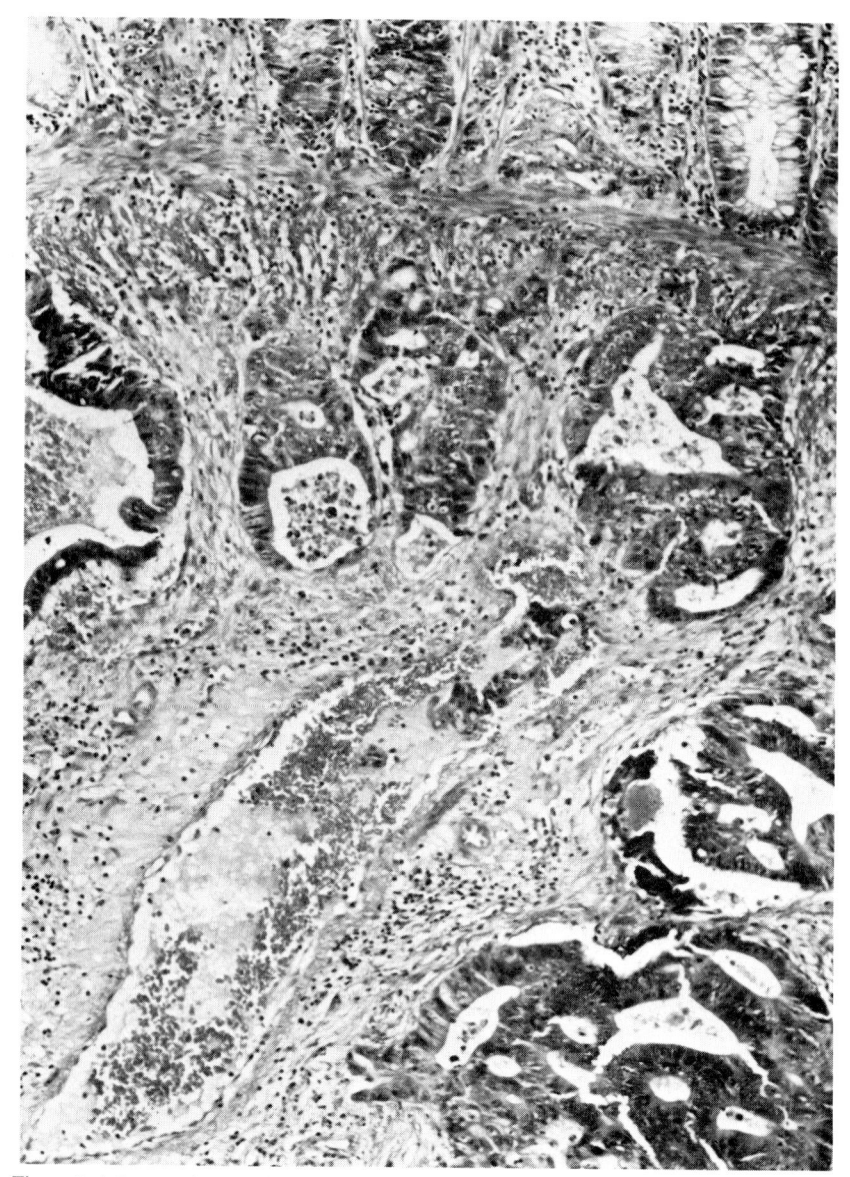

Figure 3. Adenocarcinoma of rectum invading a thin-walled submucosal (intramural) vein. The tumour cells are in contact with the venous blood. The vein wall is partially damaged. Haematoxylin and eosin, × 200.

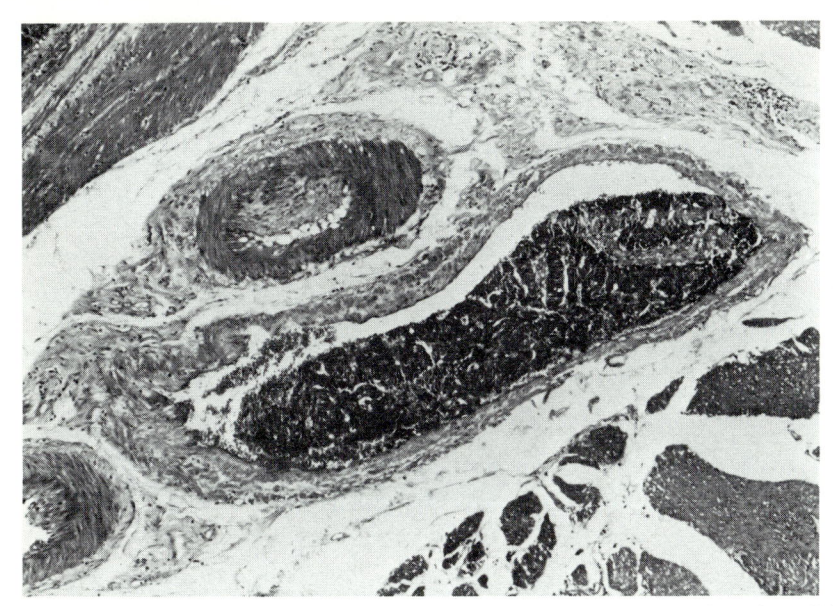

Figure 4. Invasion of an intramural vein by adenocarcinoma of rectum. The vein wall is relatively thick, with prominent smooth muscle, and is intact. Haematoxylin and eosin, × 55.

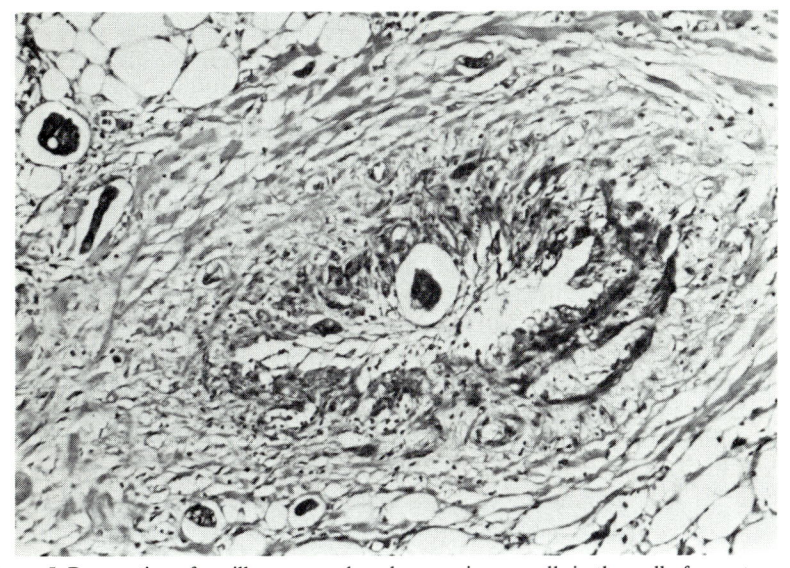

Figure 5. Permeation of capillary spaces by adenocarcinoma cells in the wall of an extramural rectal vein. Haematoxylin and eosin, × 200.

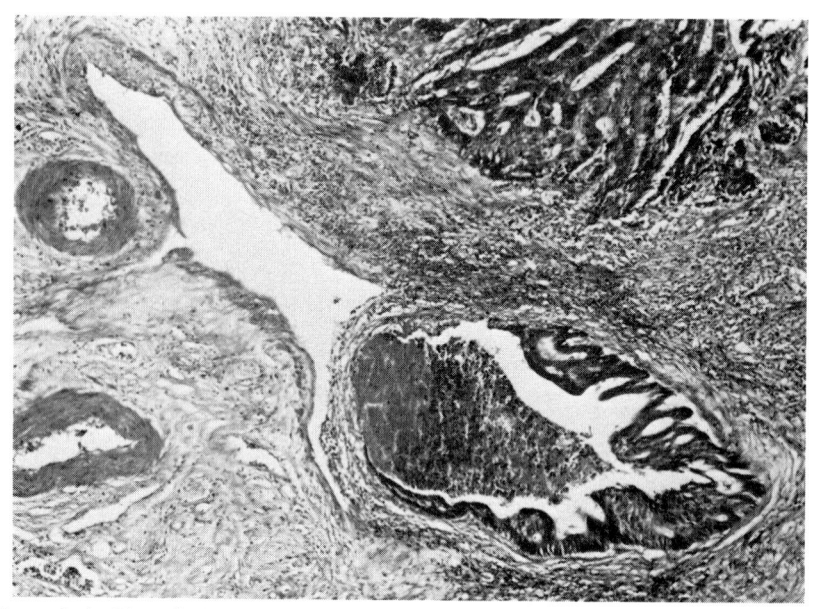

Figure 6. A thin-walled rectal vein containing adenocarcinoma. There is a central zone of necrosis, and a mantle of proliferated endothelial cells covering the 'free surface' of the growth. Haematoxylin and eosin, × 100.

survival rate when venous invasion was not demonstrated was as high as 73 per cent (Table 2). There was invasion of extramural veins in 36 per cent of the whole series and the corrected five-year survival rate of these cases was only one in three (Table 3) but when only intramural veins were involved the survival rate was almost two in three (cf. cases in which venous invasion was not demonstrated). Forty per cent of cases with extramural venous spread developed hepatic metastases (Table 4), whereas liver deposits developed in only 14 per cent of patients in whom venous invasion was not demonstrated. When only thin-walled extramural veins were invaded the corrected five-year survival rate was 41 per cent (Table 5) but only 15 of 91 patients with spread into thick-walled extramural veins survived for five years.

Necrosis of carcinoma within veins does not correlate well with prognosis (Table 6). However, there is a clear-cut relationship between the state of the walls of invaded extramural veins and survival rate; aneurysmal distension of invaded veins is associated with a better prognosis (Table 7 shows a 41 per cent five-year survival rate), although the level of significance ($P< 0.02$) is not very high. Only five out of 53 patients with extramural venous invasion survived for five years when the vein wall was intact (Table 8). When the vein wall was partially damaged the corrected five-year survival rate was nearly 30 per cent and when the wall was destroyed the survival rate was 57 per cent (similar to that of the series as a whole). Twenty-four cases showed adenocarcinoma permeating capillary channels within extramural vein walls, but only one of these survived for five years (Table 9) and it is

Table 1. *Incidence of venous invasion in operation specimens of rectal cancer*

Venous invasion	Number	%
Not demonstrated	338	48.1
Present	365 {Intramural 111, Extramural 254}	{15.8, 36.1} 51.9
	703	100.0

Table 2. *Venous invasion of rectal cancer and survival rate*

Venous invasion	Operation survivors	5-year survivors	Corrected 5-year survival rate (%)
Not demonstrated	328	206	73.0
Present	356	130	43.1

Table 3. *Extent of venous invasion of rectal cancer and survival rate*

Venous invasion	Operation survivors	5-year survivors	Corrected 5-year survival rate (%)
Not demonstrated	328	206	73.0
Intramural	108	61	64.7
Extramural	248	69	33.0

Table 4. *Venous invasion of rectal cancer and development of liver metastases*

Venous invasion	Number of cases	Liver metastases Number	%
Not demonstrated	338	48	14.2
Intramural	111	26	23.4
Extramural	254	102	40.2

Table 5. *Type of extramural venous spread and survival rate*

Invaded extramural veins	Operation survivors	5-year survivors	Corrected 5-year survival rate (%)
Thin-walled	157	54	40.9
Thick-walled	91	15	19.4

Table 6. *Necrosis with cavitation of extramural intravascular growth and corrected five-year survival rate*

Necrosis in intravascular growth	Operation survivors	5-year survivors	Corrected % survival
Absent	173	53	36.4
Present	75	16	25.2

$0.2 > P > 0.1$.

Table 7. *Aneurysmal distension of invaded extramural vein and corrected five-year survival rate*

Aneurysmal distension of invaded vein	Operation survivors	5-year survivors	Corrected % survival
Absent	142	33	27.0
Present	106	36	41.4

$P < 0.02$.

Table 8. *State of wall of invaded extramural vein and corrected five-year survival rate*

State of vein wall	Operation survivors	5-year survivors	Corrected % survival
(a) Intact	53	5	10.8
(b) Damaged	126	31	29.1
(c) Destroyed	69	33	57.1

Comparing (a) with (b) $P = < 0.02$.
Comparing (a) with (c) $P = < 0.001$.
Comparing (b) with (c) $P = < 0.001$.

Table 9. *Permeation of extramural vein wall capillaries and corrected five-year survival rate*

Permeation of capillaries in vein wall	Operation survivors	5-year survivors	Corrected % survival
Absent	230	68	36.1
Present	24	1	4.9

$P < 0.01$.

unfortunate that small numbers limit the significance of this result. Direct contact between tumour cells and venous blood was observed in 17 cases; only two of these survived for five years (Table 10). A mantle of proliferated endothelial cells covering the apex of the extramural intravenous growth was present in 60 cases and is associated with a high five-year survival rate (53 per cent; Table 11).

Finally, the relationship between venous spread and the Duke's Stage is shown in Table 12. Venous invasion was uncommon (20 per cent) in Stage A growths but was found in almost half the Stage B tumours and in most Stage C cases, extramural veins being involved in 48.4 per cent of the latter. Venous invasion does not appear to affect prognosis in patients with Stage A tumours, the survival rates being virtually identical whether venous spread was present or not. However, there is a significant lowering of the survival rate in patients with B and C Stage tumours, the five-year survival of C stage cases being halved when venous invasion is present. This trend with Stage C cases is further emphasized in Table 13, which shows a marked lowering of the survival rate to 17 per cent when extramural veins are invaded and a five-year survival rate of only 8.5 per cent when there is involvement of thick-walled extramural veins.

Table 10. *Growth in contact with blood in extramural vein and corrected five-year survival rate*

Blood in invaded vein	Operation survivors	5-year survivors	Corrected % survival
Not in contact with growth	231	67	32.8
In contact with growth	17	2	14.6

$P < 0.2$.

Table 11. *Endothelial cell mantle covering extramural intravenous tumour cells and corrected five-year survival rate*

Endothelial cell mantle	Operation survivors	5-year survivors	Corrected % survival
Absent	188	42	26.5
Present	60	27	53.3

$P < 0.001$.

Table 12. *Venous invasion and Dukes' stage: numbers of cases and survival rate*

Venous invasion	Dukes' stage: corrected 5-year survival rate (number of cases in brackets)		
	A	B	C
Not demonstrated	95.9% (76)	85.6% (140)	45.7% (122)
Present	96.8% (19)	70.4% (124)	23.2% (221)
Total	96.1% (95)	78.3% (264)	31.3% (343)

(+ 1 unclassified)

Table 13. *Invasion of extramural veins with thin and thick walls and Dukes' stage: numbers of cases and survival rate*

Extramural venous invasion	Dukes' stage: corrected 5-year survival rate (number of cases in brackets)	
	B	C
Thin-walled veins	68.3% (63)	22.8% (94)
Thick-walled veins	52.2% (23)	8.5% (67)
Total	64.0% (86)	16.8% (161)

DISCUSSION

Growth along veins is a frequent and clinically significant mode of spread in rectal cancer. Carcinoma of rectum appears to extend along venous channels as shown in Figure 7; this may well be the way in which local invasion of the tumour usually takes place and appears to have been hitherto underestimated. At a relatively 'advanced' stage extramural veins and thick-walled veins are involved and, not surprisingly, the prognosis is then rather poor. During the course of spread of tumour along a vein the lumen will become blocked, resulting in a stagnant column of blood distally. The centre of the

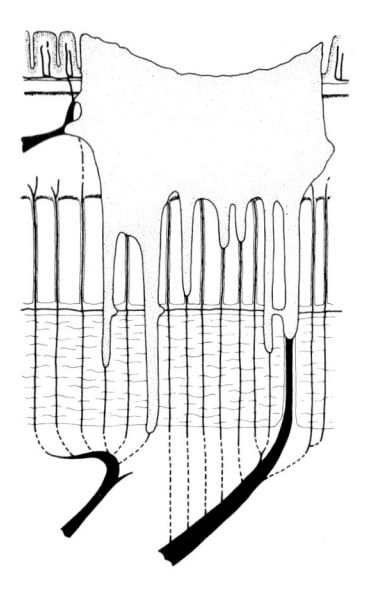

Figure 7. Diagram of suggested way in which carcinoma may invade the rectal wall via veins.

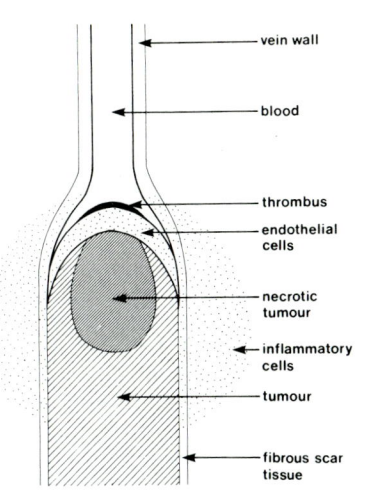

Figure 8. Diagram to show the way in which the wall of a vein permeated by tumour may become damaged by an inflammatory reaction to tumour tissue and eventually destroyed and replaced by scar tissue.

advancing tumour will then undergo ischaemic necrosis (Figure 8). An inflammatory reaction to the necrotic tumour, in and around the surrounding vessel wall, together with distension of the vein by growth, results in damage and fibrous replacement of the vein wall and the vein is not then able to function as a contractile vessel. The chance of malignant embolism occurring then appears to be reduced, thus supporting Willis's theory (Willis, 1973) that only invasion of veins with a well-developed muscular wall is of importance in dissemination of tumour by the bloodstream. These features may vary from case to case and vein to vein and, in summary (Figure 9),

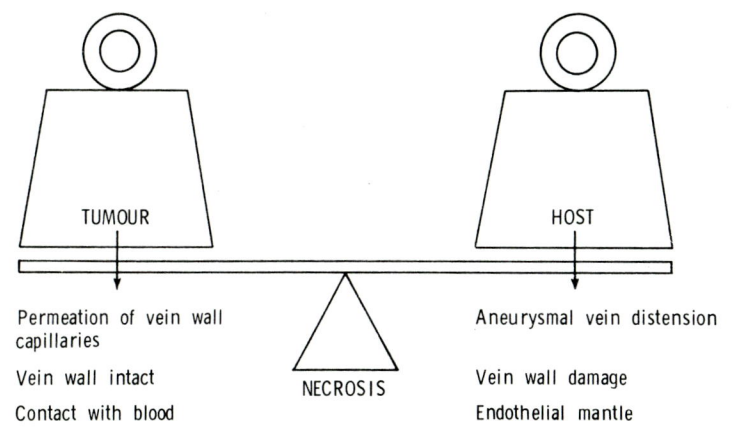

Figure 9. The tumour/host balance in rectal cancer and the principal histological features acting on it.

necrosis of intravenous tumour, alone, does not have a direct effect on survival but the balance is tipped in favour of the host if there is aneurysmal distension of the vein, or inflammatory damage to the vein wall or when endothelial cells proliferate and form a mantle covering the growth. In contrast, permeation of vein wall capillaries by carcinoma cells, or an intact wall of an invaded vein, or direct contact between tumour and venous blood, weighs heavily against the host.

CONCLUSION

Assessment of venous invasion should not supersede the Dukes' staging procedure in documenting the advancement of a tumour but is a useful adjunct to it; by taking account of both the Dukes' Stage and the presence and type of venous invasion a more precise prediction of prognosis is possible. This means that those patients who are most likely to develop metastases and who might benefit most from additional methods of treatment such as adjuvant chemotherapy can be identified. Venous spread in rectal cancer is easily detected and quantified by relatively simple pathological procedures. There is no reason why these should not be performed in any routine histopathology laboratory.

ACKNOWLEDGEMENTS

Much of this work was supported by a grant from the St Mark's Research Foundation. I gratefully acknowledge the guidance and encouragement of Dr B.C. Morson and also of Dr H.J.R. Bussey. This investigation could not have been completed without the generous help of the staff at St Mark's Hospital and the many medical practitioners, medical records officers and others elsewhere who provided me with information about the patients.

REFERENCES

Dukes, C.E. (1932) The classification of cancer of the rectum. *Journal of Pathology and Bacteriology*, **35**, 1489-1494.

Talbot, I.C. (1979) MD Thesis, University of London.

Taylor, F.W. (1962) Cancer of the colon and rectum: a study of routes of metastases and death. *Surgery* (St Louis), **52**, 305-308.

Willis, R.A. (1973) *The Spread of Tumours in the Human Body*. 3rd edn, p. 39. London: Butterworths.

Index

Note: Page numbers in *italics* refer to illustrations or tables.

AAC, *see* Antibiotic associated colitis
ABO blood group antigens, 4, 52-53
Adenocarcinoma—
　epithelial membrane antigen (EMA) and, 258
　of large bowel, *see* Colorectal carcinoma
　of stomach, *247*
　　epidemiology, 285-289
　　see also Gastric cancer
Adenomas—
　benign, colorectal cancer risk and, 314-315
　-carcinoma sequence, 303, *304*, 304-308, 331, 333, 337
　　dysplasia in, *see* Dysplasia
　　histopathology, 304, *305*
　　malignant potential, 305, *305*, *306*, 335-338, *341*
　　nature of environmental factors, 306-308
　　relative size, 304, *305*
　　see also Bacteria, carcinogen production; Colorectal carcinoma
　colorectal, definition, 331, 332
　-dysplasia sequence, 331
　　histology and grading, 333-335, *335*, *336*
　　life-history, 338
　　malignant potential, 335-338, *340*, *341*
　incidence, 305, *305*, 307, 340-341
　nuclear dehydrogeneting clostridia and, 302
　'proneness', 306
　regression, 307
Adenomatosis, *see* Polyposis coli
Adenovirus-associated virus (AAV), 109, *109*
Adenoviruses in gut, 106, *106*, 107, *108*, 114
　ecology, 117, *118*, *119*, 121
Affection, definition, 105
Alcohol, 274, 277, 278
Allograft, small intestinal, rejection, 99
Amine precursor uptake and decarboxylation (APUD) cells, 13, 27, 256
Aminopeptidase, 251
Ampicillin, 153, 166, 167
Anaemia, 59-68

Anaemia— (*contd*)
　haematinic deficiencies, *see* Folate; Iron; Vitamin B$_{12}$
　megaloblastic, 62, 63, *64*, 66, *66*
　pernicious, 61, 63, 64
　gastric cancer and, 289
Anal canal, 71, 72, 73, *73*, 86
Anal incontinence, 71
　see also Faecal incontinence
Anal reflex, 72, 87
Anal sphincter muscle, external, 71
　faecal incontinence and, 71, 74-75, 86
　histology, 76, *76*, *77*, *78*, *79*, 80, *85*, 86
　innervation, 80-81, *82*, 86-87
　normal, 71, 75, 81-82, *83*, *85*
　puborectalis muscle, separation from, 71, 75
Anal sphincter muscle, internal, 71
Anaphylactic reaction—
　in mucosa, 95
　passive, intestinal, 95-96
　systemic, small intestine, 95
Ankylosing spondylitis, 179
Ann Arbor staging system, 214-215
Anorectal angle, 71, 73-74, *74*, 86
Antibiotic-associated colitis (AAC), 131, 151, 160, 161-163, *164*, 167
Antibiotic-associated diarrhoea (AAD), 151, 167
Antibiotics, in pseudomembranous colitis, *see under* Colotis, pseudomembranous
Antibodies—
　in Crohn's disease, 180, 181
　lymphocytotoxic, 180
　tumour-specific, uptake, 262-263
　to viruses, gut, 116-117
　see also Immunoglobulins
Antigen—
　exposure in gastrointestinal tract, 93
　immunohistochemical techniques and, 12, 13
　cytoplasmic, 4, 6, 7, 12
　surface membrane, 4, 12
α-1-Antitrypsin, 15, 207, *208*
Apolipoprotein B, 3
'Appendicitis'—

365

'Appendicitis'— (contd)
   Campylobacter and, 130
   Yersinia enterocolitica and, 130
APUD cells, 13, 27, 256
Ascorbic acid, 307
Astroviruses in gut, *106*, 108, 109
   antibody, survey, 116
   diarrhoea, 113
   ecology, *118*, 119
   in lambs, calves, 114-115
Auer technique, 98
Autofluorescence, 9, 12

Bacteria—
   carcinogen production and, 297-303
      product of metabolism, 301-302, 303, 307
      substrate, 297-301
      value of FBA/NDC, 303, 307, 308
   in Crohn's disease, 183, 184-185
   gastrointestinal infections, *see* Infections, bacterial
Bacteriophage—
   diarrhoea and, 115
   in gut, 106, *106*, *110*, 111
Bacteroides fragilis, 185
Bacteroides vulgatus, 181
Barium enema, 322, 323
Beryllium, 180
Bile acids—
   faecal (FBA), 297-300, *298*, *299*, *300*
      irritant properties, 303
      value of FBA/NDC, 303, 307, 308
   nuclear dehydrogenating clostridia, 301-302
Biopsies—
   endoscopic, mucus glycoprotein and, 51-52
   faecal incontinence and, *see* Faecal incontinence
   gastric cancer and, 242, 243, *248*, *249*
   jejunal, 98, 101, 102
   multiple mucosal, 322, 323
   rectal cancer and, *see* Rectum, cancer of
Blood groups, gastric cancer and, 288, 291
Bombesin, 23, *24*, 36, 38-40
   pharmacological effects, *40*
Bombina bombina, 38
Bovine serum albumin—
   immune complex hypersensitivity and, 97
   local hypersensitivity and, 94
   reaginic hypersensitivity and, 96
Bouin's fixative, 6, 12
Bowel—
   adenocarcinoma, *see* Colorectal carcinoma
   disease, clostridial, *see* Colitis, pseudomembranous
   inflammatory disease, 179, 316

Caecitis, clindamycin-associated, 162-163
Caliciviruses in gut, *106*, *108*, *109*, 111
   diarrhoea and, 113
   ecology, *118*, *119*
Campylobacter, 125, 129-130
Cancer—
   colorectal, *see* Colorectal carcinoma
   gastric, *see* Gastric cancer
   of lung, 267, 285
   of oesophagus, *see* Oesophagus, cancer of
   of rectum, *see* Rectum, cancer of
   see also Carcinoma
Carbohydrates in mucus glycoproteins, *see* Mucus, glycoprotein
Carcinoembryonic antigen (CEA), 4
   anti-CEA uptake, 262
   in colorectal carcinoma, 257, 259-261, 323
   in pancreatic carcinoma, 261
Carcinogens—
   in colorectal cancer, 297-303
      see also under Bacteria
   in gastric cancer, 287-288
   in oesophageal cancer, 275, 276, 277, 278
Carcinoma—
   breast, 257, 263
   colorectal, *see* Colorectal carcinoma
   gastric, *see* Gastric cancer
   pancreatic, 261
   periampullary, 348, 349
   staging, 214-216
   see also Dukes' classification
Cathepsins, 251
CCK, 23, *24*, 33
Centrocytic lymphoma, *see* Multiple lymphomatous polyposis
Chagas' disease, 42, *43*
Chenodeoxycholic acid, 298
Chlamydia in Crohn's disease, 184
Chloroacetate esterase, 231
Cholecystokinin (CCK), 23, *24*, 33
Cholera, 125
Choleragen, 126
Cholesterol, 300-301
Choriocarcinoma, HCG and, 255, 257
Clindamycin—
   animal model of AAC, 161
   -associated PMC, 131, 151, 164, 167
Clostridia, nuclear dehydrogenating (NDC), 301-302, 303, 307-308
Clostridial bowel disease, 130-131
   see also Colitis, pseudomembranous
Clostridium butyricum, 130
Clostridium difficile, 131, 151, 164-165
   animal models, 161-163
   clinical studies, 163-164
   colonization of intestine, 167
   toxin of, 165, 167-168
   treatment, 131, 166
   see also Colitis, pseudomembranous

INDEX

Clostridium perfringens, 130
Clostridium sordellii, 131, 161, 162, 165, 166
Clostridium welchii, 153
Cobalamins, 60
Coeliac disease, 94
 cell-mediated immune (CMI) reactions and, 99
 diagnosis, criteria, 194
 enteroglucagon level, 34
 folate malabsorption, 67
 immune complexes and, 98
 lymphoreticular malignancy and, 227-228
 malabsorption and, 193
 MHI and, *see* Malignant histiocytosis
 secretin release, 29, 31
Colitis, 152
 acute, *Shigella* and, 128
 antibiotic, 131
 haemorrhagic, 152, 153
 ischaemic, 160, 161
Colitis, pseudomembranous (PMC), 131, 151-168
 classification and terminology, 151
 historical perspective, 152-153
 pathology, 153-156, *156, 157, 158,* 159
  biopsy diagnosis of, 156-160
  differential diagnosis, 160-161
 recent advances in study of, 161-166
  clinical studies, 163-164
  epidemiology, 164, 166
  experimental animal model, 161-163
  role of antibiotics, 163, 167, 168
   see also Clindamycin; Lincomycin
 toxin test, 165-166
 treatment, 131, 166
 see also Clostridium difficile
Colitis, ulcerative—
 antibodies in, 181
 chronic, malignant lymphomas and, 227
 colorectal cancer risk, 316, 331, 333
 Crohn's disease, 178, 179, 180
 differential diagnosis, 160, 161
 epithelial dysplasia in, 331, 338-339
 FBA/NDC, dysplasia and, 307, 308
 folate deficiency, 67
 genetic studies, 179
 mucus, 54-55
 NDC and, 302
 screening tests and, 322, 323
Colonic neo-antigens, organ-specific, 258, *259*
Colonization factor antigen (CFA), 127
Colonoscopy, 322-323
Colon-specific antigen (CSAp), 259
Colorectal carcinoma—
 aetiology, 297-308
  adenoma-carcinoma sequence, 303, 304-308, *304,* 331, 333, 337
  carcinogens, 297-303, 307

Colorectal carcinoma— (*contd*)
  see also under Bacteria
  familial component in, 306, 331, 333, 350
  nature of environmental factors, 306-308
  value of FBA/NDC, 303, 307, 308
 antibodies, specific for, 262
 antigenic changes, *256,* 258-261
 enzyme changes, 257, 258
 HCG and, 257
 histopathology, 214, 218, 226, 303-308
 incidence, *305,* 311, 324, 333
 in polyposis coli, *see* Polyposis coli
 prognosis, factors affecting, 312-313, 324
 risk factors in, 314-316, 331
 screening for, 311, 316-324
  barium enema, 322, 323
  colonic washings, 323
  colonoscopy, 322-323
  fibreoptic sigmoidoscopy, 322
  haemoccult faecal occult blood testing, 313, 317-320, 324
  numbers detected and missed, 319, 320
  occult blood tests, 316-317
  proctosigmoidoscopy, survival after, 313
  sigmoidoscopy, rigid, 320-322, 324
  tumour-associated antigens, 323
  tumour markers, 324
 steroid hormone receptor, 257
 symptoms, 313
 treatment, 324
 see also Adenomas; Dysplasia
Coronaviruses, *110,* 111, 113-114
 swine, 115
Cow's milk protein intolerance, 94, 98, 99
Coxsackie A and B viruses, 106, *106*
Crohn's disease, 67, 173-186
 colonic malignancy risk, 316
 definition, anatomical features, 173-174
 diagnosis, 174-175
 epidemiology, 179-180
 folate deficiency, 67
 future research, 186
 genetics, 179
 immunology, 181-183
 microbiology, 183-185
 pathological anatomy, 175-178
  'early' lesion, 178
  granulomas, 175-176, 177
  immunoglobulin producing cells, 177
  mucosa remote from obvious disease, 177-178
 phagocytes in, 182-183
 PMC differential diagnosis, 160, 161
 VIP nerves and, 42, *43*
 vitamin B_{12} malabsorption, *64*
Cryostat sections, 4
Crypts, cell-mediated immune reactions, 99, 100

Cyanocobalamin, 60, 63
Cystadenocarcinoma, ovarian mucinous, 259
Cystic fibrosis meconium, *see* Meconium
Cytopathic effect (CPE), faecal, 161, 163, 168
Cytotoxicity, antibody-dependent, cell-mediated, 182

Defaecation, factors leading to, 71
  see also Faecal incontinence
Deoxyribonucleic acid—
  lability, gastric cancer and, 251
  of neoplastic cell, 252
Dermatitis herpetiformis, 66, *66*
Diarrhoea—
  antibiotic-associated, 151, 167
    see also Colitis, pseudomembranous
  bacterial, 125-132
    animal, 126, 127
    see also Escherichia coli
  travellers', 126, 149
  viral infections and
    animal, 114-115
    causation, mechanisms of, 121-122
    community studies, viruses and, 116-121
    Group I viruses, *106*, 107, 114, 121
    Group II viruses, *106*, 112-114
Diet, influence on—
  cancer of oesophagus, 275, 276, 277, 278
  colorectal cancer, 297, 307
  gastric cancer, 287-288
Dimethylhydrazine, 300
DNA, *see* Deoxyribonucleic acid
Dopamine, in Type I cells, 40
Drugs, in malabsorption—
  of folate, *66*, 67
  of vitamin B_{12}, 64
Dukes' classification, 214, 215, *216*, *361*, *362*
Duodenum, cells of, *26*, *27*
Dysplasia, colorectal—
  -carcinoma sequence, 331, 338
    life-history of, 338
  epithelial, 316, 322, 331-342
    epidemiology of, *340-341*
    genetic factors in, 341-342
    histology and grading of, in colorectal adenomas, 307, 308, 333-*335*, *336*
    in juvenile polyposis, 347, 351
    malignant potential of, 307, 308, 335-338
    nomenclature, 332
    in polyposis coli, *see* Polyposis coli
    precancerous conditions, 332-333
    in ulcerative colitis, 307-308, 331, 338-339

Echoviruses, 106, *106*

Electromyography, single-fibre, 87
Electron microscopy—
  immune, 107
  of intestinal lymphomas, *204*, *205-206*
  in virus detection, 112-115
Embolism, malignant, 355, 363
  see also Rectum, cancer of
Endocrine cells of gut, morphology, 26-27, *26*, *27*
Endorphin, 5
Endoscopy—
  in Crohn's disease, 175
  in PMC, 156-157, *159*, 160
  polypectomy, 322, 324
  see also Gastric cancer; Gastrofibrescopy; Sigmoidoscopy
Enkephalins, 23, *24*, 36, 40, *41*
Enterocolitis—
  haemorrhagic, 152
  necrotizing, 131, 153
Enteroglucagon, *24*, 34-35
Enterotoxins, 126, 129
Enterovirus, *106*, *109*, *110*, 117
  see also specific viruses
Enzymes as tumour markers, *256*, 257-258, 324
Eosinophilia, malignant lymphoma with, 237-238
EPEC strains, *see under Escherichia coli*
Epithelial membrane antigen (EMA), 258, *259*, 263
Escherichia coli, 126
  987P antigen, 136, *144*
  enteroinvasive, 127
  enteropathogenic (EPEC), 127-128
    for domestic animals, 135-149
    see also E. coli, plasmid-mediated
  enterotoxigenic (ETEC), 126-127, 135, 138
  mucosal attachment, 127
  K antigens, 136, 145-147
  O antigens, 145-147
  plasmid-mediated, characteristics, 135-149
    88 antigens, 136-138
    99 antigens, 136
    in Crohn's disease, 181, 185
    effect of 88 and 99 plasmids on colonization, 141-143, *141*, *142*, *143*
    effect of 987P and 88 antigens on colonization, *144*
    effect of Ent, 88 and 99 plasmids on colonization, 138-141, *139*
    effect of O and K antigens on colonization, 145-147, *145*
    enteropathogenic *E. coli* for recently weaned pigs, effect of giving, 147-149
    experimental methods, 137-138
    raffinose utilization by 88$^+$ strains, 147

INDEX

Escherichia coli— (contd)
   susceptibility of small intestine to enterotoxin, *136*, 138
   transduction and, 115
ETEC, *see Escherichia coli*, enterotoxigenic
Ethanol procedure, cold, 5
Eubacterium, 181, 185

Faecal bile acids (FBA), *see* Bile acids, faecal
Faecal incontinence, idiopathic, 71-87
   anorectal angle and, 73-74
   biopsies
     histological observations, 76-80, *76-80*
     methods, 75
     type 1, type 2 fibre diameters, 81, 84, *85*, 86
   clinical features of, 72-73, 85, 86
   fibre hypertrophy and, 76, 81, 84, *85*, 86
   normal subjects, muscles of, 81-85, *85*
Faecal neutral steroid (FNS), *300-301*
FBA, *see* Bile acids, faecal
Ferritin, 67
Fibrescopy, *see* Gastric cancer; Gastrofibrescopy
Fixatives, 5-9, 25
Fluoroscopy, double-contrast, 250, 251
Folate, 64-67
   absorption, 64-65
   binding proteins, 65
   deficiency of, 66, 67
   enterohepatic circulation, 65
   malabsorption of, 66-67, *66*
Folate conjugase, 64, 65
Formalin fixation, 5-7, *7*, *8*, 12
Formal sublimate, 6, *8*
'Fuzzy-wuzzies' viruses, 111

Gardner's syndrome, 314, 349, 350
Gastrectomy, partial—
   iron deficiency and, 68
   vitamin B_{12} and, 61, 63
Gastric cancer—
   cytodiagnosis, 241-252
     biopsy, 243
     biopsy/cytology diagnosis, *248*, *249*
     blind tube wash, 243-244
     brush smear preparation, 245
     cytochemical DNA tests, 251-252, *251*
     cytological tumour typing, 249
     cytology of gastric smears, 245-249
     early surface cancer, 249
     efficiency of techniques, 241, *242*
     fibrescopic brush sample, 244-245
     screening, 249-251
     washing techniques, 241, *242*
   epidemiology, 267, 285-289

Gastric cancer— *(contd)*
   epidemiology-pathology studies of, 291-293
   Laurens classification, 249, 289-290, *290*, *291*
   mucus in, 53
   pathology, 289-293
Gastric inhibitory polypeptide (GIP), *24*, 33, 35
Gastric intrinsic factor (IF), 59, 60
   bicarbonate effect on competition with R binder, 61-62
   in mitochondria of enterocyte, 62
Gastric mucosal hyperplasia, 245
Gastrin, 23, *24*, 28-29, *29*, *30*
Gastrinomas, 28-29, *32*
Gastritis, atrophic, 68, 245, 246, 292
Gastritis, chronic, 228, 288
Gastroenteritis—
   infective, 125
   transmissible, 111, 115
   see also Diarrhoea
Gastrofibrescopy, 241, *242*
   see also Gastric cancer
Giardia muris, 101
GIP, *see* Gastric inhibitory polypeptide
Glicentin, *see* Enteroglucagon
Glucosamine synthetase, 178
Glucose-dependent insulinotropic peptide, *see* Gastric inhibitory polypeptide
γ-Glutamyltranspeptidase, 257, 258
Glutaraldehyde coupling techniques, 9
Glycoconjugate, 47-48
Glycoproteins, 48
   see also Mucus, glycoprotein
Goblet cells, immune complexes and, 98
Graft-versus-host disease, 99-100
Granulomas in Crohn's disease, 175-176
Growth hormone, 5
Guaiac reagent, saturated, 316, 317
Gut-associated lymphoid tissues (GALT), 93

Haemorrhage, chronic, 68
Haemorrhoidectomy, 72
Hamartomas, 345, 346, 347
HCG, *see* Human chorionic gonadotrophin
α-Heavy-chain disease, 193, 227
Helminth infections of gut, 95
Hepatitis B surface antigen, 4
Hirschsprung's disease, 42
Histiocytic medullary reticulosis, *see* Malignant histiocytosis
Histiocytosis, malignant, *see* Malignant histiocytosis
Hodgkin's disease, 234-238, *235*
Hormone(s)—
   gut, *see* Regulatory peptides

Hormone(s)— (contd)
  of 'indigestion', 35
  receptors, colorectal carcinoma and, 257
  as tumour markers, 256-257
Horseradish peroxidase, 15
Human chorionic gonadotrophin (HCG)—
  staining patterns, 17
  as tumour markers, 256-257
Hypersensitivity, small intestine and—
  cytotoxic, 96-97
  immune complex, 97-98, *102*
  local, small intestinal mucosa, 94-95
  in parasite infections, 101
  reaginic, 95-96, *102*
  T cell-mediated, 98-101, *102*
    graft-versus-host disease, 99-100
    intestinal allograft rejection, 99
    phases of, 100-101

Ia antigens, 3, 14
Imerslund-Gräsbeck's disease, 63
Immune complex—
  disease, systemic, 97-98
  goblet cells and, 98
  hypersensitivity, 97-98, *102*
Immune response—
  cell-mediated
    in Crohn's disease, 181-182
    intestinal, 94, 99
    see also Hypersensitivity
  humoral, in Crohn's disease, 181
  of small intestine, 94-102
  see also Immunoglobulins
Immune system of gastrointestinal tract, 93, 94
Immunocytochemistry, 25
  see also Immunohistochemical techniques
Immunoenzymatic procedures, 9-12
Immunofluorescent methods, 5-9, 11-12, 177
Immunoglobulin(s)—
  immunoenzymatic methods, 10
  immunofluorescent studies, 5
  plasma cell, localization, 4, 6, 7, 12, *14*
  -producing cells, in Crohn's disease, 177
  staining intensity, 17
  surface, 4, 12
  see also specific immunoglobulins
Immunoglobulin A (IgA)—
  in Crohn's disease, 177, 178
  IgA$_1$, 56, 57
  IgA$_2$, 56-57
  immunohistochemical staining and, 3, 10
  mucosal surface, secretion at, 93, 94
Immunoglobulin D (IgD), 177
Immunoglobulin E (IgE)—
  in Crohn's disease, 177
  double staining method, 10
  helminth infections, 95
  reaginic hypersensitivity and, 95-96

Immunoglobulin G (IgG)—
  in Crohn's disease, 177, 178
  in malignant histiocytes, 206
  plasma cell, staining of, 6, 7, 8, 10, *14*, 17
Immunoglobulin M (IgM), 10, 17
  in Crohn's disease, 177, 178
  mucosal surface, secretion at, 93
Immunohistochemical techniques, 3-17
  antisera specificity, 25-26
  applications, in gastrointestinal pathology, 12-17
  false negative staining, 13
  false positive staining, 13-17
  labelling techniques, 9-12
    advantages and disadvantages of, 11-12
    immunoenzymatic methods, 9-12
    immunofluorescent methods, 5, 9, 11, 12
  for neuropeptides, 25-26
  tissue preparation, 3-9
    cell suspensions, 3-4
    fixatives in, 5-9
    tissue blocks, 4-9
Immunoperoxidase technique, 5, 7, 8, 13-15, *14, 15*
  intestinal lymphomas, 206, *207, 208*
  'labelled-antigen', *14*
  lymphomas, non-Hodgkin's, 231
  in metastatic foci, detection, 263
Infections—
  bacterial, 125-132
    Campylobacter, 129
    Clostridium, 130-131
    E. coli, 126-128
    Salmonella, 129
    Shigella, 128-129
    Yersinia, 130
  definition, 105
  viral, 105-122
    causation, mechanisms, 121-122
    community studies of, 116-121
    diagnosis, 112
    evidence of excretion, 112-115
    serological surveys, 115-116
    see also Diarrhoea
Insulin stimulation, *51*
Intestinal metaplasia, 53, 245, 290, 293
Intestinal stagnant-loop syndrome, 64, 67
Intestine, small—
  E. coli colonization, *see Escherichia coli*
  immunological mechanisms in, 94-102
  mucosal pathology, *102*
  see also Malignant histiocytosis
Iron, 67-68
  absorption, 67
  deficiency, 66
  malabsorption, 67-68
Ischaemia in pseudomembranous colitis, 152, 153, 168

Jejunitis, ulcerative and MHI, 209, *210*
Jejunoileitis, non-granulomatous, 209, *210*

Kiel classification, 213, 220, 221, 222

Laurens classification, 249, 289-290
'Leakage' of proteins into cells, 15, *16*, 17
Leucocyte adherence inhibition (LAI) test, 258
Levator ani muscles, 71, *73*, 74, 86
  histological observations, *76*, 79, *80*, *85*
  innervation, 80
  normal, 81, 82, *85*
Lincomycin—
  animal model of AAC, 161
  -associated PMC, 131, 151
Lukes classification, 220, 221, 222
Lung cancer, 267, 285
Lymphocytes—
  in Crohn's disease, 181, 182
  gastrointestinal tract, 93, 94
  T cell-mediated hypersensitivity, *see under* Hypersensitivity
Lymphoid cells, 3-4
Lymphoid tissues, gut-associated, 93
Lymphokines, 'enteropathic', 100
Lymphoma—
  intestinal and malabsorption, *see* Malignant histiocytosis of the intestine
  malignant, with eosinophilia, 237-238
  Mediterranean, 193, 228
  metastatic, 215
  multifocal, primary, 218, *219*
  non-Hodgkin's, 213-238
    centrocytic type, *see* Multiple lymphomatous polyposis
    histogenesis, 226-229, *230*
    histological grading, 218-223
    Hodgkin's disease, differential diagnosis, 234-238
    immunoblastic, 220-221, *220*, *221*, 222
    lymphoblastic, 221-222, 223
    new techniques in study of, 229-234
    primary, criteria for, 214
    staging, 214-218
    survival, 223, 225-226
Lysosomes, vitamin B_{12} absorption, 62-63
Lysozyme—
  immunohistochemical staining, 9, 13, 15, 17
  in malignant histiocytosis, 206, *207*
  mucus glycoproteins and, 56

Malabsorption—
  intestinal lymphoma, *see* Malignant histiocytosis of the intestine

Malabsorption— (*contd*)
  malignant lymphoma with eosinophilia, 238
  see also Folate; Iron; Vitamin B_{12}
Malignant histiocytosis of the intestine (MHI), 194-211
  clinical features, 194
  coeliac disease, relationship, 210-211
  dissemination, 197, *201*, 202, 203, 204
  early lesion of, 207, *208*, *209*
  gross appearances, 194, *195*
  histochemistry, 202, 205
  histology, *196*, 197, *198*, *199*, *200*
  immunoperoxidase studies, 206, *207*, *208*
  plastic sections and electron microscopy, *204*, 205-206, *205*, *206*
  ulcerative jejunitis and, 209, *210*
Meconium—
  cystic fibrosis, *54*
  mucus glycoprotein, *50*, 51
Membrane antigens, 4, 12
Metastases—
  liver, cancer of rectum, 353, 358, *359*
  tumour markers in detection of, 261-263
20-Methylcholanthrene, 301
5-Methyltetrahydrofolate, 64, 65
Metronidazole, 166
MHI, *see* Malignant histiocytosis of the intestine
Minireovirus, *109*, 111
Minirotavirus, *109*, 111
Motilin, *24*, 33-34
Mucin, 47
'Mucoid', 47
Mucosa, gastric, normal cells, *246*
Mucus, gastrointestinal, 47-57
  carbohydrates, secretors and, *53*
  changes, in disease, 52-55
  components, 47, 48-52
    see also Mucus, glycoprotein
  future research on, 55-57
  glycoprotein, 47, 48-52, 56
    colonic, 49, *50*, 51
    in disease, monosaccharides, 52-55
    gastric, 49, *50*, 51
    isolation, 49-50, 56
    molecular weight, 48
    monosaccharide residues, *50*, 51-52, *52*, 55
    structure, 48-49, 51
  lysozyme interaction with, 56
  nomenclature, 47-48
  possible role of, 56-57
Multiple lymphomatous polyposis (MLP), 216-218, *217*, *218*, 222, *224*, *232*, 235-237
Multiple sclerosis, 71
Muramidase, *see* Lysozyme

Muscles—
  fibre hypertrophy, 76, 81, 84, *85*, 86
  fibre type predominance, 75
  type 1, 85, 86
  see also specific muscles
Myeloid sarcoma, 232-234

Naphthylamidase, 251
National Lymphoma Investigation (NLI) classification, 220, 221, 222
NDC, *see* Clostridia, nuclear dehydrogenating
Neuromodulators, 36-42
Neuropeptides, 5
Neurotensin, *24*, 34
Neurotransmitters, 23, 28-36
Nippostrongylus brasiliensis, 95, 101
Nitrosamines, 275, 276, 277, 288
N-Nitrosation reaction, 288
Norwalk virus, in gut, *106*, 107, *108*, *109*, 111
  antibody to, *116*
  diarrhoea and, 113
Nuclear dehydrogenating clostridia, *see* Clostridia, nuclear dehydrogenating

Oesophagitis, *280*, 281
Oesophagus—
  brush cytology, 247, *248*
  cancer of, 267-281
    aetiological hypotheses, 274-279
    in Africa, 271, *272*
    frequency changes with time, 273-274
    incidence rates of men, 267, *268-269*
    incidence rates of women, 271-272
    in Northern China, 267, *270*
    pathology, 279-281
    screening, *279*, *280*
Oldfield's syndrome, 314
Opium, 275-276
Osteomas, polyposis coli and, 349

Pancreas—
  carcinoma of, 261
  role in vitamin B_{12} absorption, 61-62
Pancreatic oncofetal antigen (POA), 261
Pancreatic polypeptide (PP), *24*, 35
Pancreatitis, chronic, 61, 62
Papanicolaou grading, 246
PAP, *see* Peroxidase-antiperoxidase
Parasite infections, 101
Penicillin, PMC and, 166
Pentagastrin stimulation, *51*
Peptides, regulatory of gut, *see* Regulatory peptides
Peptostreptococcus, 181
Periampullary carcinoma, 348, 349

Perineal descent, 72, 74
Periodate oxidation technique, 9
Peroxidase-antiperoxidase (PAP) methods, 9-10, *15*, 26
Peroxidases, occult blood tests and, 316, 317
Peutz-Jeghers syndrome, 345-346, 350-351
Phagocytes, in Crohn's disease, 182-183
6-Phosphogluconate dehydrogenase, 251
'Pig-bel', 130, 153
Pinocytosis, vitamin B_{12} absorption, 62-63
Plasmids, *see Escherichia coli*
Plastic embedding, *204*, 205-206, *205*, *206*, 231, 232, *232*, *233*
PMC, *see* Colitis, pseudomembranous
Poliovirus, *106*
Polypectomy, endoscopic, 322, 324
Polyposis coli, familial, 332-333, 347-351
  colorectal cancer risk, 314, 315, 331, 347
  dysplasia-carcinoma sequence, 338, *339*
  as experimental model, 349-350
  Gardner's syndrome and, 349
  screening tests and, 323
  small intestinal adenomas, 348-349
  treatment, 348
Polyposis, juvenile, 346-347, 350-351
Polyposis syndromes, 226-227, 345-351
  see also Multiple lymphomatous polyposis; *specific syndromes*
Polyps, colorectal cancer and, 302, 303, 314, 331
  CEA and, 323
  'mucus retention', 346
  screening tests and, *318*, 319, 320, 321-322
  see also Polyposis
Precancerous condition, 332
  definition, 332
  colorectal lesions, 332-333
Precancerous lesion, 332
Prolactin, 5
Prolylhydroxylase, 178
Proteoglycans, 48
Proteolytic digestion—
  in mucus glycoprotein isolation, 50
  prior to immunohistochemical staining, 6, 7
Pseudomembranous colitis (PMC), *see* Colitis, pseudomembranous
Pteroylpolyglutamate hydrolase, 64
Puborectalis muscles—
  external anal sphincter muscle, separation, 71, *73*, 75
  in faecal incontinence, 72, 74
  histological observations, 76, *76*, *78*, *79*, *85*, 86
  innervation, 80, 86-87
  normal, 71, *73*, 75, 81-84, *84*, *85*
Pudendal nerve, 86, 87

Radioimmunoassay (RIA), 25

INDEX

Rappaport classification, 220, 221, 222
'R' binder, 59, 60-61
  pancreatic proteases and, 61
Reaginic hypersensitivity, 95-96
Rectal prolapse, 72, 73
Rectum, cancer of—
  mucus changes, 53
  venous invasion, 353-364
    Dukes' stages and, *361, 362*
    incidence of, 358, *359*
    liver metastases, 353, 358, *359*
    methods in study, 353-355
    mode of spread, *362*
    necrosis of tumour, 358, *360, 363*
    survival rates, 358, *359, 360, 361, 362*
    tumour cell contact with venous blood, 355, *356, 361*
    tumour/host balance in, *363*
Reed-Sternberg cells, *235, 236*
Regulatory peptides of gut, 23-44
  action, 23, *24*, 28, 42-44
    hormones, circulating, 23, 35-36
    neurotransmitters/neuromodulators, 23, 36-43
  chemistry, distribution, *24*
  techniques used, 25-26
  see also specific peptides
Reovirus, *106, 108*
Rheumatoid arthritis, 66
Rhodamine, 9, 11
Radioimmunoassay (RIA), 25
Riboflavin, 275, 277, 279
Rotavirus, *106*, 107, *108*, 113
  animal diarrhoea, 114, 121-122
  antibody to, 115, *116*
  ecology of, 117, *118, 119*
  human diarrhoea, 113

Salmonella, 127, 129
Salmonella enteritidis, 129
Salmonella typhimurium, 129
Salmonellosis, 129
Sarcoma, myeloid, 232-234
Secretin, 23, *24*, 29, 31, 33
'Secretor' gene, 52-*53*
Seroconversion, 112, 113
Shigella, 127, 128-129
Shigella dysenteriae, 128
Shwartzman phenomenon, 168
Shy-Drager syndrome, 42
Sialic acid, 49
Sigmoidoscopy, 313, 320-322
  flexible, 322
  rigid, 320-322
Skin pigmentation, 346
Somatostatin, 23, *24*, 36, 39
  distribution, *24, 36, 37*
  pharmacological effects, *35*

Somatostatinomas, 36
Splenic atrophy, 66
Staphylococcus aureus, 152
Stomach, cancer of, *see* Adenocarcinoma of stomach; Gastric cancer
Substance P, 23, *24*, 36, *38, 39*, 42
Sulphomucins, 251

Toxins—
  cholera, 125-126
  C. difficile, *see* Clostridium difficile enterotoxin, 129
  E. coli, 126, 135, 136
Transcobalamin II (TCII), 59, 60
  role of, 62-63
Transduction, 106, 115
Transferrin—
  distribution, *15, 16*
  in iron absorption regulation, 67
Trichinella spiralis, 101
Tropical sprue, *64*, 67
Tumour-Node-Metastasis (TNM) system, 215, *216*
Tumour(s)—
  gastrinomas, 28-29
  islet-cell, 29, 35
  markers, 255-263
    antigens, *256*, 258-261, 323
    colorectal cancer and, 324
    in detection of metastases, 261-263
    enzymes, *256*, 257-258, 324
    hormones, 256-257, *256*
Turcot's syndrome, 314

Ulcer—
  duodenal, 52
  gastric, benign, 245, 249
  peptic, 52

Vaccines, seroconversion and, 112
Vancomycin, 131, 166
Vasoactive intestinal polypeptide (VIP), 23, *24*, 36, 40, *41, 42, 43*
Vein invasion and rectal cancer, *see* Rectum, cancer of
Verner-Morrison syndrome, 42
Vibrio cholerae, 127
VIP, *see* Vasoactive intestinal polypeptide
VIPoma syndrome, 42
Viruses in human gut, 105-111
  in Crohn's disease, 184
  group I, *106*, 107, 114
  group II, 106-107, *106*
  small round (SRV), *106, 109, 110*, 113
    ecology, *118, 119*
  see also Infections, viral; *specific viruses*

Vitamin B$_{12}$, 59-64
  absorption by pinocytotic mechanism, 62-63
  absorption tests, 63
  analogues, 60, 61
  bacterial synthesis of, 60
  congenital specific malabsorption, 63
  malabsorption, 61-62, 63-64
  radioassays versus microbiological, 61
  'R' binding proteins, 59, 60-61
  receptors, 59
  transcobalamin II, role of, 62-63

Watery diarrhoea hypokalaemia achlorhydria (WDHA) syndrome, 42
Wheat, cancer of oesophagus and, 276

Yersinia, 125
Yersinia enterocolitica, 130

Zenker's fixative, 6
Zinc glycinate marker (ZGM), 258, *259*
Zirconium, 180
Zollinger-Ellison syndrome, 28, *64*

RECENT ISSUES OF CLINICS IN GASTROENTEROLOGY

September 1977
THE GI TRACT IN STRESS AND PSYCHOSOCIAL DISORDER
Thomas P. Almy and John F. Fielding, *Guest Editors*

'... This book can be strongly recommended to all who encounter such problems in their clinical practice.' THE PRACTITIONER

January 1978
INTESTINAL PARASITES
P.D. Marsden, *Guest Editor*

'... This is a good reference book which will be an invaluable aid to gastroenterologists working in the developing world. Many gastroenterologists in the advanced countries will also find that there are plenty of parasitic diseases in their own clinics that are receiving insufficient attention.' BRITISH JOURNAL OF HOSPITAL MEDICINE, April 1978

May 1978
INVESTIGATIVE TESTS AND TECHNIQUES
R.I. Russell, *Guest Editor*

'... All clinical gastroenterologists will find this book easy reading and it should be considered a "must" for all departments.' GUT, December 1978

'... This is a useful reference book and should be in all gastrointestinal units as a guide to what is available and what results mean rather than when to do the tests.' THE LANCET, 9 September 1978

September 1978
ENDOSCOPY
K.F.R. Schiller, *Guest Editor*

'... As a whole the book is nicely put together and the topics are well chosen...' THE LANCET, 11 November 1978

'... The book is essentially for clinical gastroenterologists involved in digestive endoscopy and includes a wealth of references many of which are from the current year.' HOSPITAL UPDATE, September 1979

RECENT ISSUES OF CLINICS IN GASTROENTEROLOGY

January 1979
GI PHARMACOLOGY AND CURRENT THERAPY
James W. Freston, *Guest Editor*

'... *This book is a must for gastroenterologists and should also be bought by physicians and surgeons who deal with gastroenterological problems* ...' JOURNAL OF THE IRISH MEDICAL ASSOCIATION, 30 March 1979

May 1979
POSTSURGICAL SYNDROMES
André L. Blum and J. Rüdiger Siewert, *Guest Editors*

'... *This is a practical and imaginative edition of* Clinics in Gastroenterology *that bears a strong editorial stamp of authority* ...' GUT, February 1980

'This worthy addition to a respected series, edited jointly by a surgeon and a physician, covers the gastrointestinal tract from oesophagus to anus, and the pancreaticobiliary system; it includes surgery of portal hypertension ...' THE LANCET, 4 August 1979

September 1979
INFECTIONS OF THE GI TRACT
H.P. Lambert, *Guest Editor*

'This is a timely volume which brings together reviews in the physiology of the gastrointestinal tract to match recent advances in microbiology and virology, with special reference to infection and diarrhoea ...' GUT, February 1980

January 1980
VIRUS HEPATITIS
Sheila Sherlock, *Guest Editor*

'... *This is one of those rare occasions when one can, with a clear conscience, succumb to the temptation to say that no-one interested in liver disease can afford to be without it* ...' THE LANCET, 29 March 1980

'... *A veritable feast for the physician.*' SOUTH AFRICAN MEDICAL JOURNAL, 8 March 1980